# SEEING RED

## HIV/AIDS and Public Policy in Canada

What does it mean to think of HIV/AIDS policy in a critical manner? *Seeing Red* offers the first critical analysis of HIV/AIDS policy in Canada. Featuring the diverse experiences of people living with HIV, this collection highlights various perspectives from academics, activists, and community workers who look ahead to the new and complex challenges associated with HIV/AIDS and Canadian society.

In addition to representing a diversity of voices and perspectives, *Seeing Red* reflects on historical responses to HIV/AIDS in Canada. Among the specific issues addressed are the over-representation of Indigenous peoples among those living with HIV, the criminalization of HIV, and barriers to health and support services, particularly as experienced by vulnerable and marginalized populations. The editors and contributors seek to show that Canada has been neither uniquely compassionate nor proactive when it comes to supporting those living with HIV/AIDS. Instead, this remains a critical area of public policy, one fraught with challenges as well as possibilities.

SUZANNE HINDMARCH is assistant professor of Political Science at the University of New Brunswick.

MICHAEL ORSINI is professor in the School of Political Studies at the University of Ottawa.

MARILOU GAGNON is associate professor at the School of Nursing in the Faculty of Health Sciences at the University of Ottawa.

# Seeing Red

## HIV/AIDS and Public Policy in Canada

EDITED BY SUZANNE HINDMARCH,
MICHAEL ORSINI, AND MARILOU GAGNON

UNIVERSITY OF TORONTO PRESS
Toronto Buffalo London

ISBN 978-1-4875-0015-3 (cloth)     ISBN 978-1-4875-2009-0 (paper)

---

**Library and Archives Canada Cataloguing in Publication**

Seeing red : HIV/AIDS and public policy in Canada/edited by Suzanne
Hindmarch, Michael Orsini, and Marilou Gagnon.

Includes bibliographical references and index.
ISBN 978-1-4875-0015-3 (cloth). – ISBN 978-1-4875-2009-0 (paper)

1. AIDS (Disease) – Government policy – Canada.   2. AIDS (Disease) –
Patients – Services for – Canada.   3. AIDS (Disease) – Patients – Canada –
Social conditions.   4. Canada – Public policy.   I. Hindmarch, Suzanne, 1975–,
editor   II. Orsini, Michael, 1967–, editor   III. Gagnon, Marilou, 1980–, editor

RA643.86.C3S44 2018        362.19697'9200971        C2017-906336-7

---

This book has been published with the help of a grant from the Federation
for the Humanities and Social Sciences, through the Awards to Scholarly
Publications Program, using funds provided by the Social Sciences
and Humanities Research Council of Canada.

University of Toronto Press acknowledges the financial assistance to its
publishing program of the Canada Council for the Arts and the Ontario Arts
Council, an agency of the Government of Ontario.

**Canada Council    Conseil des Arts**
**for the Arts    du Canada**

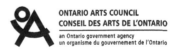

ONTARIO ARTS COUNCIL
CONSEIL DES ARTS DE L'ONTARIO
an Ontario government agency
un organisme du gouvernement de l'Ontario

Funded by the    Financé par le
Government    gouvernement
of Canada    du Canada    **Canadä**

# Contents

**Part Two: Services**

**Part Three: Populations**

# Acknowledgments

The genesis for this edited collection was a policy symposium held at the University of Ottawa in October 2013. We gratefully acknowledge the Ontario HIV Treatment Network for the financial support that made the symposium possible, and all symposium participants for their thoughtful contributions to the initial conversations that eventually, and in much different form, made their way into this book. We thank our editor at University of Toronto Press, Daniel Quinlan, for his enthusiastic support of the book; two anonymous reviewers for their careful reading and insightful recommendations, which strengthened the final manuscript; and Aaron Rudkin and Clare Bekenn for their very capable assistance with symposium logistics and manuscript preparation, respectively. We also thank Scott Treleaven for permission to use his wonderful piece of art, *Cease to Exist*, on the cover. We are deeply grateful to all contributors to this collection for their patience and commitment to this project. We recognize, with solidarity and respect, all of those living with and vulnerable to HIV who continue to live with the consequences of a flawed policy and political response to HIV, and who continue to fight for a better, more just HIV response.

SEEING RED

HIV/AIDS and Public Policy in Canada

# Introduction

MICHAEL ORSINI, SUZANNE HINDMARCH,
AND MARILOU GAGNON

The title of this collection was inspired by the anger and activism that have marked the HIV/AIDS movement since it first burst onto the political scene in North America almost four decades ago. In the early 1980s, as governments the world over turned their backs on a newly emerging illness that was striking young gay men, a grassroots movement was born. While New York and San Francisco were the epicentre of this unique brand of radical AIDS activism, Montreal, Toronto, and Vancouver were not far behind. In Toronto, for instance, *The Body Politic*, a leading monthly newspaper of record of the local gay community, published one of the first articles on what later came to be known as HIV/AIDS.[1]

Gay men mobilized quickly and effectively to build the type of communities that would sustain people living with AIDS in the face of shame, stigma, and outright rejection. It was necessary, then, to "see red": to imagine resilience, community building, support, and alliances when there was precious little of this in evidence. While literal understandings of the notion of "seeing red" might suggest someone who is so enraged as to be unable to think clearly, we view anger and rage as necessary precursors to understanding the development of HIV policy, and policymaking in general. Anger and mourning were productive, albeit complex, moral emotions in the early years of the epidemic (see Gould 2009). They gave way to forms of conventional protest as well as to bursts of creative and radical activism that dramatized and narrated the unfolding pandemic. Artist collectives such as Gran Fury in the United States and General Idea in Canada developed the first crucial artistic interventions in the epidemic. One of the most significant and well known, the inverted pink triangle of the Silence = Death slogan, became a powerful rallying cry for the fledging movement and served as a sobering reminder that policy "speaks" when it falls silent, when it leads to inaction or non-action. Even a casual observer of public policy recognizes that decisions "not" to act, or efforts to slow policy movement are fundamentally political.

Since the emergence of HIV in North America, and, as a result in large part of this early activism, there have been significant advances in HIV prevention, testing, and treatment. For some Persons Living with HIV/AIDS (PLWHAs) in industrialized countries such as Canada, access to treatment means that HIV can become chronic and manageable, even if we should stress that the discourse of "manageability" masks the complex experiences of people who are on treatment. But while the annual number of new HIV cases reported in 2014 to the Public Health Agency of Canada was the lowest since HIV first became a reportable illness in 1985, a new set of challenges has emerged on how to assist individuals who are living – and aging – with HIV, including those related to housing, disability supports, and income security, among others.

The data also obscure worrying trends, including the continued overrepresentation of Indigenous people, and specifically Indigenous women[2] among the HIV-positive population, as well as trans-identified individuals, as discussed in Duchesne's chapter in this collection. While the general decrease in new infections is cause for optimism, it is important to caution that the data are incomplete, since HIV is no longer reportable in some provinces, and even in cases where data are still reported, the information provides limited insight on the racial and ethnic background of people living with HIV/AIDS. This failure to know and appreciate the complete picture can contribute to a climate of "strategic ignorance," which can frustrate responses to the epidemic. As McGoey argues in a discussion of the mobilization of ambiguity, "Knowing the least amount possible is often the most indispensable tool for managing risks and exonerating oneself from blame" (McGoey 2012, 2–3). In addition, it is estimated that in Canada almost a quarter of people with HIV may be unaware of their status (Public Health Agency of Canada 2015), although the Centers for Disease Control recently revised this number downward to one in eight individuals (CDC 2016).

The epidemiological picture therefore masks a number of persistent challenges. Social policy responses to HIV have largely failed to address the ultimate drivers of the epidemic: poverty, racism, homophobia, and other complex, intersecting forms of social exclusion and structural inequities that make some people more vulnerable to HIV. Consequently, some populations – mainly ethno-racial and sexual minorities – continue to be disproportionately affected by HIV and to experience significant challenges in accessing appropriate services and supports. Furthermore, at the "science-policy interface" where biomedical advances and social policy meet, there continue to be complex legal and ethical debates on matters ranging from testing and treatment guidelines, to the criminalization of HIV transmission. Policymakers and community activists alike continue to struggle with the question of what an optimal set of policy responses to HIV might look like.

These debates about policy responses to an evolving HIV epidemic are occurring against the backdrop of significant demographic and political shifts, both nationally and globally. These include a global recession and the legacy of the Harper Conservatives' rollback of Canadian welfare state services; a Canadian population that is, on the whole, aging, but within which there is a young and growing Indigenous population; changing legal and social stances on sex work and drug use; and dynamic social movements advocating for LGBTQ+, Indigenous, and women's rights. Canada's HIV response is also uniquely shaped by our federal system, which has produced complex federal-provincial divisions of responsibility for health promotion and disease response, not to mention service provision to First Nations, incarcerated people, and refugees.

In this complex, dynamic policy landscape, what are the most important issues and priorities for community activists, AIDS service organizations, and policymakers involved in the Canadian HIV response? What impact have recent changes in the political and economic environment had on the HIV sector? What has been the impact of HIV policies and programming, and of broader political shifts, on the lived experiences of those people and communities most affected by HIV? What are the current issues and priorities for the HIV response in Canada? What are the causes of current policy challenges facing the sector, and how should they be addressed?

This edited collection brings together a diverse group of established and emerging academics, activists, and community organization representatives to consider these questions; to help us think creatively about the complex issues that continue to frustrate state and civil society efforts to address HIV; to promote dialogue across the HIV sector, among activists, academics, and policymakers; to encourage critical reflection on how HIV intersects with other policy areas; to identify policy priorities, gaps, and opportunities for policy change; and to catalyse discussion about opportunities and challenges in the current policy landscape. This landscape includes tensions between HIV integration and HIV exceptionalism; the growing population of older people living with HIV; the persistent over-representation of Indigenous people among those living with HIV, and the complex aetiology of this over-representation. All of these, moreover, are situated within the larger context of Canadian welfare state transformation and imminent federal and provincial shifts in the HIV response, which are poised to affect policies, service provision, and the lived experiences of HIV-positive people. These shifts include a move at the federal level and in some provinces to integrate the HIV response into wider sexually transmitted and blood-borne infection strategies; and increasing interest in "treatment as prevention" approaches that entail significant changes in testing, treatment, and support services for HIV-positive and vulnerable populations.

In the next sections, we provide a historical overview of the epidemic, our understanding of the political context that has shaped the response to HIV in Canada, and the structure of the book, including a chapter overview. But first, we discuss the multiple meanings of "seeing red" in the context of HIV in Canada.

**Seeing Red: Let Us Count the Ways**

In addition to the notion of red as synonymous with anger and rage, red is also emblazoned on one of the enduring symbols of AIDS: the red ribbon, created in the early 1990s. Its iconic status in the AIDS landscape is unmatched. The colour red was "chosen for its connection to blood and the idea of passion – not only anger, but love ... The ribbon format was selected in part because it was easy to recreate and wear. The original instructions were to 'cut the red ribbon in 6 inch length, then fold at the top into an inverted 'V' shape'" (Visual AIDS). Trendsetting and mimicked by many disease constituencies, including breast cancer advocates, the red ribbon is a recognized symbol as well as a lightning rod for criticism, viewed by some as a hollow gesture worn by celebrities that has become almost devoid of political significance.

Red is also a colour of significance for Indigenous people in Canada, who are disproportionately affected by HIV and often are framed as vulnerable to HIV because of their Indigeneity. These pathologized ways of thinking about Indigenous people's health and well-being have structured responses to a range of issues, not solely HIV, that affect Indigenous people. What is perhaps most promising in the HIV response in Canada is a growing recognition that Indigenous peoples themselves need to lead the fight against HIV in ways that recognize their power, self-determination, and will to ground their interventions in culturally appropriate ways of knowing. *Red power*, of course, is a term used to denote the Indian resurgence of the late 1960s, but it is especially timely in the wake of the resurgence characteristic of the Idle No More movement and attempts by key Indigenous scholars to challenge settler colonialism (for critical perspectives on Indigenous sovereignty and the politics of recognition, see Alfred 1999; Coulthard 2014; Simpson 2014). While some of the chapters in this collection focus specifically on Indigenous responses to the epidemic, especially as they pertain to women and aging populations, we cannot do justice to the far-reaching effects of colonialism and reconciliation processes on HIV vulnerability in and the resilience of Indigenous communities.

In the federal political context, the significance of "seeing red" also takes on a particular partisan, political relevance. Canada emerged in late 2015 from a period of Conservative federal rule under the leadership of Prime Minister Stephen Harper, who was reviled by many in the AIDS community for fighting (and eventually losing) a war against supervised injection sites in Canada, which have been shown to decrease the transmission of HIV, for stepping up a regressive criminalization "law and order" agenda, and for stalling federal efforts to support programs and policies to deal with pressing HIV/AIDS prevention needs. The election of the "red" Liberals under the leadership of Prime Minister Justin Trudeau has many seeing a different kind of red. This red is hopeful, coloured by an almost giddy optimism. Since being elected to a majority government in October 2015, Trudeau's government has already taken some impressive steps: much to the delight of AIDS activists and leading researchers with the British Columbia Centre of Excellence on HIV/AIDS, who have been mounting scientific evidence supporting safe injection sites for several years, the Trudeau government ended the war on safe injection sites that had persisted for several years under the Harper government.

While there was cause for optimism shortly after the election, one should be cautious in "seeing (Liberal) red" as somehow magically heralding a new era of progressive policy for the HIV/AIDS community and others interested in social justice and equity. The epidemic is fuelled by persistent inequalities, a longstanding failure to address enduring stigma and structural drivers, as well as logistical and functional coordination challenges. Many of these challenges transcend partisan differences between the Liberals and Conservatives, even if there is reason to hope that Liberals understand and appreciate some of these challenges and are less guided by moralistic crusades against people who make lifestyle choices with which they might disagree. It is important to recall that in 1996, it was the Liberal government of Jean Chrétien that got a frosty welcome from thousands of delegates assembled at the International Conference on AIDS in Vancouver, BC. When it was announced that the prime minister could not attend the conference as the result of a fishing vacation conflict, the crowd "welcomed" his replacement, Health Minister David Dingwall, by standing up and turning their backs to him in a dramatic show of force.

There is a risk, then, that the relief expressed by many that the punitive policies of the Harper government are now a distant memory might give way to misplaced complacency. While there are indeed promising signs and developments with the installation of a Liberal government, there are also a number of challenges that have yet to be addressed comprehensively, some of which we seek to illuminate in these pages. Moreover, we must confront the fact that previous Liberal governments' track records on HIV paint a less than rosy picture.

## Situating HIV/AIDS Historically

HIV/AIDS has been the subject of intense public fascination. First identified with gay men, today's epidemic is marked by its sheer heterogeneity, and by an increasing appreciation for the structural factors that shape vulnerability to HIV such as poverty, racism, and colonialism. This is not to say, of course, that HIV has somehow moved on from gay men. What is most disconcerting for some HIV/AIDS advocates is that legitimate concerns about the need to rethink how we view prevention strategies to meet the needs of diverse populations living with HIV could lead to a "de-gaying" of AIDS. On the contrary, we need to step up our efforts to ensure that the needs of gay men and men who have sex with men are not lost in the shuffle. After all, more than half of all new HIV infections in Canada (57 per cent) involve men who have sex with men, according to Toronto organization CATIE, the Canadian AIDS Treatment Information Exchange.

The explosion of interest in Treatment as Prevention (or TasP), which was pioneered by Dr Julio Montaner at the British Columbia Centre for Excellence in HIV/AIDS, raises important questions about what gets left out of prevention efforts that re-medicalize HIV, and potentially divert state AIDS funding from approaches or interventions that do not produce immediate results, such as efforts to tackle structural drivers including poverty, racism, and homophobia. As Kippax has asked (2012, 5), "How are those who advocate treatment as prevention going to convince governments and countries not to put all their HIV funding into treatment?" Moreover, she adds, some of the evidence about the efficacy of "treatment as prevention" applies mainly to heterosexual discordant couples and raises doubts about the ability to roll this out at a population level.

In the early years of the epidemic in Canada, where misinformation stood in the way of prevention, individuals living with HIV were shunned, stigmatized, and cast off as dirty, diseased, and literally contagious. When news spread that Canada's blood system was compromised and thousands acquired HIV, and later hepatitis C, as a result of government wrongdoing, the idea that HIV had affected so-called "innocent" blood transfusion recipients gave way to "othering" dynamics that marked them off from groups perceived as morally culpable, including gay men, people who use drugs, and sex workers.

The first AIDS cases were reported in the United States in 1978, followed a year later by the announcement in Canada of the first identified case in Windsor, Ontario. This "new" illness was identified initially as Gay-Related Immune Deficiency (GRID), much to the ire of gay rights organizations, who feared that this would further stigmatize an already marginalized population. Their concerns were well-founded: it was not long before Gaëtan Dugas, a gay flight attendant with Air Canada, was scapegoated as "Patient Zero" (Shilts 1987). Notwithstanding the lack of epidemiological evidence to support this narrative, it reflected what would become a consistent pattern of stigma, stereotyping, and scaremongering, driven by fear of those who, by virtue of their sexuality, drug use, or racialization, were designated as dangerous, morally culpable vectors of infection.

Shortly thereafter, researchers discovered that people using intravenous drugs in the New York City area were also coming down with *Pneumocystis carinii* pneumonia (PCP), which was regarded as a common marker of HIV infection; it became clear that this disease could also be transmitted through blood. By 1981, U.S. officials started investigating the first case of GRID in a heterosexual hemophiliac. Within six months, the U.S. Centers for Disease Control reported a possible link between the blood products patients were using and this new, mystery disease. Armed with new information, U.S. officials agreed, in the summer of 1982, on a new name for the condition: Acquired Immunodeficiency Syndrome (AIDS).

By December 1982, Canadian officials likewise realized that this new blood-borne illness was not restricted to gay men. *Canada Diseases Weekly Report*, a publication of the federal government's Health and Welfare Canada, released a preliminary report showing that 70 per cent of hemophiliacs had compromised immune systems. Within months the first Canadian hemophiliac had died of AIDS-related complications.

The 1980s was a period of intense interest in HIV-related research and marked the beginning of government involvement in the HIV policy domain. With the realization that three hemophiliacs in the United States were diagnosed with the same form of cancer that had been linked to a cluster of cases in gay men, the federal government struck a special committee in the fall of 1982 to study the risks of HIV transmission through blood. Almost two years later, the National Advisory Committee on AIDS was still reporting that the risk of contracting HIV from blood was extremely low. With much of the burgeoning discourse centred on the prevalence of HIV in gay men, the Canadian Red Cross Society (CRCS) decided to launch a campaign urging members of what they termed "high-risk groups" (homosexuals with multiple partners, HIV-positive people, Haitians, and intravenous drug users) to refrain from donating blood. In pamphlets and press releases, however, the CRCS adopted a less confrontational approach towards blood-donor collection, fearful that direct questioning of donors might expose the organization to human rights complaints from members of these groups.

It is difficult to think about HIV and AIDS in Canada without referring to the blood system scandal that gripped the country in the late 1980s and sparked a public inquiry into wrongdoing, resulting in a billion-dollar compensation package for people who became HIV- and HCV-positive as a result of blood transfusions. During the late 1980s, the federal government quietly acknowledged its failure to screen the blood system for the presence of HIV, and offered a four-year package to tainted-blood recipients infected with HIV. Reflecting the crude calculus and limited scientific knowledge of the time, it was presumed that the recipients would soon succumb to AIDS-related illnesses and death. Much to the surprise of the federal government, the majority of the recipients were still alive as the package was set to expire (see Orsini 2002).

The 1989 International AIDS Conference also marked a turning point in AIDS activism. It was the first time a Canadian prime minister (Brian Mulroney) spoke publicly about HIV/AIDS, saying, "Having this illness neither diminishes people's humanity nor limits their rights ... Shunning people with AIDS or attaching stigmas to the illness obscures the existence of AIDS when precisely the opposite is required" (Mulroney quoted in Picard 1998, 169). Mulroney's speech, however, was only delivered after over an hour of activist protests led by AIDS Action Now! (Toronto), ACT UP (New York), and Réaction Sida (Montreal). These activists regarded Mulroney's presence at the conference as hypocritical given his government's lack of action on AIDS, particularly when equal time had not been allocated to PHA voices. They broke through security, stormed the stage to read a list of demands for the rights of people living with AIDS, occupied VIP-reserved seats, and turned their backs on Mulroney when he finally spoke. This new brand of activism would alter the character of AIDS organizing by publicly holding governments to account and insisting on space for PHA voices in the HIV/AIDS response, including at future international AIDS conferences. (This brief summary does not capture the complexity and radical impact of early AIDS activism. For a more thorough discussion, see Kinsman's chapter in this volume.)

Regrettably, HIV policy in Canada has not been the focus of significant or recent scholarly attention, despite sustained activist mobilization (see, for example, the AIDS Activist History Project). Literature that has addressed aspects of HIV policy is largely limited to a few journal articles (Rayside and Lindquist 1992; Orsini 2002) and an edited collection addressing women and HIV prevention (Gahagan 2013). There is a significant body of sociological and public health literature examining HIV prevention and intervention strategies but this intervention research, while important, generally does not engage theoretically or empirically with larger social policy debates. Much of the North American social science literature in the field of HIV has centred on the U.S. context (Treichler 1999; Shilts 1987; Epstein 1998; Patton 1990), but the Canadian political, demographic, and social policy context differs significantly from that of the United States. Moreover, literature on Canadian social policy and on broader changes in the Canadian welfare state has typically not considered how these larger political shifts have affected the HIV/AIDS sector or people living with HIV (Dobrowolsky 2009; McBride and Whiteside 2011). By considering HIV policy through the lens of critical social science inquiry (see Mykhalovskiy and Cain 2008) and applying it to the contemporary Canadian policy context, we hope to contribute to the field of HIV policy analysis and critical praxis. Moreover, we view *Seeing Red* as contributing to and addressing the important warning that "theoretically engaged scholarly commentary on the topic is on the wane" and that there is "a certain disinterest, even closure of thought around HIV/AIDS" (Mykhalovskiy and Rosengarten 2009).

## HIV/AIDS Policy and Politics: Then and Now

HIV/AIDS is an important historical reminder of the need to take seriously the role of non-state actors in crafting innovative and life-saving responses to public health crises. Today, in the age of evidence-based policy, important questions remain about the kinds of evidence that matter most in shaping HIV policy, and the relative weight attached to lived experience in this hierarchy of evidence (see, for example, Mykhalovskiy and Weir 2004). Community-based activism is still central to the current Canadian HIV response, but this response is also characterized by a complex interplay between community groups and actors at all levels of government. The steady march of neoliberalism, and its rethinking of the welfare state and the primacy of the market, means that it is foolish to imagine that governments alone can or will lead the HIV response. An important lesson from the legacy of AIDS activism in North America is that communities can shape a grassroots response that is both effective and bold. As Epstein has demonstrated in his definitive account of US AIDS activism, people living with HIV/AIDS successfully mobilized the language and culture of medical science. They employed a range of arguments to establish themselves "as legitimate representatives of people with HIV infection and/or AIDS." In addition, they combined "methodological (epistemological) arguments and moral (political) arguments so as to monopolize different forms of credibility in different domains" (Epstein 1995, 420), including the notion that access to experimental treatments through clinical trials was a social good that must be distributed equally. A central premise of this book, therefore, is that these community activists are not merely "passive recipients" of policy, but are important policy actors in their own right.

In this respect, we depart from approaches that define policy as "whatever governments choose to do or not to do," and entailing "conscious choice that leads to deliberate action – the passage of a law, the spending of money, an official speech or gesture" (Brooks 1998, 3). Public policy, in these traditional frameworks, contains three elements: the definition of a problem, the goals to be achieved, and the means/instruments to achieve these objectives. The first element is critical because it occurs when problems are defined as "public" problems, rather than as private matters. The irony is that while problem definition is crucial to understanding public policy, it is rarely articulated in a policy statement. Second, policies identify the goals to be achieved. Is a policy intended to address behaviour change, for instance? Sometimes the goals are fuzzy or even non-existent because policymakers may be unclear themselves or are responding to public pressure or for ideological reasons. If one thinks of the clampdown on supervised injection sites under Harper's Conservative government, it is difficult to see what practical good might have been achieved by shutting down environments that reduce HIV and hepatitis C transmission, as well as overdoses and deaths. Finally, what are the instruments that will be used to address the given problem? Once actors have determined what the problem is and the goals they want to achieve, they need to choose the policy instruments that will assist in achieving these goals, which may vary in how coercive or liberty-limiting they might be.

Conventional public policy analysts also speak of policy processes or stages of decision-making (e.g., Howlett and Ramesh 1995). In the real world of policymaking, however, it is accepted that we cannot speak definitively about rational decision-making processes that move in discrete phases. And of course, the three elements discussed above presume that there is a logical movement from the definition of a problem to thinking through how to achieve the stated goals of the policy.

While we do not wish to abandon the importance of the three elements of policy identified above, we are interested in thinking about HIV policy using a critical or interpretive lens (see Orsini and Smith 2007). As Yanow reminds us, "Interpretive policy analysis asks not only *what* a policy means – a context-specific question about a specific policy – but also *how* policies mean – questions about the processes by which meanings are communicated" (Yanow 2016, 403). In addition, she notes, "Interpretive forms of policy analysis have shifted attention from the search for (and belief in the promise of finding) one correct policy formulation (correct in its definition of the policy problem, a narrative which entails the seeds for problem resolution) to engage, instead, the possible multiplicities of problem definition resulting from different interpretive communities' experiences and perceptions" (403–4). Throughout these interpretive processes of policymaking and policy analysis, community activists, as much as government representatives, are central to the meaning-making contests and dialogues through which "problems" and "solutions" in the HIV response are constructed and defined.

Now we turn to the question of how to delineate the boundaries of the field of HIV policy. Of course, if we take seriously the suggestion that a range of policies affect HIV as we know it, it seems unwise to assert that we can contain this boundary. Rather, it is best to view HIV policy as that complex of action (and inaction) that bundles a range of actors, including government, civil society organizations, and most importantly, people living with HIV. While the Federal Initiative to

Address HIV/AIDS brings together the Public Health Agency of Canada, Health Canada, the Canadian Institutes of Health Research and Correctional Services Canada to collaborate with a range of stakeholders on matters of common concern, this does not exhaust the range of policy-relevant matters in the field. For example, policies and programs that address social assistance or housing are highly significant to people living with HIV, as are legal developments that reconstitute the responsible sexual subject in the age of AIDS.

In this book, we conceive of the state as multi-vocal, complex, and in some ways, ambiguous. In her now classic formulation, Rianne Mahon spoke of the state as being held together by a "contradictory unity" (Mahon 1977). This is not intended to force a neo-Marxist lens on how we think of HIV; rather, it reminds us that how we think about and understand HIV, and policy in the name of HIV, is heavily invested in its imbrication with state authority. We need to articulate the multiple meanings of HIV and AIDS – "an epidemic of signification," to use Treichler's (1999) phrase – with a keen attention to and appreciation for the shifting nature and character of the state, as well.

This requires us to consider the larger, more daunting question of how neoliberalism relates to HIV in contemporary Canada. Wendy Larner explores three ways in which neoliberalism is articulated in a range of social science literature: as policy, as ideology, and as governmentality. While the first and second are self-evident, denoting neoliberalism as either a policy response to the exigencies of the global economy, or the capturing of the policy agenda by the "New Right," Larner exhorts us to dig deeper. She suggests that viewing neoliberalism solely in the first two senses runs "the risk of under-estimating the significance of contemporary transformations in governance." Neoliberalism, she counters, "is both a political discourse about the nature of rule and a set of practices that facilitate the governing of individuals from a distance" (Larner 2000, 6). It is a mode of governing that exhorts "people to see themselves as individualized and active subjects responsible for enhancing their own well-being. This conception of the 'active society' can also be linked to a particular politics of self in which we are all encouraged to 'work on ourselves' in a range of domains" (13). In the context of HIV, Kinsman wrote a prescient article in 1996 in which he warned of the dangers of a focus on individual responsibility, and the false distinction between "responsible" and "irresponsible" PLWA/ HIV (see Kinsman 1996).

Reflecting the complexity of defining "policy" and the relationship between the HIV response and broader neoliberal forces, contributors to this book offer diverse perspectives on these matters.

## Book Structure, Synopsis, and Themes

The book is organized in three sections and structured by level of analysis. The first section is mainly conceptual and theoretical, focused on the systems level, while the other two sections, exploring service provision and policy impact at the level of populations and individuals, are more applied and empirical. The latter two sections include reflective pieces, narrative reflections from service providers and people living with HIV that centre contributors' own lived experiences with HIV policy, programming, and service provision. These contributions are intended to ground and contextualize the theoretical and systems-level analyses, by illustrating the "real world" consequences of particular modes of policy and political thought and action.

The first section of the book, "Systems," focuses on the overarching systems and structures that organize the HIV response in Canada, asking how these legal, political, and economic systems and structures work to construct different categories of HIV-positive and vulnerable citizens, who then have unequal abilities to make claims upon the state. Focusing specifically on HIV exceptionalism, integration, and criminalization, this section introduces the overarching theoretical and policy problems that are then explored through applied policy analysis in the subsequent two sections.

In chapter 1, Richard Elliott, the executive director of the Canadian HIV/AIDS Legal Network, tackles the controversial notion of "HIV exceptionalism." The debate has often ended up unhelpfully – and inaccurately – pitching human rights concerns against (often narrowly defined) public health objectives. In recent years, a new push for "integration" of the response to HIV with other health issues has arisen, with renewed calls for an end to so-called HIV exceptionalism. The new backdrop for this debate is the intensified interest in HIV "Treatment as Prevention," a related push for more routine approaches to HIV testing, and often-facile discussions about "the end of AIDS." But Elliott suggests that it is incorrect to claim that HIV exceptionalism and integration are mutually exclusive. HIV certainly is exceptional in that it has highlighted fault lines of socio-economic injustice in a way that few

other communicable diseases have. As a result, and because of the political context in which the epidemic emerged, it has also provoked an
exceptional activist response – including demands for action on fronts
that governments were often reluctant to address, basic human rights
for those living with HIV and those at risk of infection, and ultimately
an understanding that the epidemic is not merely a public health issue
but also one of social justice.

In chapter 2, Marilou Gagnon and Christine Vézina use structural
stigma as a conceptual entry point for thinking about the criminalization of HIV non-disclosure and its effects on people living with HIV.[3]
The authors take an interdisciplinary approach, based partly on the legal analysis of criminal cases, partly on the theoretical work of Hannem
and Bruckert (2012), and finally through a Foucauldian perspective, all
in an attempt to understand the ways in which stigmatizing assumptions about people living with HIV work to produce new categories
of (potentially) dangerous offenders and create a need for regulation
– and exclusion.

Chapter 3, by criminologist Jennifer Kilty, explores how carceral
spaces institutionalize risk, expose inmates to various forms of state
violence, and deprive them of basic human rights. Kilty focuses on how
neoliberal approaches to governance have affected Canada's evolving
approach to public health and penality. Drawing on Wacquant's (2010)
notion of the "daddy-state," which she contrasts with the idea of the
nanny state, Kilty argues that federal responses to HIV as they pertain
to prisons and penality combine aspects of legal moralism, legal paternalism, and the politics of blame.

Finally, Francisco Ibáñez-Carrasco, a long-time AIDS advocate, offers
a provocative meditation on life in the shadow of public health paternalism. He asks pointedly if our own public health systems are bad
for our collective health, and for PWAs in particular. Weaving personal
narrative with trenchant analysis, Ibáñez-Carrasco's reflections on life
as a positive man are interspersed with sharp social commentary.

The second section, "Services," zooms in one level of analysis, examining trends and challenges in service provision. Drawing attention
to the emerging and closely related issues of aging with HIV, and the
move towards approaching HIV as an episodic disability, this section
asks how emerging challenges in the HIV/AIDS sector should be understood and addressed. The section also considers a key challenge
faced by service providers at this "middle level": how to balance the

often-competing demands and needs of state funders, community members, and people living with HIV.

In chapter 5, Kate Murzin and Charles Furlotte tackle the impact of aging on access to health resources for older adults and marginalized people living with HIV. They argue that the erosion of Canada's social safety net is creating increasing challenges for older PHAs, ranging from age-based eligibility criteria for "seniors" programming and benefits to funding and bureaucratic structures that limit intersectoral collaboration and integrated care. Drawing from the results of a recent community-driven national environmental scan, Murzin and Furlotte show that program planners have managed to creatively circumvent some of the organizational and social policies that restrict access to rehabilitation services by older adults with HIV.

Next, Nicole Greenspan's chapter takes us inside the AIDS service organization (ASO) sector, providing insight into how ASOs evaluate their HIV prevention work and how changes in evaluation policy have affected practice at these organizations. These practices – both formal and tacit – assist in a collective "sense-making" of HIV prevention work with diverse communities, but in ways that cannot be fully captured in or reflected through funder-mandated evaluation metrics.

Long-time activist Ron Rosenes, a recipient of the Order of Canada, provides personal reflections on life as a gay man living with HIV for several decades. His unique portrait of aging with HIV offers a rich springboard for a discussion of far-ranging policy reforms, including guaranteed income supplements, that would improve the well-being of people aging with HIV.

Finally, the section ends with a reflective chapter on HIV, employment, and income security by Wendy Porch and Tammy C. Yates from Realize (formerly the Canadian Working Group on HIV and Rehabilitation). As they explain, while there is good news about increased life expectancy for people living with HIV, focusing solely on life expectancy as an indicator of well-being disregards the complicated and topsyturvy reality of what it means to live, day by day, year by year, with HIV. Focusing on disease outcomes ignores the emotional, social, financial, and employment-related challenges associated with living with an unpredictable, stigmatized, and invisible episodic disability. This chapter examines some of the challenges people living with HIV have faced, and continue to confront, related to employment and income security. This chapter also reflects on the often-limited role played by social policy and examines how new ways of thinking about HIV and disability might transform individual lives. Building from a case study, the chapter develops a larger analysis of the evolution of HIV-related employment and income security issues, as well as the opportunities and constraints these social policies create for people living with HIV.

The third and final section, "Populations," focuses on the impact of HIV policy and welfare state transformation on some of the populations disproportionately affected by HIV. Contributors to this section ask how people and communities interact with, and mobilize in response to, state policy decisions. With particular focus on trans and Indigenous women, immigrants, and refugees, the section draws attention to variation in policy and community organizing in response to these effects. Invariably, the inclusion of specific groups comes at the expense of other groups or populations that are not explicitly discussed in this section. It is important to stress, however, that these seeming exclusions are in no way intended as normative statements about which groups or populations deserve attention. We are interested, rather, in the policy challenges inherent in efforts to explicitly address the complex identities and experiences of groups or populations – as well as the ways in which these populations are themselves constructed in and through state policies. Epidemiologic data about risk groups or risk categories, regrettably, leave intact many of the problematic assumptions about behaviour that are associated with membership in a particular group; when these assumptions then form the basis for policy and program responses to HIV, the result can, as chapters in this section demonstrate, be policies that fail to address the complex lived realities of people living with HIV.

In chapter 9, Alex McClelland, Adrian Guta, and Nicole Greenspan train a critical lens on a key challenge in a range of policy areas, that is the meaningful participation of citizens and specifically affected individuals who bring "lived experience" to the table. Their chapter offers a trenchant critique of key international and Canadian texts that purport to promote the Greater Involvement of People Living with HIV & AIDS (GIPA). Examining key GIPA policy and programmatic documents with an eye to what forms of participation these texts enable or constrain, the authors offer a critical interpretation of what they represent for the engagement of people living with HIV in the Canadian and global response.

In chapter 10, Natalie Duchesne draws on the notion of "policy mess" to describe the experience of trans women living with HIV in

Montreal and Toronto. The encounters trans women have with a range of policies – be it in the fields of housing, social assistance, or immigration – provide a window into the complex challenges associated with responding to the specific needs of individuals who are vulnerable to and living with HIV. In addition, it is an important reminder that the perspectives of trans people are still under-represented in public policy development and research.

In chapter 11, Tracey Prentice, Doris Peltier, Elizabeth Benson, Kerrigan Johnson, Kecia Larkin, Krista Shore, and Renée Masching present an innovative framework and methodology for understanding how Indigenous women living with HIV think about and understand the connections among HIV, broader social determinants of health, and the cumulative impact of colonization. Mainstream public health approaches continue to emphasize behavioural determinants and are frequently framed by a biomedical perspective that pathologizes Indigenous women, sacrifices cultural diversity, and hinders Indigenous self-determination. The authors put forward an approach that is culturally grounded, decolonizing, and strengths-based, which community participants described as "damn good medicine."

Chelsea Gabel, Randy Jackson, and Chaneesa Ryan bring together two HIV-related policy issues that have often proceeded on separate tracks: aging with HIV, and Indigenous people. The authors begin with the observation that Indigenous people make up the second-largest ethnic group among older Canadians living with HIV. Studies of aging and HIV provide important information about the general experience of aging with HIV, but provide limited culturally appropriate knowledge. This chapter draws on decolonizing and Indigenous methodologies to guide future research, policy and program development that is grounded in the perspectives of Indigenous peoples.

Chapter 13, by Teresa Chulach, Marilou Gagnon, and Dave Holmes draws on a qualitative study of the experience of pregnancy among HIV-positive refugee women. Focusing on the narratives of three HIV-positive women, the chapter explores what pregnancy means for these women and challenges it poses at the micro, meso, and macro levels. Their analysis draws attention to the intersection of various dimensions of identity, and how these intersections influence the ways in which HIV-positive refugee women define themselves and are defined by others. The analysis ultimately sheds light on social relationships and the broader context in which HIV-positive refugee women are located. The chapter concludes by offering key policy recommendations, with particular emphasis on mandatory HIV testing policies.

Chapter 14 is a reflective piece by Colleen Price that explores the challenges associated with HIV-HCV co-infection. In it the author discusses her early encounters with medical providers and community supports and how they became the catalyst for her subsequent advocacy and activist work.

Finally, sociologist and HIV/AIDS historian Gary Kinsman offers a distinctive perspective on the contemporary AIDS crisis, one that is grounded in his own experience as an AIDS activist and intellectual. He compels us to resist the urge to forget the legacy of AIDS activism, arguing that these previous struggles continue to inform and shape the present. There is no greater time to "remember resistance," he argues, especially critical as we confront a "more consolidated neoliberal capitalism" characterized by cuts in social assistance and health care and criminalization.

In our conclusion, we reflect on the main themes and situate the historical response to HIV in relation to the contemporary context.

NOTES

1   As Robertson recounts in an analysis of the impact of the publication, the paper's coverage of HIV embodied four approaches: "Skepticism of scientific and media authority; the need to resist panic and hysteria both within and beyond the gay community; the need to seek information on which we can make informed judgments about sexual practices; and, most recently, the need to preserve what is best and most distinctive about gay erotic culture in the face of a disease which apparently threatens its very roots" (Bébout quoted in Robertson 2002, 416).

2   According to the Public Health Agency of Canada (2015), more than 16 per cent of all reported cases in 2014 were among Indigenous people, and Indigenous women represented more than 30 per cent of all cases reported among women for that year.

3   A word about terminology is in order here. Recognizing the importance of self-naming and person-first language, we chose not to require standardization of terms to describe people living with HIV/AIDS, instead respecting the language and terminology employed by each contributor. Therefore, some authors use PLWH, PWA, or PHA, or eschew acronyms entirely. This

variation reflects ongoing debates about the politics of language, labelling, and naming in the HIV response. Similarly, we have respected each contributor's choice to use Indigenous, Aboriginal, First Nations, or other terms to denote the original inhabitants of "Canadian" territory.

REFERENCES

"AIDS Activist History Project." http://www.aidsactivisthistory.ca.

Alfred, T. 1999. *Peace, Power, Righteousness: An Indigenous Manifesto*. Don Mills, ON: Oxford University Press.

Brooks, S. 1998. *Public Policy in Canada*. 3rd ed. Toronto: Oxford University Press.

Centers for Disease Control. 2016. "HIV in the United States: *At a Glance*." https://www.cdc.gov/hiv/statistics/overview/ataglance.html.

Coulthard, G. 2014. *Red Skin, White Masks: Rejecting the Colonial Politics of Recognition*. Minneapolis: University of Minnesota Press. https://doi.org/10.5749/minnesota/9780816679645.001.0001.

Dobrowolsky, A. 2009. *Women and Public Policy in Canada: Neoliberalism and After?* New York: Oxford University Press.

Epstein, S. 1995. "The Construction of Lay Expertise: AIDS Activism and the Forging of Credibility in the Reform of Clinical Trials." *Science, Technology & Human Values* 20 (4): 408–37. https://doi.org/10.1177/016224399502000402.

– 1998. *Impure Science: AIDS, Activism and the Politics of Knowledge*. Berkeley: University of California Press.

Gahagan, J., ed. 2013. *Women and HIV Prevention in Canada: Implications for Research, Policy, and Practice*. Toronto: Women's Press.

Gould, D. 2009. *Moving Politics: Emotion and ACT UP's Fight against AIDS*. Chicago: University of Chicago Press.

Hannem, S., and C. Bruckert, eds. 2012. *Stigma Revisited: Implications of the Mark*. Ottawa: University of Ottawa Press.

Howlett, M., and M. Ramesh. 1995. *Studying Public Policy: Policy Cycles and Policy Subsystems*. Toronto: Oxford University Press.

Kinsman, G. 1996. "'Responsibility' as a Strategy of Governance: Regulating People Living with AIDS and Lesbians and Gay Men in Ontario." *Economy and Society* 25 (3): 393–409. https://doi.org/10.1080/03085149600000021.

Kippax, S. 2012. "Effective HIV Prevention: The Indispensable Role of Social Science." *Journal of the International AIDS Society* 15 (17357). http://dx.doi.org/10.7448/IAS.15.2.17357.

Larner, W. 2000. "Neo-liberalism: Policy, Ideology, Governmentality." *Studies in Political Economy* 63:5–25.

Mahon, R. 1977. "Canadian Public Policy: The Unequal Structure of Representation." In *The Canadian State: Political Economy and Political Power*, edited by Leo Panitch, 165–98. Toronto: University of Toronto Press.

McBride, S., and H. Whiteside. 2011. *Private Affluence, Public Austerity: Economic Crisis and Democratic Malaise in Canada*. Halifax: Fernwood.

McGoey, L. 2012. "Strategic Unknowns: Towards a Sociology of Ignorance." *Economy and Society* 41 (1): 1–16. https://doi.org/10.1080/03085147.2011.637330.

Mykhalovskiy, E., and R. Cain. 2008. *Critical Work: Invigorating Critical Social Sciences and Humanities Research on HIV/AIDS in Ontario*. Report prepared for the Ontario HIV Treatment Network.

Mykhalovskiy, E., and M. Rosengarten. 2009. "HIV/AIDS in Its Third Decade: Renewed Critique in Social and Cultural Analysis." *Social Theory & Health* 7 (3): 187–95. https://doi.org/10.1057/sth.2009.13.

Mykhalovskiy, E., and L. Weir. 2004. "The Problem of Evidence-Based Medicine: Directions for Social Science." *Social Science & Medicine* 59 (5): 1059–69. https://doi.org/10.1016/j.socscimed.2003.12.002.

Orsini, M. 2002. "The Politics of Naming, Blaming and Claiming: HIV, Hepatitis C and the Emergence of Blood Activism in Canada." *Canadian Journal of Political Science* 35 (3): 475–98. https://doi.org/10.1017/S0008423902778323.

Orsini, M., and M. Smith, eds. 2007. *Critical Policy Studies*. Vancouver: University of British Columbia Press.

Patton, C. 1990. *Inventing AIDS*. New York: Routledge.

Picard, A. 1998. *The Gift of Death: Confronting Canada's Tainted Blood Tragedy*. Rev. ed. Toronto: HarperCollins Publishers.

Public Health Agency of Canada. 2015. *HIV and AIDS in Canada. Surveillance Report to December 31, 2014*. Ottawa: Minister of Public Works and Government Services Canada.

Rayside, D., and E. Lindquist. 1992. "AIDS Activism and the State in Canada." *Studies in Political Economy* 39 (1): 37–76. https://doi.org/10.1080/19187033.1992.11675417.

Robertson, M.L. 2002. "AIDS Coverage in the Body Politic, 1981–1987: An Annotated Bibliography." *American Review of Canadian Studies* 32 (3): 415–31. https://doi.org/10.1080/02722010209481669.

Shilts, R. 1987. *And the Band Played On: Politics, People and the AIDS Epidemic*. New York: Penguin Books.

Simpson, A. 2014. *Mohawk Interruptus: Political Life across the Borders of Settler States*. Durham, NC: Duke University Press. https://doi.org/10.1215/9780822376781.

Treichler, P.A. 1999. *How to Have Theory in an Epidemic: Cultural Chronicles of AIDS*. Durham, NC: Duke University Press.

Visual AIDS. "The Red Ribbon Project." https://www.visualaids.org/projects/detail/the-red-ribbon-project.

Wacquant, Loïc. 2010. "Crafting the Neoliberal State: Workfare, Prisonfare, and Social Insecurity." *Sociological Forum* 25 (2): 197–220. https://doi.org/10.1111/j.1573-7861.2010.01173.x.

Yanow, D. 2016. "Making Sense of Policy Practices: Interpretation and Meaning." In *Handbook of Critical Policy Studies*, edited by F. Fischer et al., 401–21. Cheltenham, UK: Edward Elgar Publishing.

# PART ONE

## Systems

# 1 The Rights Response Is (Still) Required: Preserving the Human Rights Core of HIV Exceptionalism in Pursuing the End of AIDS

RICHARD ELLIOTT

Halfway through the fourth decade of the HIV pandemic, there has been substantial scientific progress in both prevention and treatment – welcome developments that have led some political leaders and key global institutions, including all member states of the UN General Assembly, to declare that the world should strive for "an end to AIDS" within a generation (White House 2011). Yet there is also recognition, albeit too often only rhetorical, that such biomedical advances will be insufficient without also creating an "enabling environment," including a policy environment that protects and promotes human rights (UNAIDS 2011; Schwartländer et al. 2011). To successfully achieve both HIV prevention and treatment goals, this must include the rights of both people already living with HIV (PLHIV), and "key populations" and communities most heavily affected by the epidemic. This, of course, reflects the reality that these populations and communities are so affected in part because of social inequities and the denial or infringement of their human rights. Without creating such an environment, the gaps in the HIV response will mean those most at risk and most in need will be "left behind" (UNAIDS 2014a, 2014b). This would be an ethical failure and a failure to comply with numerous widely endorsed commitments under international human rights law; it should also be of concern to policymakers on public health grounds because it will ultimately frustrate the goal of ending the epidemic.

In this chapter, I argue that this insistence on human rights – and their implications for transforming policy and practice in responding to a public health challenge – is the necessary core of what is too often derided as "HIV exceptionalism." Despite important successes, that transformative project remains very much a work in progress: in many countries, punitive policies undermining effective HIV prevention and treatment remain firmly in place, and Canada has its share of examples. Addressing the human rights drivers of the epidemic remains imperative if there is to be an "end to AIDS." In addition, in recent years there has been a growing demand, including by government funders, for "integration" of the HIV response with other public health efforts – which impetus carries potential benefits, depending on how it is implemented, but also carries further risk of a simplistic, misguided dismissal of HIV exceptionalism. It would be a mistake in Canada and elsewhere to ignore a key lesson of the HIV pandemic and, in the name of such integration to prematurely jettison the insistence on human rights that lies at the heart of an appropriately exceptional approach to HIV, particularly when the legal and policy environment continues to be exceptionally hostile to effective HIV responses and to PLHIV and communities affected by HIV.

## Regressive Policy Environment as Disabling for the HIV Response

Despite the recognition that it is an essential element of the response, creating the necessary "enabling environment" through protecting and fulfilling human rights remains a challenge. On many HIV-related fronts, the relevant and necessary public policy measures remain hotly contested – and too often, public policy creates barriers and causes entirely avoidable harm, instead of protecting and promoting health and other human rights. To note but a few key examples: it is a constant struggle to close the persistent, iniquitous gap in equitable access to affordable medicines, globally and at the country level (even in some wealthy countries, including Canada). This gap widens with each new "free trade" agreement containing ever more restrictive rules on intellectual property, which further limits countries' flexibility to adapt policy to serve public interests (e.g., UNDP & UNAIDS 2012; Global Commission on HIV and the Law 2012). Law reform and other advocacy efforts to protect and advance women's equality, bodily integrity, and economic autonomy remain urgently needed in order to reduce women's risk of HIV infection and to ensure equitable access to care, treatment, and support for women living with HIV (Chu et al. 2014). Stigma, discrimination, and violence continue to play a key role in driving the HIV epidemic among people who use illegal drugs (Jürgens et al. 2010), gay men and other men who have sex with men (MSM) (Altman et al. 2012), sex workers (Decker et al. 2015), and transgender people (WHO 2015b); in many countries, such stigma, discrimination, and violence are rooted in, and fostered by, punitive laws that criminalize these populations or otherwise deny or impede their access to services. Meanwhile, correctional statutes, prison policies, and practices routinely infringe on the human rights of incarcerated people in ways that undermine their health, including denial of adequate access to health goods, services, and information equivalent to those outside prison, a clear breach of long-settled international human rights standards (UNAIDS 2014c; Chu and Elliott 2009; UN General Assembly 2015b). Overly broad use of criminal law to prosecute PLHIV for transmission, exposure, or even non-disclosure – often with little regard for available scientific evidence about the actual risk of transmission – is an unfortunate phenomenon that has spread globally since first emerging in North America in the late 1980s (Bernard and Cameron 2013). Ensuring the rights to informed consent to HIV testing and treatment, to freedom from discrimination, and to protection of private health information remains a systemic challenge in many settings, even when law and stated policy ostensibly guarantee such standards, while young people, including those most affected by the epidemic, are often denied access to health services and information they need to protect and promote their health (WHO 2015c, 2015d, 2015e, 2015f).

Canada has not been immune to these contests over public policy in the response to HIV. Indeed, the last decade has been a particularly turbulent period in which federal government policy on numerous aspects of the HIV response has been widely criticized by community organizations, human rights advocates, and health experts as being divorced from – and even flatly contradicting – the best available evidence, as well as disregarding or breaching human rights standards, including rights ostensibly guaranteed by the constitution. Three examples of hotly disputed developments in federal law and policy stand out as illustrative, all of them affecting various dimensions of the HIV response and of both domestic and international interest.

First, with respect to illegal drugs, between 2007 and 2015, the federal government: completely excised harm reduction from a new (and newly named) National Anti-Drug Strategy; actively attempted to terminate or block harm reduction measures such as safer consumption services and opposed such measures in international forums; intensified a prohibitionist response to drugs by legislating mandatory minimum sentences for certain drug offences (including for possession in certain circumstances); refused to implement needle and syringe programs as part of comprehensive harm reduction services in federal prisons, as well as cancelled a pilot safer tattooing program in prisons despite positive evaluations; and adopted new regulations directly aimed at preventing the continued prescription of pharmaceutical-grade heroin for medical purposes to a subset of opioid-dependent patients, despite the great benefits of this treatment option demonstrated in a clinical trial.[1] At this writing, some of these harmful legislative and policy measures have been successfully resisted by advocates, and some shifts in tone and approach have been signalled by a government elected in 2015 – to a degree. The Supreme Court has struck down one aspect of mandatory minimum sentencing for drug offences (*R v Lloyd* 2016), and the government has made a groundbreaking commitment to legalizing and regulating cannabis (the scope and details of which are under active discussion at this writing).[2] However, the extent to which a promised review of federal criminal justice policy will lead to broader repeal and revision of prohibitionist drug policy is unclear, and advocates' calls for more broadly decriminalizing the possession of drugs (beyond cannabis) for personal use have been rebuffed, despite the growing number of countries moving in this direction and the growing body of evidence of benefits (Eastwood et al. 2016). Meanwhile, statements of support for harm reduction measures such as safer consumption services are welcome, and in May 2017, at the urging of advocates, the federal government repealed the restrictive Respect for Communities Act – the legal regime that was enacted by the previous government, against the urgings of the vast majority of health experts and human rights advocates, with the deliberate objective of erecting numerous hurdles to securing the exemptions that enable such health services to operate without the risk of criminal prosecution of clients or staff for drug offences such as possession.[3] Similarly, in response to questions about prison-based needle and syringe programs, during the 2015 federal election campaign, the Liberal Party stated its general support for evidence-based policy (see Canadian HIV/AIDS Legal Network 2015b), and after it was elected to power, newly elected federal ministers and departmental spokespeople have subsequently made encouraging statements to the same effect – but at this writing, there has been no commitment to implement such programs (or to reintroduce the safer tattooing program cancelled by the previous government). In December 2016, the National Anti-Drug Strategy adopted by the previous government was renamed the Canadian Drugs and Substances Strategy and the federal health minister declared that harm reduction was being reinstated as a key element of said strategy; it remains to be seen just how extensively there will be a real shift – including in resources allocated under the strategy – away from a prohibitionist, law-enforcement-heavy response towards an evidence-based, health-focused response to drugs.

A second contentious area has been sex work–related law and policy, as evidenced in part by court challenges to several Criminal Code provisions related to "prostitution" on the basis that they unconstitutionally endangered sex workers' health and safety, in breach of the Charter right to security of the person. The federal government staunchly (and unsuccessfully) defended those provisions – and, after a landmark Supreme Court of Canada ruling in December 2013 striking them down as unconstitutional (*R v Bedford* 2013), enacted the so-called Protection of Communities and Exploited Persons Act (PCEPA) in 2014, which largely replicates the substance of those damaging provisions and even extends the scope of criminalization (Canadian HIV/AIDS Legal Network et al 2014). Despite public expressions of "grave concern" at the time by the Premier of Ontario about the potential harms of such legislation, and calls for non-enforcement by sex worker advocates and their allies, that province's attorney general declared a few months later that her office would enforce the law. Meanwhile, no other provincial premier or attorney general has expressed such concerns. Since the new law was enacted, there have been crackdowns in cities across Canada, and sex workers have documented various ways in which the new legal regime perpetuates the harms of the former one (Canadian Alliance for Sex Work Law Reform 2015; Footer et al. 2016).[4] Again, there may be some hope for legislative reform: during the 2015 election, the Liberal Party declared that it was "committed to replacing this flawed, unconstitutional legislation," and said it would "deliver on prostitution reforms laws [*sic*] formed in consultation with experts and civil society, including sex workers themselves, which includes rigorous examination of supporting facts and evidence" (see Canadian HIV/AIDS Legal Network 2015a). At this writing, initial discussions with federal government ministers and policy advisors elicited further statements of interest by government in examining the concerns and proposals for reform, but it is too early to tell whether the government has the appetite to introduce and advocate for legislative amendments that have been urged by the Canadian Alliance for Sex Work Law Reform (a national alliance of sex worker groups and allied human rights organizations). In the meantime, in response to ongoing urging by HIV advocates, in launching a somewhat redesigned federal HIV funding program in 2016, the federal government finally identified sex workers as a "priority population" in the HIV response.

Finally, intellectual property law reforms and developing-country access to affordable medicines has been a site of contention between HIV (and other) activists and the federal government over nearly two decades. Advocates began lobbying in 2001 for Canada to take a more development-friendly position at the World Trade Organization (WTO), in the context of bitter debates over barriers to affordable medicines created by WTO treaty rules on pharmaceutical patents and other aspects of intellectual property (IP). This advocacy flowed into a nine-year effort to convince Canada to adopt and implement a simple, straightforward means of using flexibility under WTO rules to enable the compulsory licensing of patented medicines so that lower-cost, generic versions could be exported to eligible developing countries. While legislation creating Canada's Access to Medicines Regime (CAMR) was adopted unanimously in Parliament in 2004, with the stated objective of supporting countries in acquiring more affordable medicines, the regime proved sufficiently user-unfriendly that it has been used but a single time (in 2007 and only as a result of years of effort) (Canadian HIV/AIDS Legal Network 2012). Yet despite widespread public support, and endorsement by international legal experts, proposed legislative reforms to strengthen CAMR were met with hostility and blatant misrepresentation by patented pharmaceutical companies and federal government ministers, with proposed reforms finally being defeated by the then-majority government in a whipped vote in Parliament in 2012 (Elliott 2013). At this writing, indications are that, despite stated support in 2012 for CAMR reform by the current prime minister and the large majority of MPs from his party then sitting in the House of Commons, the government elected in 2015 has little interest in introducing the reforms needed if CAMR is to deliver on Parliament's unanimous pledge to developing countries. Meanwhile, under the new government, Canada has agreed in principle to yet further trade agreements with restrictive IP provisions (e.g., the Trans-Pacific Partnership), despite growing expressions of concern about the "incoherence" between such rules and stated commitments to health, human rights, and development (see UNDP and UNAIDS 2012; Global Commission on HIV and the Law 2012; Office of the UN High Commissioner for Human Rights 2015; UNAIDS 2015; UN Secretary-General's High-Level Panel on Access to Medicines 2015). Since then, the Trump administration in the United States has demanded renegotiation of NAFTA; it remains to be seen whether Canada will reject the more restrictive intellectual property and investment provisions that are virtually certain to be advanced by the United States in those negotiations, at the behest of the patented pharmaceutical industry (among others).

During this same period the legal situation also worsened in some respects for people living with HIV. After some initially encouraging developments in provincial appellate courts suggesting that the judiciary was willing to entertain important limitations on the scope of criminal prosecutions against PLHIV, some prosecutors pursued more vigorous application of aggravated sexual assault charges for HIV non-disclosure, and in a substantial setback in 2012, the Supreme Court of Canada appears to have agreed – which rulings have provoked further concern on the part of human rights advocates (Canadian HIV/AIDS Legal Network et al. 2012) including feminist legal academics and other women's rights advocates (see Athena Network 2009; Grant 2011, 2013; Buchanan 2014)[5] and leading HIV scientists (Loutfy et al. 2014). More recently, some lower-court judges have also expressed concerns about the Supreme Court rulings, in some cases echoing concerns that advocates have been raising for many years (see *R v JTC* 2013; *R v Thompson* 2016). At this writing, more than 180 PLHIV in Canada have been prosecuted for alleged non-disclosure, exposure, and/or transmission of HIV, one of the highest per capita rates in the world.[6]

Meanwhile, lacking sufficient independence from the government of the day, the Public Health Agency of Canada (PHAC) and the Chief Public Health Officer were substantially silent as the federal government's financial commitment to an HIV response steadily eroded and its policy prescriptions worsened various social determinants of health. Amidst much talk of "aligning" the Federal Initiative to Address HIV/AIDS in Canada with government priorities, the government's public health agency refused to take – at least publicly – any position or steps that supported evidence-based harm reduction policy or programs (including in prisons, despite its own research report on the subject) or sex workers' health (refusing to even name them as a "priority population"), or to engage with community organizations in any collaboration to address growing concern about the over-extension of the criminal law to PLHIV (e.g., a proposal to convene community experts, PLHIV, prosecutors, and public health practitioners). Instead, the chief activities of PHAC during most of the last decade seem to have been to maintain its (limited) capacity for epidemiological surveillance, produce a handful of "status reports" documenting the state of the HIV epidemic among certain key populations, and develop new guidance that seeks to "normalize" HIV testing as a part of "routine medical care" and encourages disclosure of results (Public Health Agency of Canada 2013). Meanwhile, demands for scaling up testing and treatment have intensified in light of the well-established body of evidence demonstrating both the clinical benefits for PLHIV of early treatment with highly active antiretroviral therapy (HAART) (INSIGHT START Study Group 2015; WHO 2015a) and the broader HIV prevention benefits of suppressing viral load and thereby dramatically reducing the prospects of onward transmission of the virus (Rodger et al. 2014;[7] Loutfy et al. 2013; Baggaley et al. 2013; Cohen et al. 2011; Anglemyer et al. 2011) – a "treatment as prevention" (TasP) strategy, the benefits of which Canadian researchers have played a key role in demonstrating and advocating (yet the implementation of which raises important human rights concerns regularly ignored or dismissed).

It seems cruelly ironic that the legal and (federal) policy environment should have become so hostile, for such a sustained period, precisely when there are such promising pathways to ending the epidemic. Yet this should not cause advocates and policymakers to lose sight of the broader global context, or to abandon efforts to articulate a sound response to HIV in Canada that is based on evidence and on human rights, and that engages PLHIV, affected communities, and community organizations in that response – for this is ultimately necessary for a successful response, political winds do shift, and policy environments can and do change as a result. As noted above, in October 2015 a federal election led to a change in government, and at the time of writing in early 2017, we have witnessed important reforms in a number of areas of federal law and policy, removing at least some of the more punitive policy approaches adopted during the previous government's tenure. However, early indications also suggest the need for sustained advocacy, even with a seemingly more sympathetic government, to secure needed legislative, policy, and funding changes.

## "HIV Exceptionalism" and the Growing Push for "Integration"

It is against this backdrop that the federal government – and in particular the Public Health Agency of Canada – began in 2011 to actively pursue "integrating" the HIV response with the response to other sexually transmitted and/or blood-borne infections (STBBIs), including hepatitis C virus (HCV). Most concretely, this has been embedded in discussions of a new funding model for the federal strategy on HIV. It is therefore no surprise that this, coupled with the enhanced drive to "test and treat," has led to renewed discussion of what has been labelled "HIV exceptionalism."

The term *HIV exceptionalism* is tossed around in a variety of ways – often pejorative. Recently, the term *integration* is, to some degree, being presented in contra-distinction to exceptionalism – i.e., exceptionalism is bad; integration, the supposed opposite, is good. However, it is incorrect and simplistic to claim that exceptionalism and integration are antonyms or mutually exclusive; rather, it depends on what is understood and meant by each. Therefore, we must define these shorthand terms with more precision for there to be a productive consideration of (1) whether HIV exceptionalism is a good or bad phenomenon, and hence whether the supposed opposite, integration, is desirable or undesirable, and (2) what it might or should mean for policy and programmatic responses to HIV.

Not surprisingly, "HIV exceptionalism" has always been contested. Historically, there have been two particular (and occasionally overlapping) sources of opposition: (1) those invested in "traditional" public health strategies and systems (i.e., chiefly health professionals and government officials tasked with public health responsibilities and the often inadequate budgets that accompany them), who have derided HIV exceptionalism as impeding their public health goals; and (2) political conservatives who see the phenomenon as a manifestation in public policy of an approach that is too respectful of human rights, particularly of groups and populations whose rights they have historically opposed, whether because of personal (often religious) conviction or a more crass, political calculus (or sometimes both). The latter camp is far less likely to be familiar with or use the language of "HIV exceptionalism," which has emerged mainly in discussions among academics, public health and community actors engaged in the HIV response. Rather, conservatives are more likely to deride the phenomenon in the language of "special" rights, privileges, or funding for "special interest groups" (e.g., gay people, persistently targeted by the religious right) or in other coded, often hateful language of moral judgment deriding the very notion of rights for populations seen as undeserving (e.g., people who use drugs, sex workers, prisoners, migrants, and racialized people).

Both of these perspectives persist in the contemporary attack on so-called HIV exceptionalism. The political, often religious conservatives have not significantly updated or refined their criticisms – perhaps because it has been unnecessary to do so in light of their significant political influence. But in more recent years the backlash led by public health "traditionalists" has been more sophisticated, whether criticizing human rights concerns in HIV policy and practice directly or, at other times, taking on an ostensibly more beneficent gloss – and even in some cases attempting to couch a return to traditional public health approaches in co-opted "human rights" language. This has been particularly evident in the last decade as scientific advances in both HIV testing (e.g., rapid, point-of-care testing) and treatment (e.g., the use of antiretrovirals as prevention) have been invoked by health professionals – and even some PLHIV and AIDS organizations – to justify their demands for an end to "HIV exceptionalism," by which they chiefly seem to mean any laws, policies, or programmatic requirements that they perceive as impediments to the goal of detecting every single person living with HIV and getting all on treatment. However, HIV exceptionalism has never been quite as firm or dominant a paradigm as its critics contend (and as some of its supporters might wish). Rather, the practical human rights underpinnings of what is derided as "HIV exceptionalism" are not firmly rooted and are therefore particularly vulnerable to this latest, more sophisticated – but ultimately misguided – critique.

Therefore, it is worth asking more carefully, What does "HIV exceptionalism" mean? On one level, it refers to the existence of separate strategies, funding streams, organizations, services, and programs that are focused primarily or exclusively on HIV, and that sometimes exist as entirely stand-alone initiatives or at a remove from other initiatives addressing (public) health issues. In this narrow sense, it could be said that "integration" is indeed the opposite of "exceptionalism" – in the sense of collapsing dedicated HIV-specific funding into larger health-funding envelopes, having organizations address not just HIV but also other related health concerns, having a clinic or health centre provide not just HIV care but instead embrace a more holistic approach, etc.

But having a national (or provincial/local) AIDS strategy, a government advisory committee on HIV, dedicated HIV funding, or community-based service organizations focused exclusively or primarily on HIV is not unique. Consider, after all, such things as national strategies (with associated funding, research initiatives, community organizations, etc.) on other health concerns such as cancer, smoking, mental health, drug use, bullying, housing, unhealthy diets, and lack of fitness, etc. It makes perfect sense that a response to a significant public health concern be organized by identifying the concern and coming up with steps, funding, and initiatives to tackle it. The question ought to be, Is the response informed by evidence, and does it consider the multiple facets that need to be addressed? The existence of HIV strategies, HIV-dedicated funding, and HIV organizations cannot per se be considered objectionable "exceptionalism," because they single out and "favour" a particular disease or health concern for "special treatment," unless having a Canadian Partnership against Cancer or a Canadian Drugs and Substances Strategy or a Mental Health Commission of Canada is also somehow objectionable. It follows that "integrating" the HIV response with other initiatives cannot automatically be a good measure required to cure the supposed ailment of HIV exceptionalism, because there is nothing really exceptional about so-called HIV exceptionalism if it is understood in this simplistic sense.

But to consider "HIV exceptionalism" as simply meaning the existence of HIV-specific strategies, funding, organizations, etc. is not only factually inaccurate (because this is not really exceptional); it also overlooks its deeper, more fundamental significance, the value of which should be better appreciated and not forgotten amidst the clamour for "integration" on the road to "ending AIDS." In a deeper sense, the term means that HIV is exceptional as a public health challenge in ways that have warranted and produced – and continue to warrant and should produce – an exceptional response that in some fundamental and valuable respects deviates from a "traditional" public health approach.

## Human Rights as the Valuable Core of HIV Exceptionalism

HIV is exceptional – albeit not unique – because it (1) travels along, highlights, and is fuelled by social fault lines and inequalities in ways, or to a degree, that is unusually pronounced, (2) has an overlay of moralism that is uncommon, and (3) has been and is marked by an unusual degree of stigma and prejudice, with all the resulting human rights violations. I say HIV is unusual, rather than unique, because many diseases travel along socio-economic fault lines – indeed, this is embedded in the notion of a population health approach that tackles various determinants of health, including social determinants – but HIV has highlighted them in a way that relatively few diseases have in the modern era. And of course, disease of all sorts has often been entwined with moral judgment; certainly any disease whose transmission is associated with sexual or drug-using practices deemed deviant, sinful, or criminal carries this burden particularly heavily. But even among this subset of diseases, it seems that HIV has carried a particular stigma exceeding that associated with other sexually transmitted infections, presumably because of its potential, especially pre-HAART, to cause very visible "stigmata" (e.g., Kaposi's sarcoma lesions, wasting, lipodystrophy), followed relatively quickly by death. The stigmatizing, discriminatory, and punitive responses that HIV provoked, whether in the delivery of health services, the epidemic of human rights–violating laws, or the shameful refusal of political leaders to even acknowledge the problem – all of which were facilitated by HIV's association with "undesirable" populations – has not generally been seen (at least in the context of high-income welfare states of the West[8]) in response to other sexually transmitted or blood-borne infections.

The fact that HIV has highlighted such fault lines and human rights concerns in a way rarely seen with other communicable diseases has also generated an exceptional activist response. "HIV exceptionalism" arose out of this activist response – one that demanded action on fronts that governments were often reluctant to address, that demanded basic human rights for those living with HIV, and that ultimately evolved from an immediate crisis response to save the lives of those devalued by politicians and others in power to an ongoing response that has recognized, at least in principle, that HIV is fundamentally not only a public health issue but also a social justice issue.

That activist response has been lauded as creating a paradigm shift in how the political and research establishments responded to a communicable disease. For example, it was eventually accepted that PLHIV and communities particularly affected by HIV needed to be active participants in shaping the response, rather than simply being the objects of that response.[9] One marker of this paradigm shift is activists' challenge to such stigmatizing, medicalized language as "HIV sufferers/ patients" or "AIDS carriers" that reduces people to their virus and status as perceived public health threats; activists demanded to be identified instead as "people (living) with HIV/AIDS," thereby insisting on the dignity of personhood (and the human rights claims this implies or entails) and on the need for action so that people can *live* with the virus rather than die from it.[10] Beyond simply changing the use of language, demands for actualizing the principle of the "greater involvement of people with AIDS" (GIPA) gained important traction, changing substantially how "business got done" in responding to this new public health crisis and, indeed, changing the course of the epidemic. Exceptional activism mobilized what has been an exceptional response – including funding for research and services, challenging discrimination by health-care workers, demanding safer sex education, access to condoms, and clean needles, campaigning for more affordable access to medicines, etc. – without which in the last thirty-five years we would not have seen important scientific advances in treatment, changes in law and policy to respect and protect human rights, and infections averted and lives saved. Indeed, mobilization in response to HIV has had numerous spillover benefits for public health more broadly: consider the scaling up of responses to TB and malaria, or the broader, strengthening health systems, via the Global Fund to Fight AIDS, Tuberculosis and Malaria, which first arose largely out of the efforts of HIV activists.

Beyond mobilizing funds and creating a critical infrastructure of services and programs – which, as I have argued above, cannot legitimately be seen as constituting "special," privileged treatment for HIV/ AIDS or even as only benefiting HIV – the activist response that is the core of "HIV exceptionalism" has been the insistence on human rights and how those norms must transform policy and practice in responding to a public health concern. The basic proposition is that, in the HIV response, human rights are critical at both the individual and population health level.[11] This is not to claim that human rights and public health are never in tension – that would be too simplistic and easily shown to be incorrect – but rather that, as a general matter, for both principled and pragmatic reasons, efforts to protect and promote public health ought to be premised on protecting and promoting the human rights of PLHIV and communities particularly affected by HIV. And furthermore, any infringement or limitation of human rights requires strict justification by the state, including when such limitation is done in the name of public health.

What might such a human rights approach entail? For example, recognizing that the stigma and discrimination surrounding HIV have been barriers to HIV testing, anonymous testing was implemented in some jurisdictions – something that public health traditionalists resisted fiercely and have never fully embraced. Similarly, recognizing that testing positive for HIV is qualitatively different from testing positive for high cholesterol or even for another sexually transmitted infection, steps were taken (at least on paper) to ensure that properly informed consent to HIV testing was obtained and documented. I mention these two examples because it is in the context of HIV testing (and related "surveillance" and "disease control" techniques organized around HIV testing) that the pushback against "HIV exceptionalism" has been perhaps the most focused and sustained, particularly by public health traditionalists seeking simultaneously to discredit HIV exceptionalism by framing human rights as an obstacle to "sound" or "effective" public health responses, while also dressing up efforts to routinize testing in ostensible human rights language (e.g., invoking "the right to know one's status" as somehow a justification for disregarding the right to give informed consent in deciding whether to find out one's status).[12] A classic instance is the 2002 *Lancet* commentary by DeCock et al. (2002), in which the authors suggested, as part of their argument for routinely testing people for HIV, that concern for human rights was a barrier to effective public health responses.

But it is not just a human rights challenge to policies and practices related to HIV testing that could be considered a manifestation of "HIV exceptionalism." Rather, one way in which the HIV response has been exceptional is in the articulation of a broader, human rights–based approach to a public health challenge – such as is found in the *International Guidelines on HIV and Human Rights*, promulgated by UNAIDS and the Office of the UN High Commissioner for Human Rights (2006) to assist states in ensuring their HIV prevention and care efforts are more effective, more ethical, and in conformity with international law by respecting, protecting, and fulfilling human rights.[13]

In this sense, beyond asserting GIPA as a new norm, the HIV pandemic and response has been at the core of an invigorated "health and human rights" movement that explores the multiple ways in which health and human rights are intimately connected. It has led to the emergence of a significant (if still too small) number of organizations and researchers dedicated to tackling the human rights abuses that make HIV exceptional, and that must be addressed if HIV prevention and care are ultimately to be successful (see UNHR, UNDP, and UNAIDS 2009). Such efforts have shown that the violation of human rights (e.g., criminalizing of populations already at risk, violating privacy, unethical medical research practices, denying evidence-based health services, keeping medicines unaffordable) can undermine HIV prevention and care. Conversely, they have also shown that protecting and promoting rights (e.g., protecting against discrimination or violence, protecting confidentiality, ensuring access to services, realizing the right to adequate housing, etc.) can strengthen prevention and care. The demand that lies at the heart of HIV exceptionalism – to take human rights concerns into account in making policy and implementing programs – is relevant to myriad policy areas, from immigration law to housing policy to income security programs; from a wide range of criminal justice policy concerns (HIV criminalization, illicit drug laws, criminalization of sex work[ers] and of LGBT people, prison regulations) to intellectual property policy and international trade law; from privacy law to access to the legal services and support needed to defend human rights.

### Challenging HIV Exceptionalism: The Case of HIV Testing Policy and Practice

As noted above, the project of embedding human rights principles and approaches in HIV policies and programs remains very much a work in progress – and even where it has had some important impact, it has not taken root so firmly that it could not be shifted again. Indeed, there is a concerted effort to turn the clock back, to undo the recognition that respecting, protecting, and fulfilling human rights is central to an ultimately effective (and ethical) HIV response. The fight over approaches to HIV testing – revived in part by welcome advances in testing technology and treatment – has been the principal terrain so far in which this has been manifest.

It is true that in some parts of the world, thanks largely to wider availability of HAART, living with HIV is "different now" from the way it was in the 1980s or early 1990s – as is claimed by a recent campaign launched in BC[14] specifically to market the aggressive push for more routine HIV testing by health authorities. Their materials weaken what is considered satisfactory for informed consent and actively dissuade testing providers from encouraging too many questions by patients. Their complementary initiatives include such measures as "testing fairs" on public streets (raising serious questions of respect for privacy) (Vonn 2012). But the social and clinical phenomenon of HIV is not so different in the era of HAART that it warrants doing away with human rights as a cornerstone of policy and programming – and their relevance remains equally important in the context of efforts to scale up access to HIV testing (which of course is a desirable objective from the vantage point of both public health and human rights). Yet attention to human rights is conspicuously and persistently absent from the push by public health professionals and institutions to scale up testing. In November 2015, a leading HIV public health researcher, clinician, and advocate for "treatment as prevention" called for "universal testing" of all Canadians for HIV (CBC 2015; Duran 2015). Aside from the eerie echoes of similar (but less well-intentioned) calls in the early years of the epidemic, what was also striking was the absence of any discussion, including in the media, of the human rights implications of such a strategy – which, if recent history is any indication, would very likely give short shrift to notions of informed consent in the testing process.

Furthermore, there is something perverse about the implicit claim that respect for human rights in health policies and programs is warranted only if, and as long as, there is significant stigma surrounding a particular condition. For example, even if, by some magical means, tomorrow the stigma surrounding HIV – and all related stigmas surrounding LGBT people, sex workers, people who use drugs, as well as the racism and xenophobia that often are part of how HIV is constructed as the problem of the "other," and the gender inequality that puts women at greater risk of HIV and impedes their access to HIV care – were to disappear, how would this justify the claim that we no longer need be concerned about ensuring informed consent to testing? Securing informed consent is good, ethical health practice, regardless of whether HIV and those living with it are subject to widespread stigma and discrimination (although the presence of such potential harms certainly further underscores the importance of testing being done only with informed consent). It is troubling that what is perceived as "exceptional" in the HIV context – in this case, the insistence on ensuring a medical procedure is performed only with truly informed consent of a patient – is too often the exception, rather than being widely implemented good, ethical practice. That manifestation of HIV exceptionalism is disappointing – because a human rights success achieved in the HIV context (albeit only to a limited and increasingly threatened degree) has not been extended to solidify respect for the human rights of patients in other contexts.

To remain for a moment with the debate over HIV exceptionalism in HIV testing, there is also questionable thinking in the proposal to do away with the "exceptional" approach to HIV testing. When proponents attempt to justify routine testing as a benefit to the individual patient or to the public good, they claim that HIV and HIV testing need to be "normalized" because the stigma surrounding HIV (among other things) creates a barrier to testing. By some strange alchemy, making HIV testing routine – by which they mean essentially watering down measures for ensuring informed consent – will dispel stigma.[15]

If (1) providers *presume* patients' consent to testing in a clinical encounter unless, against all the overt and subtle pressures to accede, a
patient expressly refuses an HIV test, and (2) in that same setting, patients are provided little information about the risks and benefits of an
HIV test and are given little opportunity to ask questions, before testing
is performed on the basis of that presumed consent, the unsurprising
outcome will be a high "uptake" of HIV testing. But this does not *do
away* with HIV stigma; rather, it *works around it* to achieve the goal of
testing, by diminishing or even ignoring a patient's right to make an
informed choice about whether to get tested. How such an approach
– which involves *less* education of patients, not more – will eliminate
deep-seated prejudices and stigma, including at the population level, is
a mystery that proponents have never been able to explain. It exposes
more people, with less preparation, to the HIV stigma that proponents
of routine testing acknowledge exists – and that is central to their argument that testing should be made more routine. (Performing tests
without fully informed consent – particularly when the result may be
as life-altering as an HIV diagnosis – also undermines patient trust in
the provider who has subjected them to such treatment.) Nor can we
ignore the broader legal context of such efforts to routinize HIV testing,
because a concern for human rights means that, when considering HIV
testing policy and practice, we cannot limit our concern just to stigma
and the adverse consequences engendered by such stigma that people
testing HIV-positive may encounter. In Canada, even more than some
other jurisdictions, testing HIV-positive now also exposes someone to
the potential for criminal prosecution in a wide array of circumstances
(Canadian HIV/AIDS Legal Network and HIV & AIDS Legal Clinic
Ontario 2017).

In any event, we are a long way from the happy situation of a world
free of HIV stigma, and routinely testing people without ensuring informed consent will not bring it about. Let us be clear: nobody suggests
that scaling up access to HIV testing should wait until we have completely eliminated stigma and discrimination. That would be foolish,
and also a human rights violation, because people do indeed have a
right to know their status and gain access to services, *as long as it is of
their own free will* – that is, in conformity with the basic bioethical principle of respect for autonomy and with the legal requirement to respect
informed consent.[16] But what has changed so substantially that would
render the *International Guidelines on HIV and Human Rights*, and the recommended actions under them, irrelevant? On at least one front (i.e.,

overly broad criminalization), the potential risks of testing HIV-positive have worsened, even as the benefits (e.g., more effective treatment) have also increased. And while major advances in treatment, if diagnosed with HIV, have certainly changed the risk/benefit calculus of getting tested much for the better, it doesn't follow that the basic ethical and human rights requirement of securing an individual's informed consent to testing can be set aside.

## Conclusion: Making Human Rights Unexceptional

It would be profoundly premature to eject "HIV exceptionalism" – in the sense of heightened commitment to human rights–respecting policies, programs, and practices – from the future HIV response. Rather than abandon the human rights gains and principles embodied in HIV exceptionalism, we should insist that they be spread beyond the HIV response. In this sense, the agenda of "integration" offers an important opportunity, if implemented correctly. There are good reasons to integrate HIV prevention into efforts to prevent diseases communicable in similar ways and affecting the same populations. And it makes good sense for the health of PLHIV that HIV care, treatment, and support should be coordinated or delivered alongside other health care required by PLHIV (e.g., sexual and reproductive health services and harm reduction services). In the interests of "treating the whole person," HIV-specialist health professionals should appreciate other health needs of their patients living with HIV, and non-HIV specialists should have adequate knowledge of HIV to provide respectful, non-judgmental, non-discriminatory, and informed care within their field to their patients living with HIV. To the extent that "integration" is an effort to harmonize and coordinate research, policies, programs, and services so as to achieve fewer new HIV infections and better care for PLHIV, including by addressing comorbidities and social determinants of health, that impetus should be welcomed.[17] In this sense, integration is the means to important, worthwhile ends – i.e., better health through more effective prevention and care – not an end in itself. In such a scenario, "integration" and "HIV exceptionalism" are – or at least need not be – in opposition; rather, the human rights core of HIV exceptionalism can and should inform and be integrated into that broader, more holistic response.

But to the extent that "integration" cloaks an effort to roll back the human rights gains made by "HIV exceptionalism," this agenda should be resisted. When calls for "integration" emanate from government decision-makers who attempt to erode and eliminate the welfare state, and refuse to base public policies applicable to the HIV response on evidence and on human rights, we should be sceptical of the "real" agenda. On the one hand, government claims that the HIV response should be integrated with the response to other public health concerns (e.g., STBBIs, including HCV; mental health; health issues associated with aging; and other determinants of health). And yet the impact on the HIV epidemic (or other public health concerns) is not factored into public policymaking in a host of areas (e.g., excising harm reduction from a National Anti-Drug Strategy – an ill-advised decision of the previous government recently corrected by the current government), and governments often pursue policy that undermines HIV prevention and care and public health more broadly (e.g., by worsening income inequality; putting more people with addictions in prisons and denying adequate HIV/HCV prevention services in prisons; pursuing trade agreements that further limit access to medicines by making them costlier for longer; resisting in international fora the advancement of women's rights, the rights of indigenous peoples, or economic, social, and cultural rights generally; etc.). Meanwhile, over the last decade, according to figures provided and confirmed by the Public Health Agency of Canada itself, nearly $104 million in funds committed to the federal HIV strategy – in keeping with implementing a unanimous recommendation from an all-party parliamentary committee – has been diverted from that strategy or simply gone unspent – and as of early 2017, there is as yet no commitment from the government elected in 2015 to restore those lost funds.[18] In such a context, the call for "integration" is suspect. This should signal that integration could simply be the latest guise of a project that, whether deliberately or not, further erodes human rights in the name of advancing public health and weakens the HIV response, rubbing off the "sharp edges" of human rights activism that have helped define it and have led to signal advances in responding to one of the world's greatest public health challenges.

The history of HIV and the response to it demonstrates the critical importance of respecting, protecting, and fulfilling human rights, as a matter of ethics and social justice and of good public health policy. At the heart of "HIV exceptionalism" lies the proposition that respecting, protecting, and fulfilling human rights is a touchstone of the HIV response. This need not entail rejection of calls to "integrate" the HIV response with other public health concerns; where and how it makes sense to improve health outcomes, such integration can be a positive evolution in the HIV response. But "integration" should not mean or become justification for funding cuts, nor is it a justification for an end to HIV exceptionalism – i.e., an abandonment of the principles, policies, and practices in the response to HIV that are rooted in the correct recognition that HIV remains qualitatively different from other health conditions. The exceptional nature of HIV as a public health phenomenon, and of the response to it, should offer lessons for improving the response to similar public health challenges, rather than weakening the HIV response by lowering standards back down to those that had been considered acceptable public health practice until challenged by HIV advocates. In the words of the UNAIDS Reference Group on HIV and Human Rights,

> The HIV response has been exceptional compared to other health and development issues – in the degree to which communities have mobilized, resources have been invested, and realization of human rights has had a central role in achieving results for people, including those most at the margins. The lessons already learned from this exceptional response, and why and how that exceptionalism has been necessary, must be carried through right to the end of the epidemic and beyond. Otherwise, we risk falsely declaring "the end of AIDS" with AIDS becoming another disease of those who are poor and marginalized … We must all speak boldly and honestly not only of the successes of the HIV response, but also of the failures – including the ongoing human rights failures – because both successes and failures offer key lessons to galvanize future commitment and action, not only to end AIDS eventually but also to transform and advance global health more broadly. (UNAIDS Reference Group on HIV and Human Rights 2014)

NOTES

1  For a summary and additional citations, see Canadian HIV/AIDS Legal Network et al. (2015).
2  See the work of the federal Task Force on Legalizing and Regulating Cannabis (http://healthycanadians.gc.ca/task-force-marijuana-groupe-etude/index-eng.php), and the bills introduced in Parliament in April 2017 to legalize and regulate cannabis.

3  For an overview and critique of the bill eventually enacted as the Respect for Communities Act, see Kazatchkine et al. (2014).

4  See also the forthcoming compilation of accounts from sex workers by the Canadian Alliance for Sex Work Law Reform.

5  See also the perspectives articulated in the documentary film *Consent: HIV Non-Disclosure and Sexual Assault Law* (2015).

6  Data provided by the Canadian HIV/AIDS Legal Network (www.aidslaw .ca) archive of all known cases of prosecutions for HIV transmission, exposure, or non-disclosure in Canada (data current to December 2016); Bernard and Cameron (2016).

7  See description of the findings in CATIE (2014).

8  In China, which is a different case, there is widespread stigmatization and discrimination against people with hepatitis B virus (HBV) or hepatitis C virus (HCV), akin to that faced by PLHIV.

9  This is not unique. Feminists in the 1960s and 1970s had already begun to demand women's empowerment in shaping policies and programs to protect and promote women's health (including reproductive health), a precedent that informed the AIDS activist movement.

10  The influence of HIV activism in asserting this principle has been felt beyond the HIV response. In the 1990s, people with disabilities began to demand to be referred to as such, rather than "the disabled," and the slogan "Nothing about Us without Us" began to gain currency as a slogan of the disability rights movement. More recently, people who currently use illegal drugs have challenged their description as "addicts" or "drug users," demanding recognition of their personhood and similarly adopting "Nothing about Us without Us" as a demand – a process that human rights advocates have facilitated (see Canadian HIV/AIDS Legal Network 2005).

11  It's important to stress that "human rights" encompasses civil and political rights *and* economic, social, and cultural rights, all of which are undergirded by the basic cross-cutting principle of non-discrimination.

12  When challenged, proponents of routine testing will sometimes – not always – protest that they mean routinely *offering* HIV testing (and they will come up with phrases such as "provider-initiated testing and counselling," which is exactly what happened with WHO/UNAIDS. But upon closer examination, this is not really what many of them mean: in fact they want to see HIV testing not just offered routinely, but performed routinely, based on simply presuming "consent" to testing (which is what opt-out testing is intended to achieve).

13  The guidelines were first elaborated in 1996, then updated a decade later
    to reflect important developments on access to treatment. For more recent
    guidance on incorporating human rights standards into HIV prevention,
    testing, and treatment, see UNAIDS (2017).
14  See http://itsdifferentnow.org.
15  It invites the question of how proponents can explain the persistence
    of deeply rooted stigma in many countries where there is a much higher
    prevalence of HIV than in Canada, with millions of people having been
    tested – including under regimes of questionable ethical calibre, given the
    strong push for "routine," opt-out testing – and diagnosed as HIV-positive.
16  Some have suggested that insisting on informed consent in HIV testing
    could undermine human rights, but the concerns seem unpersuasive upon
    closer examination. For example, one stated concern is that procedures
    for counselling (especially pre-test counselling) and record-keeping (e.g.,
    some explicit written documentation of specific consent to HIV testing)
    are onerous. Most troubling about this claim is the underlying notion that
    ethical conduct with patients should be secondary to efficiency: can it re-
    ally be credibly claimed that having to tick an additional box or two on a
    form, explicitly confirming informed consent in particular to an HIV test,
    is so onerous on a testing provider that it outweighs a patient's right to
    bodily autonomy? The very proposition signals the problematic thinking
    underlying demands for "routine testing" – i.e., the low value too often
    assigned to respecting patient autonomy. It is also usually a "straw man"
    argument, resting on the misconception that advocates for informed con-
    sent in HIV testing insist on a simple, inflexible, one-size-fits-all approach,
    that cannot be adapted (within certain bounds) to the circumstances, there-
    by wasting time and valuable health-care system resources. But this is not
    the case. As with any encounter between health-care provider and service
    user, part of the service provider's task is to assess the level of knowledge
    of the service user and to tailor the provision of information accordingly.
    There is nothing inherently inflexible or unjustifiably inefficient in requir-
    ing HIV testing providers to secure the informed consent of a given service
    user before proceeding with a test.
        A second concern is that requiring testing providers to secure informed
    consent to HIV testing could require counsellors to engage in intrusive
    questioning that violates personal privacy. This is not logical. The key to
    ensuring informed consent is to ensure the *provision* of information by the
    testing provider to the person considering testing, including creating the
    opportunity for questions by the service user. A counsellor might pose
    some general questions to assess the level of the service user's knowledge,

but nothing in that exchange should compel the service user to provide information they wish to keep private, nor does it require a counsellor to subject the person to an intrusive cross-examination about personal matters (e.g., sexual or drug-use practices). Providing information to a service user about various means of HIV transmission and prevention, or about the efficacy of available HIV treatment, does not require the service user to divulge anything.

Finally, concern has been expressed that requiring informed consent to HIV testing could result in counsellors acting as gatekeepers to testing. Again, this is not a persuasive concern. Testing providers keen to increase uptake of HIV testing, to the point that they seek to relax requirements for truly informed consent, are unlikely to be inclined to act as gatekeepers *denying* HIV testing to a service user who has sought out the service. Aside from the question of whether this is likely to be a common occurrence, the notion that *some* testing providers might act as unethical gatekeepers, denying HIV testing for inappropriate reasons, cannot serve as a valid argument for adopting an unethical approach to testing that waters down or does away with the requirement for informed consent. One potential wrong does not justify another, wider wrong.

17 In fairness, many service providers (and researchers, advocates, etc.) have been practising an "integrated" approach to HIV from the outset, whether because of necessity in responding to the varied health needs of their HIV-positive or at-risk populations, or conscious recognition of the multiple determinants that affect HIV risk and care.

18 Letter from National Partners to Prime Minister Justin Trudeau, Health Minister Jane Philpott, and Finance Minister Bill Morneau, 20 December 2016 ("Re: Adequately Funding Canada's Federal HIV Strategy"), on file.

REFERENCES

Altman, Dennis, et al. 2012. "Men Who Have Sex with Men: Stigma and Discrimination." *Lancet* 380 (9839): 439–45. http://dx.doi.org/10.1016/ S0140-6736(12)60920-9.

Anglemyer, Andrew, et al. 2011. "Antiretroviral Therapy for Prevention of HIV Transmission in HIV-Discordant Couples." *Cochrane Database Systematic Review* 10 (8): CD009153.

Athena Network. 2009. "Ten Reasons Why Criminalization of HIV Exposure or Transmission Harms Women." http://www.athenanetwork.org/our-work/promoting-sexual-and-reproductive-health-and-rights/10-reasons-why-criminalization-harms-women.html.

Baggaley, Rebecca F., et al. 2013. "Heterosexual HIV-1 Infectiousness and Antiretroviral Use: Systematic Review of Prospective Studies of Discordant Couples." *Epidemiology* 24 (1): 110–21.

Bernard, Edwin J., and Sally Cameron. 2013. *Advancing HIV Justice: A Progress Report of Achievements and Challenges in Global Advocacy against HIV Criminalization*. Amsterdam: Global Network of People Living with HIV and HIV Justice Network.

– 2016. *Advancing HIV Justice 2: Building Momentum in Global Advocacy against HIV Criminalisation*. Brighton: HIV Justice Network and GNP+. http://www.hivjustice.net/advancing2/.

Buchanan, Kim Shayo. 2014. "When Is HIV a Crime? Sexuality, Gender and Consent." *Minnesota Law Review* 99 (4): 1231–1342. http://www.minnesotalawreview.org/wp-content/uploads/2015/05/Buchanan_pdf.pdf.

Canadian Alliance for Sex Work Law Reform. 2015. "Violence against Sex Workers Is Violence against Everyone." Ricochet, 15 December. https://ricochet.media/en/824/violence-against-sex-workers-is-violence-against-everyone.

Canadian HIV/AIDS Legal Network. 2005. "'Nothing about Us without Us': Greater, Meaningful Involvement of People Who Use Illegal Drugs: A Manifesto by People Who Use Illegal Drugs." http://www.aidslaw.ca/site/nothing-about-us-without-us-greater-meaningful-involvement-of-people-who-use-illegal-drugs-a-manifesto-by-people-who-use-illegal-drugs/.

– 2012. "Fixing Canada's Access to Medicines Regime (CAMR): 20 Questions & Answers." Toronto: Canadian HIV/AIDS Legal Network. http://www.aidslaw.ca/site/fixing-canadas-access-to-medicines-regime-camr-20-questions-answers/?lang=en.

– 2015a. "Election 2015: Bill C-36 and Sex Workers' Rights – Canada's Major Federal Parties Respond." 7 October. http://www.aidslaw.ca/site/election-2015-bill-c-36-and-sex-workers-rights-canadas-major-federal-parties-respond/?lang=en.

– 2015b. "Election 2015: Prisoners' Right to Health – Canada's Major Federal Parties Respond." http://www.aidslaw.ca/site/election-2015-prisoners-right-to-health-canadas-major-federal-parties-respond/?lang=en.

Canadian HIV/AIDS Legal Network and HIV & AIDS Legal Clinic Ontario. 2017. "Exploring Avenues to Address Problematic Prosecutions against People Living with HIV in Canada." http://www.aidslaw.ca/site/exploring-avenues-to-address-problematic-prosecutions-against-people-living-with-hiv-in-canada/?lang=en.

Canadian HIV/AIDS Legal Network et al. 2012. "Unjust Supreme Court Ruling on Criminalization of HIV Major Step Backwards for Public Health and Human Rights." www.aidslaw.ca/site/unjust-supreme-court-ruling-on-criminalization-of-hiv-major-step-backwards-for-public-health-and-human-rights/?lang=en.

– 2015. "Drug Policy and Human Rights: The Canadian Context – Submission to the Office of the UN High Commissioner for Human Rights." Toronto. http://www.aidslaw.ca/site/drug-policy-and-human-rights-ohchr/?lang=en.

Canadian HIV/AIDS Legal Network, Pivot Legal Society and Maggie's. 2014. "Reckless Endangerment – Q&A on Bill C-36: Protection of Communities and Exploited Persons Act." Toronto: Canadian HIV/AIDS Legal Network, Pivot Legal Society, Maggie's. http://www.aidslaw.ca/site/reckless-endangerment-qa-on-bill-c-36-protection-of-communities-and-exploited-persons-act/?lang=en.

CATIE. 2014. "Insight into HIV Transmission Risk When the Viral Load Is Undetectable and No Condom Is Used." 10 April.

CBC. 2015. "It's Time to Test Everyone in Canada for HIV/AIDS, Says Dr Julio Montaner." CBC News, 24 November. http://www.cbc.ca/news/canada/british-columbia/julio-montaner-universal-hiv-aids-testing-1.3332164.

Chu, Sandra, et al. 2014. "Strengthening the Enabling Environment: Advancing Human Rights and Access to Justice for Women and Girls." In *What Works for Women and Girls: Evidence for HIV/AIDS Interventions*, edited by J. Gay, M. Croce-Galis, and K. Hardee, 2nd ed. Washington, DC: Futures Group, Health Policy Project. http://www.whatworksforwomen.org/chapters/21-Strengthening-the-Enabling-Environment.

Chu, Sandra Ka Hon, and Richard Elliott. 2009. *Clean Switch: The Case for Prison Needle and Syringe Programs in Canada*. Toronto: Canadian HIV/AIDS Legal Network.

Cohen, Myron S., et al. 2011. "Prevention of HIV-1 Infection with Early Antiretroviral Therapy." *New England Journal of Medicine* 365:493–505.

*Consent: HIV Non-Disclosure and Sexual Assault Law*. 2015. Goldelox Productions & Canadian HIV/AIDS Legal Network. Film.

Decker, Michelle, et al. 2015. "Human Rights Violations against Sex Workers: Burden and Effect on HIV." *Lancet* 385 (9963): 186–99. http://dx.doi.org/10.1016/S0140-6736(14)60800-X.

DeCock, Kevin M., Dorothy Mbori-Ngacha, and Elizabeth Marum. 2002. "Shadow on the Continent: Public Health and HIV/AIDS in Africa in the 21st Century." *Lancet* 360 (9326): 67–72.

Duran, Estefnia. 2015. "General HIV Testing Only Solution to Stop Epidemic: Vancouver Doctor." Global News, 26 November. http://globalnews.ca/news/2363750/general-hiv-testing-only-solution-to-stop-epidemic-vancouver-doctor/.

Eastwood, Niamh, Edward Fox, and Ari Rosmarin. 2016. *A Quiet Revolution: Drug Decriminalization Policies in Practice across the Globe*. 2nd ed. London: Release. http://www.release.org.uk/publications/drug-decriminalisation-2016.

Elliott, Richard. 2013. "Government of Canada Misleads Parliament and Public, Kills Bill on Access to Medicines for Developing Countries." *Policies for Equitable Access to Health*, 4 March. http://www.peah.it/2013/03/government-of-canada-misleads-parliament-and-public-kills-bill-on-access-to-medicines-for-developing-countries/.

Footer, Katherine H.A., et al. 2016. "Policing Practices as a Structural Determinant for HIV among Sex Workers: A Systematic Review of Empirical Findings." *Journal of the International AIDS Society* 19, S3: 20883. doi: 10.7448/IAS.19.4.20883.

Global Commission on HIV and the Law. 2012. *Risks, Rights & Health*. New York: UNDP.

Jürgens, Ralf, et al. 2010. "People Who Use Drugs, HIV, and Human Rights." *Lancet* 376 (9739): 475–85. http://dx.doi.org/10.1016/S0140-6736(10)60830-6.

Grant, Isabel. 2011. "The Prosecution of Non-Disclosure of HIV in Canada: Time to Rethink *Cuerrie*." *McGill Journal of Law and Health* 5 (2): 7–59.

– 2013. "The Over-Criminalization of Persons with HIV." *University of Toronto Law Journal* 63 (3): 475–84.

INSIGHT START Study Group. 2015 "Initiation of Antiretroviral Therapy in Early Asymptomatic HIV Infection." *New England Journal of Medicine* 373:795–807.

Kazatchkine, Cécile, Richard Elliott, and Donald MacPherson. 2014. *An Injection of Reason: Critical Analysis of Bill C-2 (Q&A)*. Toronto: Canadian HIV/AIDS Legal Network and Canadian Drug Policy Coalition. http://www.aidslaw.ca/site/wp-content/uploads/2014/10/C2-QA_Oct2014-ENG.pdf.

Loutfy, Mona R., et al. 2013. "Systematic Review of HIV Transmission between Heterosexual Serodiscordant Couples Where the HIV-Positive Partner Is Fully Suppressed on Antiretroviral Therapy." *PLoS ONE* 8 (2): e55747. https://doi.org/10.1371/journal.pone.0055747.

Loutfy, Mona, et al. 2014. "Canadian Consensus Statement on HIV and Its Transmission in the Context of the Criminal Law." *Canadian Journal of Infectious Diseases & Medical Microbiology* 25 (3): 135–40.

Office of the UN High Commissioner for Human Rights. 2015. "UN Experts Voice Concern over Adverse Impact of Free Trade and Investment Agreements on Human Rights." News release, 2 June. www.ohchr.org/EN/NewsEvents/Pages/DisplayNews.aspx?NewsID=16031.

Office of the United Nations High Commissioner for Human Rights and
  the Joint United Nations Programme on HIV/AIDS. 2006. *International
  Guidelines on HIV/AIDS and Human Rights*. 2006 Consolidated Version.
  Geneva.
Public Health Agency of Canada. 2013. *Human Immunodeficiency Virus: HIV
  Screening and Testing Guide*. Ottawa: Public Health Agency of Canada.
  http://www.phac-aspc.gc.ca/aids-sida/guide/hivstg-vihgdd-eng.php.
Rodger, Alison, et al. 2014. "HIV Transmission Risk through Condomless Sex
  if HIV+ Partner on Suppressive ART: PARTNER Study." In *Program and
  Abstracts of the 21st Conference on Retroviruses and Opportunistic Infections,*
  3–6 March, Boston, abstract 153LB. http://www.croiconference.org/
  sessions/hiv-transmission-risk-through-condomless-sex-if-hiv-partner-
  suppressive-art-partner-study.
Schwartländer, Bernhard, et al. (on behalf of the Investment Framework Study
  Group). 2011. "Towards an Improved Investment Approach for an Effective
  Response to HIV/AIDS." *Lancet* 377 (9782): 2031–41. http://dx.doi.org/
  10.1016/S0140-6736(11)60702-2.
UN General Assembly. 2015. "United Nations Standard Minimum Rules for
  the Treatment of Prisoners" (the Nelson Mandela Rules). UN Doc.
  A/RES/70/175.
UN Secretary-General's High-Level Panel on Access to Medicines:
  2015. *Terms of Reference*. https://static1.squarespace.com/
  static/562094dee4b0d00c1a3ef761/t/568d535a1c12106651299f
  6e/1452102490740/TOR+on+new+template+5Jan16+FINAL.pdf.
UNAIDS. 2011. *A New Investment Framework for the Global HIV Response*.
  Geneva: UNAIDS.
– 2014a. *Fast-Track: Ending the AIDS Epidemic by 2030*. Geneva: UNAIDS.
  http://www.unaids.org/en/resources/documents/2014/JC2686_
  WAD2014report.
– 2014b. *The Gap Report*. Geneva: UNAIDS.
– 2014c. *Guidance Note: Services for People in Prisons and Other Closed Settings*.
  Geneva: UNAIDS.
– 2015. "UNAIDS Calls on Trade Negotiators to Uphold Governments'
  Commitments to Public Health and Access to Medicines." News release,
  28 July. http://www.unaids.org/en/resources/presscentre/
  pressreleaseandstatementarchive/2015/july/20150728_trips_plus.
– 2017. *Guidance Note: Fast-Track and Human Rights: Advancing Human Rights
  in Efforts to Accelerate the Response to HIV*. Geneva: UNAIDS.

UNAIDS Reference Group on HIV and Human Rights. 2014. "Defeating AIDS: The Role of Human Rights." In *Commonwealth Health Partnerships 2014*, edited by A. Robertson, with R. Jones-Parry, 25–7. London: Commonwealth Secretariat. http://www.hivhumanrights.org/statements/defeating-aids-the-role-of-human-rights-published-in-commonwealth-health-partnerships-2014/.

UNDP and UNAIDS. 2012. *Issue Brief: The Potential Impact of Free Trade Agreements on Public Health.* New York: UNDP, UNAIDS.

UNHR, UNDP, and UNAIDS. 2009. "Human Rights and HIV/AIDS: Now More Than Ever: 10 Reasons Why Human Rights Should Occupy the Center of the Global AIDS Struggle." 4th ed. http://www.hivhuman rightsnow.org/downloads/nmte_20090923_0.pdf.

Vonn, Michael. 2012. "British Columbia's 'Seek and Treat' Strategy: A Cautionary Tale on Privacy Rights and Informed Consent for HIV Testing." *HIV/AIDS Policy & Law Review* 16 (2012): 15–18.

White House. 2011. "Fact Sheet: The Beginning of the End of AIDS." Washington, DC: Office of the Press Secretary.

WHO. 2015a. *Guideline on When to Start Antiretroviral Therapy and on Pre-Exposure Prophylaxis for HIV.* Geneva: WHO.

– 2015b. *Policy Brief: Transgender People and HIV.* Geneva: WHO.

– 2015c. *Technical Brief: HIV and Young Men Who Have Sex with Men.* Geneva: WHO.

– 2015d. *Technical Brief: HIV and Young People Who Inject Drugs.* Geneva: WHO.

– 2015e. *Technical Brief: HIV and Young People Who Sell Sex.* Geneva: WHO.

– 2015f. *Technical Brief: HIV and Young Transgender People.* Geneva: WHO.

**Legal Cases**

*Canada (Attorney General) v Bedford*, 2013 SCC 72, [2013] 3 SCR 1101.
*R v JTC*, 2013 NSPC 10.
*R v Lloyd*, 2016 SCC 13.

## 2 HIV Criminalization as "Risk Management": On the Importance of Structural Stigma

MARILOU GAGNON AND CHRISTINE VÉZINA

In recent years, criminal laws have been increasingly applied in matters related to HIV non-disclosure, HIV exposure, and/or HIV transmission. In North America, we have witnessed a dramatic increase in the number of people charged for allegedly not disclosing their serological status before engaging in sexual activities, exposing others to HIV, and/or sexually transmitting HIV. In fact, Canada is now known as a criminalization "hotspot" (Global Network of People Living with HIV [GNP+] and HIV Justice Network 2013) – a country where criminal laws are systematically used to prosecute people living with HIV (PLWH) primarily for failing to disclose their serological status to sexual partners and, in some instances, for potentially exposing others to the virus (e.g., by spitting or biting). As of 2015, there had been 185 HIV non-disclosure cases in Canada (Mykhalovskiy 2015). Of this number, the vast majority resulted in a conviction, although it remains difficult to determine exactly how many PLWH have been convicted, because the figures do not account for the cases settled before going to court (Canadian HIV/AIDS Legal Network 2014).

A number of Canadian scholars have studied and analysed the implications of HIV criminalization. The bulk of this work has taken place over the past decade, largely because most HIV non-disclosure cases have occurred after 2004 (Mykhalovskiy 2015). The Canadian literature on this topic can be divided into three categories: (1) public health (i.e., counselling, testing, prevention, and treatment) and professional practice implications of HIV criminalization,[1] (2) sociological and critical approaches to the problem of HIV criminalization,[2] and (3) legal analyses of HIV criminalization based on feminist, human rights, and criminal law frameworks.[3] In addition to the scholarly literature, many events have been organized (i.e., with clinicians, researchers, feminists, and so forth) and documents produced by lawyers, advocates, clinicians, and policy experts to expose the harmful consequences of HIV criminalization in the Canadian context.

While there is a general agreement that HIV criminalization is "bad policy," new theoretical approaches are needed to move beyond analyses that take singular categories (i.e., gender or race) and consequences (i.e., on the person, the clinicians, and the service providers) as their starting point. Such new approaches could help us understand the structural dimensions of HIV criminalization, which remain largely overlooked in the literature. For example, they could help us move beyond the understanding that HIV criminalization further increases stigma of PLWH and allow us to take a closer look at stigma as the very core of HIV criminalization. By turning our attention to the structural dimensions of HIV criminalization, we seek to uncover assumptions embedded within the criminal justice system – assumptions that make it possible to construct risk, produce crime (and a new class of criminals), and engage in various forms of capture, including incarceration, voluntary and involuntary solitary confinement, dangerous offender designation, conditions of parole, and surveillance in the form of the National Sexual Offender Registry.

This chapter uses structural stigma as a conceptual entry point for thinking about the criminalization of HIV non-disclosure and its effects on PLWH in Canada. Our interdisciplinary approach is based on the legal analysis of criminal cases, the theoretical work of Hannem and Bruckert (2012), and the work of key scholars on criminalization and stigma, all in an attempt to understand the ways in which stigmatic assumptions about PLWH work to produce new categories of criminals and create a need for regulation – and exclusion through imprisonment and surveillance. We begin with a brief presentation of our theoretical framework, followed by an overview of the state of HIV criminalization in Canada. This is followed by a critical analysis of structural stigma, with particular emphasis on the construction of PLWH as a "collective risk" and a new category of criminals. Lastly, we look at the functions of imprisonment and surveillance as calculated "risk management" strategies.

**Theoretical Framework**

Our analysis of HIV criminalization is guided by a theoretical framework that combines the work of Goffman (1963) and Foucault (1980, 1990, 1995, 2003). According to Hannem and Bruckert (2012), this framework offers a point of entry for studying stigma at the level of individual interactions and thinking about the systematic application of stigma at a structural level.

Goffman (1963) defines stigma as an attribute (or symbol) that casts strong disfavour on people or groups that do not conform to social norms. This attribute is not inherent to an individual or a group. Rather, it is produced during social interactions when a person who possesses certain physical traits, displays specific behaviours, or belongs to a social group is labelled and stereotyped, producing status loss and discriminatory behaviours (Goffman 1963). These behaviours are often reported as "the observable evidence of stigma" (Hannem 2012, 15) by people who experience prejudicial treatment, limited opportunities, and social exclusion.

Hannem and Bruckert's Foucauldian revision of stigma exposes the stigmatic assumptions embedded in policies, practices, and discourses as well as the institutional responses to particular stigmatized groups. These assumptions are often "systematically applied by agencies, institutions and individuals to particular group[s] of people or populations as a whole" (Hannem 2012, 23) as a way to target such groups or populations, manage the risk they pose, and govern their interactions with the state. Through the language of risk, particular groups can become stigmatized in such a way as to allow surveillance and interventions to be deployed on a larger scale (Hannem and Bruckert 2012).

This framework is particularly relevant when seeking insight into the criminal prosecution of PLWH who fail to disclose their serological status to sexual partners. Through the language of risk, this particular group has become the target of more aggressive forms of surveillance, reporting, and punishment through the use of criminal law. This framework offers a more accurate depiction of HIV-related stigma as both a "negative" attribute that is produced through social interactions and a "positive" or "productive" (in the Foucauldian sense) attribute that serves a particular purpose within structures of power (i.e., criminal justice, health care [Gagnon 2015], social assistance, and so forth).

Increasingly, HIV scholars are recognizing the importance of paying closer attention to structural stigma and power to better understand the experience of PLWH. As such, it is no longer deemed sufficient to study stigma from the viewpoint of the individual (Parker and Aggleton 2003). Stigma does not exist outside of context. It does not exist without power (Link and Phelan 2001). In fact, "it is entirely contingent on access to social, economic, and political power that allows for the identification of differentness, the construction of stereotypes, the separation of labelled persons into distinct categories, and the full expression of disapproval, rejection, exclusion, and discrimination" (363–85). This approach to stigma is consistent with intersectionality-based policy analysis, which recognizes that the social locations of PLWH are shaped by processes and structures, which, in turn, are shaped by power (Hankivsky et al. 2014). Attention to such processes and structures is essential to fully comprehend the nature and impact of "bad policies" (including HIV criminalization).

## A Review of HIV Criminalization in Canada[4]

The evolution of criminal law in HIV criminalization in Canada can be divided into two periods. The first period began with the Supreme Court of Canada's ruling in *R v Cuerrier* in 1998. The second period began in 2012 with the Supreme Court's rulings on "companion cases" *R v Mabior* and *R v DC*.

### 1998–2012: The Cuerrier Era

The *R v Cuerrier* decision (henceforth *Cuerrier*) introduced the criminalization of HIV non-disclosure in Canadian law. With this ruling, the Supreme Court introduced a significant change in criminal law by conceptualizing the crime of HIV non-disclosure when there is a significant risk of serious bodily harm. The Court based its reasoning on the offences of assault and aggravated assault, which requires the Crown to demonstrate beyond all reasonable doubt that (1) the PLWH's actions endangered the victim's life (subsection 268 [1] Criminal Code); and (2) the PLWH intentionally applied force without the victim's consent (paragraph 265 [1] [a] Criminal Code).

Concerning the first component of the burden of proof, the Court ruled that the victim need not be infected, because "endangerment" itself – in this case, exposure to a significant risk of HIV transmission – was sufficient. For the second component, the majority of the Court called upon the concept of fraud as provided for in paragraph 265 (3) (c). It was judged on this basis that HIV non-disclosure constituted a fraudulent act vitiating the partner's consent and that, in these circumstances, an otherwise consensual sexual act could be seen as a form of assault, i.e., a non-consensual use of force. In the Court's opinion, circumstances involving "a significant risk of serious bodily harm" (*R v Cuerrier*, para. 128) required absolute disclosure of HIV status by a PLWH. In the absence of disclosure, true consent to sexual activity (para. 127) could not be given because it was vitiated by fraud.

To illustrate the relevance of expanding the concept of fraud, the Court relied upon a historical analysis of fraud in Canadian jurisprudence. Specifically, the Court cited the restrictive interpretation of fraud that had prevailed since the 1888 Court of Queen's Bench decision in *R v Clarence*. In this decision, the nature and character of the act itself had to be fraudulent in order to enforce criminal law in cases of rape and indecent assault. According to this criterion, only deceit and deception regarding the character of the act – for example, deceiving a woman by claiming to conduct a gynaecological exam in order to assault her sexually – or the partner's identity – for example, an assailant presenting himself to a woman as a gynaecologist – could be criminalized in terms of fraud vitiating consent to sexual activity.

Following this reasoning, the Supreme Court judged that HIV non-disclosure constituted a fraudulent act, vitiating a sexual partner's consent. As a result, consent no longer applied to the sexual act itself but, rather, to consent to sexual activity with an HIV-positive person. The Court, however, did not strictly impose absolute disclosure. As previously mentioned, the degree of risk associated with sexual activity was identified as the key criterion (*R v Cuerrier*, para. 127), but a more precise definition of such a degree of risk was not provided. The potential consequences of linking disclosure of HIV-positive status to the degree of risk were well illustrated by Judge Cory's famous *obiter*, in which he suggested that the careful use of condoms could reduce risk to the point of eliminating the obligation to disclose (para. 129).

Although the relationship described by the Supreme Court in *R v Cuerrier* is conceptually straightforward, the Court's vague definition and measurement of "significant risk of serious bodily harm" created confusion and inconsistencies in its application (Grant 2011). In the *Cuerrier* decision, the Court stated that vaginal penetration without a condom by an HIV-positive partner poses a "significant risk of serious bodily harm." But what of other sexual practices? For example, should the risk associated with oral sex without a condom with an HIV-positive person be considered sufficiently significant to require disclosure? Should disclosure after a condom has broken – which gives the HIV-negative partner an opportunity to obtain post-exposure prophylaxis[5] – constitute grounds for criminal prosecution? The Supreme Court did not explore these questions and instead limited itself to stating that, when non-disclosure can lead to a "devastating illness with fatal consequences," the obligation to disclose one's serological status is absolute (*R v Cuerrier*, para. 127).

Consequently, courts of first instance were faced with the difficult task of applying the law to facts distorted by ignorance, fear, and prejudice. Some courts cited Judge Cory's *obiter* to conclude that disclosure does not apply to sexual activities in which condoms are used. However, in the absence of a ruling on this specific question from the country's highest court, grey areas persisted in the definition and scope of the concept of "significant risk of serious bodily harm." The vagueness of this statement caused considerable confusion, both legally and socially, and led to many injustices (Symington 2013). Crown prosecutors across Canada adopted a variety of positions,[6] and contradictory jurisprudence was developed in courts of first instance.[7] Although there is a tendency to recognize that neither oral sex nor sex with condoms poses the degree of risk required to meet the standard of "significant risk of serious bodily harm" (Factum 2012), some rulings have nonetheless criminalized PLHIV in situations of minimal risk (Symington 2013). Moreover, in other cases, HIV-positive people have pleaded guilty, even though they may not have been legally required to do so (ibid.). Very often, courts criminalized PLWH in cases where HIV was not transmitted.

More recently, however, the law has demonstrated increasing openness to scientific and therapeutic advances (*R v Mabior* 2010). At the time of *Cuerrier*, therapeutic advances were in their infancy. Today, living with HIV is entirely different. Advances in HIV science and medical care have improved understanding of HIV transmission, increased the life expectancy of PLWH to match, or nearly match, that of the general population, and transformed treatment into a prevention strategy (Montaner et al. 2014; Cohen et al. 2011). The effect of these advances is that criminal law is now faced with a new paradigm in the fight against HIV. The major turning point in this confrontation occurred in 2012, when the Supreme Court was tasked with clarifying the concept of "significant risk of serious bodily harm" in companion cases *R v Mabior* and *R v DC*.

## 2012: Mabior *and* DC *Impose a New Direction*

In the *Mabior* decision, the Supreme Court of Canada had to determine whether the approach used in *Cuerrier* were still appropriate to analyse fraud vitiating consent to sexual relations with an HIV-positive person.

Specifically, the Court needed to address two problematic aspects of the *Cuerrier* decision: the vagueness of the concept of "significant risk of serious bodily harm" and the scope of the concept of fraud under sections 265, 268, and 273 of the Criminal Code.

The vagueness of the offence attracted criticism as a result of the inconsistent interpretation of the idea of significant risk of serious bodily harm in Canadian jurisprudence (Grant 2011). Clearly identifying the line separating criminal and non-criminal acts required a more accurate definition of this criterion. A more transparent definition was also required to make it easier for PLWH to know beforehand which acts could or could not lead to criminal prosecution. With regards to the scope of the offence, the Court was faced with the task of defining a framework of application capable of maintaining a balance between unduly increasing criminalization and protecting informed consent in light of the values of equality, autonomy, and dignity enshrined in the Canadian Charter of Rights and Freedoms (*R v Mabior*, paras 44–8).

Noting the need to clarify the law, the Supreme Court unanimously decided to uphold the principles established in the *Cuerrier* decision. However, the Court also judged that the time had come to accurately define the specific circumstances that pose a "significant risk of serious bodily harm." To do this, it was decided that the significant risk of serious bodily harm is established and the criterion of deprivation is respected in cases where a "realistic possibility of transmission of HIV" is demonstrated (*R v Mabior*, para. 84). In the opinion of the Court, this standard avoids criminalizing PLWH in situations of minimal risk (para. 78) while simultaneously requiring disclosure of HIV-positive status in situations of high risk (para. 87). The decision also specifies that the "realistic possibility of transmission" test applies only to the possible transmission of HIV, to the exclusion of all other sexually transmitted infections.

For these reasons, and on the basis of facts presented in *Mabior*, the Court ruled that the test of "realistic possibility of transmission" is not met when viral load is low and a condom is used. Without actually establishing clear guidelines that would permit lower courts to apply this new standard to the variety of practices that constitute sexual life – those other than vaginal penetration by an HIV-positive partner[8] – the Court adhered to an inflated vision of risk that does not sufficiently take into account current knowledge on transmission and treatment. Given that the relationship between the degree of risk and the seriousness of harm or risk of bodily harm should, theoretically, be inversely proportional (*R v Mabior*, paras 86 and 92), and in light of scientific and therapeutic advancements lessening the seriousness of bodily harm or risk of bodily harm, one could logically expect that the risk required to necessitate disclosure would be lower than in previous jurisprudence. And yet the *Mabior* decision closed the door Judge Cory had begun to open in his *obiter* in *Cuerrier*, which suggested the possibility of aligning the application of criminal law with the existence of certain practices, such as condom use, that reduce risk to such a degree that public health authorities consider them preventive.

In attempting to create greater transparency, the Court developed a position that not only leaves many questions unanswered, but also rejects an approach that would limit the scope of sexual assault and aggravated sexual assault, which, it bears repeating, are among criminal law's most serious offences. Although the Court is careful to argue convincingly against over-criminalization[9] and absolute disclosure, regardless of the degree of risk involved (*R v Mabior*, paras 66, 67, and 85), paradoxically, it also introduces a new norm that permanently expands the scope of criminal law. This inconsistency is present throughout the decision (Symington 2013) and results in a rule of law that contributes to the very same adverse effects denounced by the Court by increasing HIV-related stigma and vulnerability, exposing PLWH who act responsibly and whose conduct causes no harm to the risk of criminal prosecutions, and contributing to the further widening of social inequities (*R v Mabior*, para. 67).

Following this line of reasoning, the Court simultaneously positions itself against absolute disclosure in cases where risk is minimal (*R v Mabior*, para. 85) and requires disclosure in all cases of non-negligible risk (para. 99). It is therefore difficult to establish the Court's true intention. While negligible or "speculative" (para. 101) risk does not necessitate absolute disclosure, the Court's interpretation of the degree of "realistic" risk seems quite low. And although the Court recognizes that Canada's approach to HIV criminalization goes far beyond that of other common law jurisdictions, it nonetheless continues in this vein (para. 43).

Following the *Mabior* and *DC* verdicts, many decisions have been rendered by lower courts across the country. Although the tendency is to apply the test of realistic possibility of transmission according to the requirements set out in *Mabior*, the case of *R v JTC* shows that expert testimony can have an impact on how the test is interpreted. In this case, after hearing expert testimony demonstrating that the viral load of the accused was undetectable at the time of the events, the Nova Scotia Provincial Court ruled (*R v JTC* 2013 NSPC 105) that the risk presented by the sexual activities in question was close to zero. In light of this important information, the trial judge stated that, even when a condom is not used, the Court cannot assert the existence of a realistic possibility of transmission when there is evidence of an undetectable viral load. According to the judge, concluding otherwise is equivalent to criminalizing individuals who are no different from the rest of the population (para. 88). Although this decision thus far remains in the minority, the fact that it provides the basis for an argument founded on the right to equality makes it worthy of closer examination, particularly within the current context.

To conclude, it must be remembered that, in *Mabior*, the Supreme Court recognized that the test of a realistic possibility of transmission can "[adapt] to future advances in treatment and to circumstances where risk factors other than those considered in this case are at play" (*R v Mabior*, para. 95). Since this decision, a group of over eighty experts has produced the "Canadian Consensus Statement on HIV and Its Transmission in the Context of Criminal Law" (Loutfy et al. 2014). This statement presents a detailed account of the degree of risk of HIV transmission associated with a variety of practices, including spitting, biting, and other sexual practices, and takes condom use and low viral loads into account. Practices are placed on a scale from low to negligible to no risk. This document could be useful for courts called upon to participate in the evolution of current law according to the Supreme Court's recommendations in the *Mabior* decision.

### Analysis[10]

At its essence, structural stigma is "productive." In other words, it allows us (as a society) to achieve particular ends, namely to "keep people down," "keep people in," and "keep people away" (Phelan, Link, and Dovidio 2008; Link and Phelan 2014). Stigmatic assumptions about groups of people and populations make it possible to keep them "down" through exploitation and domination (Phelan, Link, and Dovidio 2008). They also make it possible to enforce social norms to ensure they stay "in" – in their place and within the boundaries of what is considered to be socially acceptable (ibid.; Link and Phelan 2014). Lastly, they justify the need to contain disease by keeping certain groups "away" using strategies that range from subtle, institutionalized forms of exclusion to more coercive forms of isolation (i.e., segregation, quarantine, compulsory detention, compulsory treatment, etc.) (Phelan, Link, and Dovidio 2008; Link and Phelan 2014).

Using structural stigma as a conceptual entry point for thinking about HIV criminalization allows us to do three things: first, to recognize that HIV criminalization meets particular ends, to "keep down," "keep people in," and "keep people away"; second, to think critically about the ways in which these ends are achieved within the criminal justice system; and third, to challenge the underlying assumptions that make it possible for PLWH to be constructed in such a way as to warrant the reinforcement of social norms and the containment of a perceived risk to others. For the purpose of this analysis, we are interested in what structural stigma has to offer to the analysis of HIV criminalization as a phenomenon that draws on the relations among social norms, social constructions of risk and crime, and structures of power.

### Breaking Norms: Non-Disclosure and Risk

We cannot fully understand structural stigma in the context of HIV criminalization unless we appreciate the extent to which, and the ways in which, risk has been constructed in legal texts. For the purpose of this analysis, we focused primarily on the legal texts of *R v Cuerrier*, *R v Aziga*, *R v DC*, and *R v Mabior*. These cases (as discussed above) made it possible to construct HIV non-disclosure as a risk to others and justify the use of the criminal law to "manage" this risk. As such, these cases should be understood as textual expressions of the power of the law and its capacity to produce risk – even when an actual risk does not exist.

HIV criminalization is concerned with risks that are both "real" *and* symbolic. On one hand, it focuses on the "real" risk of contracting HIV; this is captured in the legal concepts of "significant risk" (*R v Cuerrier*) and "realistic possibility" (*R v DC,* and *R v Mabior*) of HIV transmission. This type of risk can be calculated, estimated, debated, and challenged in court in light of scientific evidence. Consensus (Loutfy et al. 2014) on the exact nature of this risk and how it should be interpreted in court can also be achieved as a way to decrease the likelihood that it will be somewhat amplified, misinterpreted, or disconnected from the state of scientific knowledge on HIV transmission. Based solely on this risk, which approaches zero when PLWH are treated with antiretroviral combination therapy and achieve an undetectable viral load (ibid.), further criminalization would cease. However, this is unlikely to occur because HIV criminalization is also driven by the need to manage a risk that is neither tangible nor calculable (known as symbolic risk) (Hannem 2012).

Weait (2007) argues that a broader approach to risk is necessary to expose the underlying drivers of HIV criminalization. When risk is framed in legal (i.e., risk of bodily harm) and public health (i.e., risk of HIV transmission) terms, it provides only a partial picture of what criminalization hopes to achieve and limits our ability to challenge its very foundation. Structural stigma offers another way to look at HIV criminalization by focusing on the assumption that PLWH are intrinsically "risky" and "dangerous" to others (Hannem 2012). The cases of *R v Cuerrier*, and subsequently the cases of *R v DC* and *R v Mabior*, demonstrate that this assumption permeates the criminal justice system. These cases suggest that by virtue of being HIV-positive, people are systematically seen as posing a risk to others for two reasons: first, because they have the potential to transmit the virus to others, and second, because they have the potential to withhold that information from others.

In the context of criminalization, it is important to understand that such a risk is constructed in legal texts and media representations. It feeds on our collective imagination and stereotypical representations of PLWH as problematic, promiscuous, dishonest, and careless. It also serves a clear purpose. Risk, as a precursor of structural stigma, works by creating a need to intervene (Hannem 2012). In fact, it provides the necessary justification for the development of policies, laws, and programs that are intended to "manage" certain groups of people, including prisoners, sex workers, migrants, and people with mental illness (ibid.). Within the Canadian context, it is important to emphasize that the risk posed by PLWH is socially constructed (or symbolic) rather than the result of objective facts and scientific evidence (ibid.). Because such a risk does not depend on actual harms being realized (i.e., HIV transmission), it is a powerful tool with a very broad reach.

Despite the way it has been portrayed in criminal cases, HIV nondisclosure does not pose a risk to others. Disclosing or not does not prevent the further transmission of HIV. In fact, people have been shown to engage in unprotected sex after disclosure takes place (Simoni and Pantalone 2004). Moreover, the likelihood of PLWH transmitting the virus to others once they know their serological status and take antiretroviral combination therapy is close to zero (Loutfy et al. 2014). Yet PLWH continue to be constructed, in the popular imagination, as posing a risk to others. In reality, people who are unaware of their serological status are responsible for 23 per cent of all new cases of HIV infection (Frieden, Foti, and Mermin 2015). If we follow the logic of risk here, this group should be the target of criminal prosecutions, as opposed to people who have already been diagnosed and are less likely to transmit because of HIV treatment. While our intention is not to advocate for new forms of criminalization, we want to challenge the logic at play here. In doing so, we wish to point out that HIV criminalization in its current form has more to do with "keeping people in" than having a real impact on HIV transmission.

Criminal law plays an important role in targeting people who do not perform and conform to the normative standards of society (Mason and Mercer 1999). When the criminal law is applied to HIV, it reinforces social norms around sexuality – who is allowed to have sex, what should be said before sex, what is consensual sex, who is responsible for ensuring safe sex, and so on. In the absence of actual harms (i.e., HIV transmission), the social construction of risk relies on a potential threat to others (ibid.). In the context of HIV, the threat is that PLWH will not conform to such norms; they will not stay in their place and within the boundaries of what is considered to be socially acceptable for PLWH. In this sense, HIV criminalization sends a clear message about these boundaries and what happens when one crosses them. By making non-disclosure a crime, it is then possible to manage those who fail to "stay in" and to remind others of their responsibilities.

*Making Crime: Criminal Law and Risk Management*

As we have argued elsewhere, court decisions have played an important role in the making of HIV as a disability (Gagnon and Stuart 2009). The case of *Bragdon v Abbott* in the United States is a salient example of how these decisions have been used to broaden and generalize the scope of what constitutes a disability (ibid.). In the same way, the case of *R v Cuerrier*, and subsequently the cases of *R v DC* and *R v Mabior*, have played a key role in framing HIV non-disclosure as a crime. Because Canada does not have HIV-specific laws, the making of this new crime required the broadening of sexual assault law and reframing of non-disclosure as a fraud that invalidates consent to sex.

The concept of crime is dynamic, not static: "Laws are constantly changing, evolving, being formed, and being abolished: and they are always relative to the particular society that upholds them" (Mason and Mercer 1999, 5). In Canada, sexual assault law was not developed with non-disclosure in mind. Yet it has helped define non-disclosure as a crime by establishing that consent to sex cannot be fully obtained if information is withheld by the HIV-positive person. In order to challenge HIV criminalization, it is essential to return to the idea that crime (like risk) is a social construction (ibid.). It always emerges at a particular time, in a particular context, and for a particular purpose (ibid.). As such, we need to ask why non-disclosure became a crime in Canada when it did and what purpose it served – and still serves today.

The case of *R v Cuerrier* went before the Supreme Court of Canada in 1998, two years after the introduction of antiretroviral combination therapy. At the time of the hearing, the judges were well aware that antiretroviral combination therapy was allowing PLWH to stay healthier and live longer. Yet HIV was still considered a deadly disease with devastating physical consequences (hence the notion of bodily harm). The fact that PLWH were starting to live longer and were gradually returning to a "normal life" gave rise to a new social problem. Returning to a "normal life" meant that PLWH could put other members of society at risk, say in the context of sexual intercourse, by failing to disclose their status (i.e., breaking norms) and/or by transmitting the virus to sexual partners (i.e., posing a threat). Making non-disclosure a crime became an institutional response to this social problem. As such, it became a risk management strategy at a time when PLWH were reintegrating into society.

Structural stigma not only allows us to think critically about the ways in which PLWH are systematically constructed as "risky," but it also provides a lens to understand criminalization as a form of "risk management" (Hannem 2012; Kinsman 1996). Criminalization is one institutional response to one particular problem; and yet it is justified by the same rhetoric of risk-management that is common to all forms of structural stigma, whether it is targeted at men who have sex with men, sex workers, migrants, racialized groups, or people living with mental illness (Hannem 2012). Under the guise of risk management, criminalization does not necessarily stand out as a "bad policy." In fact, most people believe that it is a reasonable response to a foreseeable risk – one that needs to be contained, reduced, and ideally eliminated. However, when this belief circulates within the criminal justice system, it produces structural discrimination and unjust effects on PLWH (ibid.).

Structural discrimination materializes when PLWH are treated differently and unjustly within the criminal justice system (Hannem 2012). Structural discrimination often begins at the moment of the arrest and continues at every stage of the process. PLWH have seen their confidentiality breached and personal lives exposed from the moment of the arrest and onward. They have also experienced bias in the courtroom, resulting in more severe charges, longer sentences, and harsher detention conditions. In addition, it has become common practice to deny bail to PLWH because of the presumed risk they pose to society and to pressure them into pleading guilty before the case goes to trial. By virtue of its impact on the outcomes of non-disclosure cases, the most striking manifestation of structural discrimination is the conviction rate. Conviction rates are unusually high in cases of HIV non-disclosure. For example, "by the end of 2010, 78% of cases had ended in a conviction on at least one charge related to HIV non-disclosure" (Canadian HIV/AIDS Legal Network 2014).

The conviction rates and severity of punishments for PLWH who are found guilty of non-disclosure shed light on the inherent structural stigma that permeates the criminal justice system. This stigma (and the discrimination that ensues) is very problematic for all the reasons listed above. It is also problematic because it often intersects with structural homophobia and racism. Wilson argues that HIV criminalization can act as a form of oppression by keeping particular groups of PLWH "down." This is particularly true for African, Caribbean, and Black (ACB) Canadian communities. Over 90 per cent of non-disclosure cases in Canada have been against men. ACB men continue to account for a higher proportion of the men charged in these cases. The overrepresentation of ACB men is symptomatic of other structural influences that contribute to racial oppression within the criminal justice system (Wilson 2013).

*Throwing away the Keys: Capture and Surveillance*

By making non-disclosure a crime, we have created a new class of criminals. PLWH can now be charged for aggravated sexual assault and sentenced to jail time if found guilty of non-disclosure, up to a maximum sentence of life imprisonment. They can also be charged with murder and sentenced to life imprisonment without parole if found guilty of non-disclosure resulting in HIV transmission and death of a sexual partner (Canadian HIV/AIDS Legal Network 2014).

Generally speaking, structural stigma helps to justify the existence of systems that keep people "away." In the context of HIV criminalization, these systems serve a clear purpose by minimizing a perceived threat to the social body *and* social order. In other words, they work to ensure that PLWH who are found guilty of a crime do not pose a risk to the health of others and behave in a way that is consistent with a set of pre-determined rules. The carceral system puts people away and isolates them from the rest of society (Mason and Mercer 1999). After all, it is the most powerful system of capture in our society.

However, as we have seen in numerous non-disclosure cases – including the case of *R v Aziga* – there are additional forms of capture within the carceral system, including, but not limited to, voluntary and involuntary solitary confinement, dangerous offender designation, conditions of parole, and surveillance in the form of the National Sexual Offender Registry. The case of *R v Aziga* is a landmark case for many reasons. First, it illustrates how public health, law enforcement, and criminal law intersect in particular ways. Prior to his arrest in 2003, Aziga had been in contact with public health for approximately a year. He had been issued a Section 22 Order under the Health Protection and Promotion Act,[11] as well as a court order to reiterate the terms of the section 22 order and summon him to a court hearing. Second, it illustrates the severity of the crimes PLWH face in Canada. Following his arrest, Aziga was charged with two counts of first-degree murder and thirteen counts of aggravated sexual assault. He was convicted of two counts of first-degree murder, ten counts of aggravated sexual assault, and one count of attempted aggravated sexual assault in 2009. Third, it clearly shows how various forms of capture operate within the carceral system.

Like many other PLWH who face charges of sexual assault for non-disclosure, Aziga spent lengthy periods of time in voluntary solitary confinement (known as protective custody placement) before and during his trial. Because of the nature of his crimes, Aziga has since remained in protective custody placement, where he will most likely have to spend the rest of his indeterminate sentence. This form of capture is a direct outcome of the broadening of sexual assault law to include an act (non-disclosure) that has nothing to do with sexual assault. Like other convicted sexual offenders, PLWH are typically placed in solitary confinement for their own protection. This form of capture has little to do with the threat they pose to others and more to do with their identity as criminals – an identity that puts them in great danger within the carceral system. Yet it is rarely (if ever) discussed in the Canadian literature, despite having a significant impact on the experience of PLWH who become captives of their own criminal identity.

In the case of *R v Aziga*, a number of experts were consulted to determine if Aziga should be designated as a dangerous offender. As per the Criminal Code, this designation is intended "to protect society from the most dangerous violent and sexual predators." As such, it can be used only when "the offender constitutes a threat to the life, safety or physical or mental well-being of the public." During his testimony, one expert acknowledged that the usual tools used by psychiatrists to assess risk and the likelihood of serious future crimes were irrelevant to this particular case, because Aziga was not a "typical sex offender." While he was unable to use instruments or provide any assistance to the court to determine future risk or likelihood of criminal offences, he nevertheless considered that Aziga presented a substantial threat to society and insisted that risk management for this type of offender would be nearly impossible.

Even if Aziga was placed in long-term supervision with strict conditions, experts argued, these conditions would not ensure that he would never be left alone with a woman or that he would always disclose his serological status prior to sexual activity. For this reason, experts made a strong case for adding another form of capture to Aziga's sentence – one that would make him make him part of the "system" for life and allow the carceral system to keep him "away" for as long as needed. Surveillance, in the form of the National Sexual Offender Registry, is another form of capture that is commonly used in non-disclosure cases. Independently of the sentence, the designation of PLWH as sexual offenders allows authorities to limit their movements, conduct regular check-ups, and warn others about the risk they may pose. Along the same lines, conditions of parole act as a form of capture by imposing a predetermined structure and a set of fixed rules to PLWH who are returning to the community.

In sum, these various forms of capture equate to "locking PLWH up and throwing away the keys." They work by keeping PLWH away physically through imprisonment and confinement as well as socially through special designations, rules, and surveillance. Most importantly, they work because they provide the means to manage the risk and crime that is non-disclosure.

## Conclusion

In this chapter, we proposed structural stigma as a conceptual entry point for thinking about the criminalization of HIV non-disclosure and its effects on PLWH in Canada. Using an interdisciplinary approach combining legal and critical studies, we provided an overview of the state of HIV criminalization in Canada and proposed three ways of problematizing this phenomenon. First, we argued that HIV non-disclosure is seen as a breach of social norms and a risk to others. Second, we described how the construction of HIV non-disclosure as a crime and the designation of PLWH as criminals serve to manage this risk. Last, we exposed the fact that imprisonment and surveillance function as calculated "risk management" strategies.

Minimal attention has been paid to structural stigma as it relates to HIV criminalization in the literature. Parker and Aggleton brought structural stigma to the attention of HIV scholars and researchers more than a decade ago in a call for more attention to structure and power. This analysis has sought to demonstrate that structural stigma is indeed a useful entry point to think differently about complex socio-political-legal issues in the field of HIV (including HIV criminalization) and challenging "bad policies" that affect the lives of PLWH.

## NOTES

1 Patrick O'Byrne and Marilou Gagnon, "The Ramifications of the Current Context of Criminal Prosecutions for Non-Disclosure of HIV Status on Nursing Practice: Meeting Report," *Aporia: The Nursing Journal* 4, no. 2 (2012): 5–34; Patrick O'Byrne, "HIV, Nursing Practice, and the Law: What Does HIV Criminalization Mean for Practicing Nurses?" *Journal of the Association of Nurses in AIDS Care* 22, no. 5 (2011): 339–44; O'Byrne, "Criminal Law and Public Health Practice: Are the Canadian HIV Disclosure Laws an Effective HIV Prevention Strategy?" *Sexuality Research and Social Policy* 9, no. 1 (2012): 70–9; Patrick O'Byrne, Alyssa Bryan, and Marie Roy, "HIV Criminal Prosecutions and Public Health: An Examination of the Empirical Research," *BMJ Medical Humanities* 39, no. 2 (2013): 85–90; Bryan, O'Byrne, and Roy, "Sexual Practices and STI/HIV Testing among Gay, Bisexual, and Men Who Have Sex with Men in Ottawa, Canada: Examining Nondisclosure Prosecutions and HIV Prevention," *Critical Public Health* 23, no. 2 (2013): 225–36; Patrick O'Byrne, Dave Holmes, and Marie Roy, "Counselling about HIV Serological Status Disclosure: Nursing Practice or Law Enforcement? A Foucauldian Reflection," *Nursing Inquiry* 22, no. 2 (2015): 134–46; Patrick O'Byrne, Jacqueline Willmore et al., "Do HIV Status Nondisclosure Prosecutions Affect Population Health Goals? Examining HIV Testing and Diagnosis and the Attitudes/Behaviours of

Men Who Have Sex with Men in the Context of Media Coverage about Nondisclosure Prosecutions," *BMC Public Health* 13 (2013): 94; Patrick O'Byrne, Alyssa Bryan, and Cody Woodyatt, "Nondisclosure Prosecutions and HIV Prevention: Results from an Ottawa-Based Gay Men's Survey," *Journal of the Association of Nurses in AIDS Care* 24, no. 1 (2013): 81–7; Eric Mykhalovskiy, "The Problem of 'Significant Risk': Exploring the Public Health Impact of Criminalizing HIV Non-Disclosure," *Social Science & Medicine* 73, no. 5 (2011): 668–75; J. Craig Phillips, Allison Webel et al., "Associations between the Legal Context of HIV, Perceived Social Capital, and HIV Antiretroviral Adherence in North America," *BMC Public Health* 13, no. 1 (2013): 736; Chris Sanders, "Discussing the Limits of Confidentiality: The Impact of Criminalizing HIV Non-Disclosure on Public Health Nurses' Counseling Practices," *Public Health Ethics* 7, no. 3 (2014): 253–60; Sanders, "Examining Public Health Nurses' Documentary Practices: The Impact of Criminalizing HIV Non-Disclosure on Inscription Styles," *Critical Public Health* 25, no. 4 (2015): 398–409; Martin French, "Counselling Anomie: Clashing Governmentalities of HIV Criminalisation and Prevention," *Critical Public Health* 25, no. 4 (2015): 427–40.

2  Marilou Gagnon, "Toward a Critical Response to HIV Criminalization: Remarks on Advocacy and Social Justice," *Journal of the Association of Nurses in AIDS Care* 23, no. 1 (2012): 11–15; J. Craig Phillips, Jean-Laurent Domingue, and Duane A.G. Morrisseau-Beck, "'I Need My Nurse!' Nurses and the Criminalization of HIV in North America," *Journal of the Association of Nurses in AIDS Care* 24, no. 6 (2013): 471–2; Barry D. Adam, Patrice Corriveau et al., "HIV Disclosure as Practice and Public Policy," *Critical Public Health* 25, no. 4 (2015): 386–97; Barry D. Adam, Richard Elliott, Patrice Corriveau et al., "Impacts of Criminalization on the Everyday Lives of People Living with HIV in Canada," *Sexuality Research & Social Policy* 11, no. 1 (2014): 39–49; Barry D. Adam, Richard Elliott, Winston Husbands et al., "Effects of Criminalization of HIV Transmission in Cuerrier on Men Reporting Sex with Men," *Canadian Journal of Law and Society* 23, nos 1–2 (2008): 143–59; Mary S. Petty, "Social Responses to HIV: Fearing the Outlaw," *Sexuality Research & Social Policy* 2, no. 2 (2005): 76–88; Gary Kinsman, "Vectors of Hope and Possibility: Commentary on Reckless Vectors," *Sexuality Research & Social Policy* 2, no. 2 (2005): 99–105.

3  Ciann Wilson, "The Impact of the Criminalization of HIV Non-Disclosure on the Health and Human Rights of 'Black' Communities," *Health Tomorrow* 1 (2013): 109–43; Isabel Grant, "The Over-Criminalization of Persons with HIV," *University of Toronto Law Journal* 63, no. 3 (2013):

475–84; Isabel Grant, Martha Shaffer, and Alyson Symington, "Introduction," *University of Toronto Law Journal* 63, no. 3 (2013): 462–5; Martha Shaffer, "Sex, Lies, and HIV: Mabior and the Concept of Sexual Fraud," *University of Toronto Law Journal* 63, no. 3 (2013): 467–74; Alyson Symington, "Injustice Amplified by HIV Non-Disclosure Ruling," *University of Toronto Law Journal* 63, no. 3 (2013): 485–95; Eric Mykhalovskiy and Glenn Betteridge, "Who? What? Where? When? And with What Consequences? An Analysis of Criminal Cases of HIV Non-Disclosure in Canada," *Canadian Journal of Law and Society* 27, no. 1 (2012): 31–53; Isabel Grant, "Rethinking Risk: The Relevance of Condoms and Viral Load in HIV Nondisclosure Prosecutions," *McGill Law Journal* 54, no. 2 (2009): 389–404; Grant, "The Prosecution of Non-Disclosure of HIV in Canada: Time to Rethink Cuerrier," *McGill Law Journal* 5, no. 1 (2011): 7–59.

4  This section was translated from the French by Catriona LeBlanc.

5  Post-exposure prophylaxis refers to the preventive use of HIV medications after an exposure to HIV.

6  For example, in *DC v R*, 2010 QCCA 2289 (at para. 84), the Quebec attorney general conceded that vaginal intercourse with a condom did not present a significant risk of transmission, while the Manitoba attorney general argued that "even protected sex may be caught" in *R v Mabior* 2012 SCC 47, [2012] SCR 584. As reported in the Factum of the Interveners of the Supreme Court of Canada in the case of R v Mabior, court file nos. 33976/34094, http://www.aidslaw.ca/site/wp-content/uploads/2013/04/Mabior-DC_SCCfactum2012.pdf (at para. 8).

7  A man with HIV was prosecuted in 2010 in Ontario for performing oral sex, which poses at most an infinitesimal risk of transmission. See Canadian HIV/AIDS Legal Network, "AIDS Organization Welcomes Crown Decision to Stay Criminal Charges in Hamilton HIV Case," news release, Toronto, 22 April 2010. Some people have also been convicted despite condom use or the fact that the Crown could not establish beyond a reasonable doubt that sex was unprotected, while others have been acquitted in the same circumstances: e.g., *R v Mekonnen*, 2009 ONCJ 643 (overturned on appeal; *R v Mekonnen*, 2013 ONCA 414); *R v Felix*, 2010 ONCJ 322 (at para. 71–2); *R v Felix*, 2013 ONCA 413. See Factum of the Interveners, at para. 8, note 20.

8  These are the facts presented in *Mabior.*

9  Ibid., para. 19.

10 Subtitles for this section were inspired by T. Mason and D. Mercer, *A Sociology of the Mentally Disordered Offender* (London: Longman, 1999).

11  Under Section 22 of the Health Protection and Promotion Act (HPPA),
    if the legal requirements of that section are met, medical officers of health
    (MOHs) have the legislative authority to issue a written order to, among
    other things, require a person to take or to refrain from taking any action
    with respect to a communicable disease. PIDAC (2009).

REFERENCES

Adam, Barry D., et al. 2015. "HIV Disclosure as Practice and Public Policy."
    *Critical Public Health* 25 (4): 386–97. https://doi.org/10.1080/09581596.2014
    .980395.
Adam, Barry D., et al. 2014. "Impacts of Criminalization on the Everyday
    Lives of People Living with HIV in Canada." *Sexuality Research & Social
    Policy* 11 (1): 39–49. https://doi.org/10.1007/s13178-013-0131-8.
Adam, Barry D., et al. 2008. "Effects of Criminalization of HIV Transmission in
    Cuerrier on Men Reporting Unprotected Sex with Men." *Canadian Journal of
    Law and Society* 23 (1–2): 143–59. https://doi.org/10.1017/S0829320100009613.
Canadian HIV/AIDS Legal Network. 2010. "AIDS Organization Welcomes
    Crown Decision to Stay Criminal Charges in Hamilton HIV Case." News
    release, Toronto, 22 April 2010.
–  2014. "Criminal Law & HIV Non-Disclosure in Canada." http://www
    .aidslaw.ca/site/wp-content/uploads/2014/09/CriminalInfo2014_ENG.pdf.
Cohen, Myron S., et al. 2011. "Prevention of HIV-1 Infection with Early
    Antiretroviral Therapy." *New England Journal of Medicine* 365:493–505.
Factum of the Interveners of the Supreme Court of Canada: R v Mabior and
    R v DC (2012), court file nos 33976/34094. http://www.aidslaw.ca/site/
    wp-content/uploads/2013/04/Mabior-DC_SCCfactum2012.pdf.
Foucault, Michel. 1980. *Power/Knowledge: Selected Interviews and Others Writings
    (1972–1977)*. New York: Pantheon Books.
–  1990. *The History of Sexuality*, vol. 1. New York: Vintage Books.
–  1995. *Discipline and Punish: The Birth of the Prison*. New York: Vintage Books.
–  2003. "Govermentality." In *The Essential Foucault: Selections from Essential
    Works of Foucault 1954–1984*, edited by Paul Rabinow and Nickolas Rose,
    229–45. New York: New Press.
French, Martin. 2015. "Counselling Anomie: Clashing Governmentalities of
    HIV Criminalisation and Prevention." *Critical Public Health* 25 (4): 427–40.
    https://doi.org/10.1080/09581596.2015.1046814.
Frieden, T.R., K.E. Foti, and J. Mermin. 2015. "Applying Public Health Principles
    to the HIV Epidemic: How Are We Doing?" *New England Journal of Medicine*
    373 (23): 2281–7. https://doi.org/10.1056/NEJMms1513641.

Gagnon, Marilou. 2012. "Toward a Critical Response to HIV Criminalization: Remarks on Advocacy and Social Justice." *Journal of the Association of Nurses in AIDS Care* 23 (1): 11–15. https://doi.org/10.1016/j.jana.2011.08.012.

– 2015. Re-Thinking HIV-Related Stigma in Health Care Settings: A Qualitative Study. *Journal of the Association of Nurses in AIDS Care* 26 (6): 703–19. https://doi.org/10.1016/j.jana.2015.07.005.

Gagnon, Marilou, and Meryn Stuart. 2009. "Manufacturing Disability: HIV, Women and the Construction of Difference." *Nursing Philosophy* 10 (1): 42–52. https://doi.org/10.1111/j.1466-769X.2008.00380.x.

Global Network of People Living with HIV (GNP+) and HIV Justice Network. 2013. *Advancing HIV Justice: A Progress Report of Achievements and Challenges in Global Advocacy against HIV Criminalisation.* http://www.hivjustice.net/wp-content/uploads/2013/05/Advancing-HIV-Justice-June-2013.pdf.

Goffman, Erving. 1963. *Stigma: Notes on the Management of Spoiled Identity.* New Jersey: Prentice-Hall.

Grant, Isabel. 2009. "Rethinking Risk: The Relevance of Condoms and Viral Load in HIV Nondisclosure Prosecutions." *McGill Law Journal/Revue de Droit de McGill* 54 (2): 389–404. https://doi.org/10.7202/038659ar.

– 2011. "The Prosecution of Non-Disclosure of HIV in Canada: Time to Rethink Cuerrier." *McGill Law Journal/Revue de Droit de McGill* 5 (1): 7–59.

– 2013. "The Over-Criminalization of Persons with HIV." *University of Toronto Law Journal* 63 (3): 475–84. https://doi.org/10.3138/utlj.63.3.0301-2.

Grant, Isabel, Martha Shaffer, and Alyson Symington. 2013. "Introduction." *University of Toronto Law Journal* 63 (3): 462–5. https://doi.org/10.3138/utlj.0302.

Hankivsky, Olena, et al. 2014. "An Intersectionality-Based Policy Analysis Framework: Critical Reflections on a Methodology for Advancing Equity." *International Journal for Equity in Health* 13 (1): 119–35. https://doi.org/10.1186/s12939-014-0119-x.

Hannem, Stacey. 2012. "Theorizing Stigma and the Politics of Resistance." In *Stigma Revisited: Negotiations, Resistance and the Implications of the Mark,* edited by Stacey Hannem and Chris Bruckert, 10–28. Ottawa: University of Ottawa Press.

Hannem, Stacey, and Chris Bruckert. 2012. *Stigma Revisited: Negotiations, Resistance and the Implications of the Mark.* Ottawa: University of Ottawa Press.

Kinsman, Gary. 1996. "'Responsibility' as a Strategy of Governance: Regulating People Living with AIDS and Lesbians and Gay Men in Ontario." *Economy and Society* 25 (3): 393–409. https://doi.org/10.1080/03085149600000021.

– 2005. "Vectors of Hope and Possibility: Commentary on Reckless Vectors." *Sexuality Research & Social Policy* 2 (2): 99–105. https://doi.org/10.1525/srsp.2005.2.2.99.

Link, Bruce G., and Jo C. Phelan. 2001. "Conceptualizing Stigma." *Annual Review of Sociology* 27 (1): 363–85. https://doi.org/10.1146/annurev .soc.27.1.363.

– 2014. "Stigma Power." *Social Science & Medicine* 103:24–32.

Loutfy, Mona, et al. 2014. "Canadian Consensus Statement on HIV and Its Transmission in the Context of Criminal Law." *Canadian Journal of Infectious Diseases and Medical Microbiology* 25 (3): 135–40. https://doi.org/10.1155/ 2014/498459.

Mason, Tom, and David Mercer. 1999. *A Sociology of the Mentally Disordered Offender*. London: Longman.

Montaner, Julio S.G, et al. 2014. "Expansion of HAART Coverage Is Associated with Sustained Decreases in HIV/AIDS Morbidity, Mortality and HIV Transmission: The 'HIV Treatment as Prevention' Experience in a Canadian Setting." *PloS ONE* 9 (2): e87872. https://doi.org/10.1371/journal.pone .0087872.

Mykhalovskiy, Eric. 2011. "The Problem of 'Significant Risk': Exploring the Public Health Impact of Criminalizing HIV Non-Disclosure." *Social Science & Medicine* 73 (5): 668–75. https://doi.org/10.1016/j.socscimed.2011.06.051.

– 2015. "The Public Health Implications of HIV Criminalization: Past, Current, and Future Research Directions." *Critical Public Health* 25 (4): 373–85. https://doi.org/10.1080/09581596.2015.1052731.

Mykhalovskiy, Eric, and Glenn Betteridge. 2012. "Who? What? Where? When? And with What Consequences? An Analysis of Criminal Cases of HIV Non-Disclosure in Canada." *Canadian Journal of Law and Society* 27 (1): 31–53. https://doi.org/10.3138/cjls.27.1.031.

O'Byrne, Patrick. 2011. "HIV, Nursing Practice, and the Law: What Does HIV Criminalization Mean for Practicing Nurses." *Journal of the Association of Nurses in AIDS Care* 22 (5): 339–44. https://doi.org/10.1016/j.jana.2011 .02.002.

– 2012. "Criminal Law and Public Health Practice: Are the Canadian HIV Disclosure Laws an Effective HIV Prevention Strategy?" *Sexuality Research & Social Policy* 9 (1): 70–9. https://doi.org/10.1007/s13178-011-0053-2.

O'Byrne, Patrick, Alyssa Bryan, and Marie Roy. 2013a. "HIV Criminal Prosecutions and Public Health: An Examination of the Empirical Research." *BMJ Medical Humanities* 39 (2): 85–90. https://doi.org/10.1136/medhum-2013-010366.

– 2013b. "Sexual Practices and STI/HIV Testing among Gay, Bisexual, and Men Who Have Sex with Men in Ottawa, Canada: Examining Nondisclosure Prosecutions and HIV Prevention." *Critical Public Health* 23 (2): 225–36. https://doi.org/10.1080/09581596.2012.752070.

O'Byrne, Patrick, Alyssa Bryan, and Cody Woodyatt. 2013. "Nondisclosure Prosecutions and HIV Prevention: Results from an Ottawa-Based Gay Men's Survey." *Journal of the Association of Nurses in AIDS Care* 24 (1): 81–7. https://doi.org/10.1016/j.jana.2012.01.009.

O'Byrne, Patrick, and Marilou Gagnon. 2012. "The Ramifications of the Current Context of Criminal Prosecutions for Non-Disclosure of HIV Status on Nursing Practice: Meeting Report." *Aporia: The Nursing Journal* 4 (2): 5–34.

O'Byrne, Patrick, Dave Holmes, and Marie Roy. 2015. "Counselling about HIV Serological Status Disclosure: Nursing Practice or Law Enforcement? A Foucauldian Reflection." *Nursing Inquiry* 22 (2): 134–46. https://doi.org/10.1111/nin.12075.

O'Byrne, Patrick, et al. 2013. "Nondisclosure Prosecutions and Population Health Outcomes: Examining HIV Testing, HIV Diagnoses, and the Attitudes of Men Who Have Sex with Men Following Nondisclosure Prosecution Media Releases in Ottawa, Canada." *BMC Public Health* 13 (1). https://doi.org/10.1186/1471-2458-13-94.

Parker, Richard, and Peter Aggleton. 2003. "HIV and AIDS-Related Stigma and Discrimination: A Conceptual Framework and Implications for Action." *Social Science & Medicine* 57 (1): 13–24. https://doi.org/10.1016/S0277-9536(02)00304-0.

Petty, Mary S. 2005. "Social Responses to HIV: Fearing the Outlaw." *Sexuality Research & Social Policy* 2 (2): 76–88. https://doi.org/10.1525/srsp.2005.2.2.76.

Phelan, Jo C., Bruce G. Link, and John F. Dovidio. 2008. "Stigma and Prejudice: One Animal or Two?" *Social Science & Medicine* 67 (3): 358–67. https://doi.org/10.1016/j.socscimed.2008.03.022.

Phillips, J. Craig, Jean-Laurent Domingue, and Duane A.G. Morrisseau-Beck. 2013. "'I Need My Nurse!' Nurses and the Criminalization of HIV in North America." *Journal of the Association of Nurses in AIDS Care* 24 (6): 471–2. https://doi.org/10.1016/j.jana.2013.08.004.

Phillips, J. Craig, et al. 2013. "Associations between the Legal Context of HIV, Perceived Social Capital, and HIV Antiretroviral Adherence in North America." *BMC Public Health* 13 (1): 736. https://doi.org/10.1186/1471-2458-13-736.

Provincial Infectious Diseases Advisory Committee (PIDAC). 2009. *Sexually Transmitted Infections Case Management and Contact Tracing Best Practice Recommendations.* Ministry of Health and Long-Term Care. https://www.publichealthontario.ca/en/eRepository/STIs%20Case%20Management%20Contact%20Tracing.pdf.

Sanders, Chris. 2014. "Discussing the Limits of Confidentiality: The Impact of Criminalizing HIV Non-Disclosure on Public Health Nurses' Counseling

Practices." *Public Health Ethics* 7 (3): 253–60. https://doi.org/10.1093/phe/phu032.
– 2015. "Examining Public Health Nurses' Documentary Practices: The Impact of Criminalizing HIV Non-Disclosure on Inscription Styles." *Critical Public Health* 25 (4): 398–409. https://doi.org/10.1080/09581596.2015.1019834.
Shaffer, Martha. 2013. "Sex, Lies, and HIV: Mabior and the Concept of Sexual Fraud." *University of Toronto Law Journal* 63 (3): 466–74. https://doi.org/10.3138/utlj.63.3.0301-1.
Simoni, Jane M., and David W. Pantalone. 2004. "Secrets and Safety in the Age of of AIDS: Does Disclosure Lead to Safer Sex?" *Topics in HIV Medicine* 12 (4): 109–18.
Symington, Alyson. 2013. "Injustice Amplified by HIV Non-Disclosure Ruling." *University of Toronto Law Journal* 63 (3): 485–95. https://doi.org/10.3138/utlj.0302-3.
Weait, Matthew. 2007. *Intimacy and Responsibility: The Criminalisation of HIV Transmission*. New York: Routledge.
Wilson, Ciann. 2013. "The Impact of the Criminalization of HIV Non-Disclosure on the Health and Human Rights of 'Black' Communities." *Health Tomorrow* 1:109–43.

## Case Law

*DC v R*, 2010 QCCA 2289.
*The Queen v Clarence* (1888), 22 QBD 23.
*R v Cuerrier*, [1998] 2 RCS 371.
*R v DC*, 2012 SCC 48, [2012] 2 SCR 626.
*R v Felix*, 2010 ONCJ 322.
*R v Felix*, 2013 ONCA 413.
*R v JTC* 2013 NSPC 105.
*R v Mabior*, 2012 SCC 47, [2012] SCR 584.
*R v Mabior* (CL), 2010 MBCA 93.
*R v Mekonnen*, 2009 ONCJ 643 (overturned on appeal).
*R v Mekonnen*, 2013 ONCA 414.

# 3 Institutionalizing Risk in the "Daddy State": Carceral Spaces as HIV Risk Environments

JENNIFER M. KILTY

People living with HIV/AIDS (PHAs) are some of the most vulnerable and stigmatized members of carceral populations worldwide; they experience an increased risk of isolation, violence, and human rights abuses (Lines 2007). Fear about HIV is magnified in the carceral environment due to factors including: misinformation about HIV transmission; the closed nature of this total institution; and the stigma and discrimination of already vulnerable groups (e.g. sex workers, people who use drugs and homosexuals) within the prisoner population (Lines 2007, 61). While it is widely recognized that, despite institutional prohibition, prisoners engage in sex and drug taking (Jürgens 2007a, 2007b), many prison administrations around the world, including in Canada, fail to provide access to life-saving harm-reduction technologies. This policy failure contributes to the production of carceral spaces as elevated HIV risk environments that can facilitate rather than prevent HIV and other infections.

The fact that carceral spaces are elevated HIV risk environments suggests the possibility of a "carceral syndemic," where HIV is not only linked to other comorbid sexually transmitted infections (notably HCV) (Zakaria, Thompson, and Borgatta 2010), substance use (Rhodes 2009), mental illness/distress (OCI 2012, 2014), poor psychosocial coping skills, and forms of structural violence (e.g., poverty, racism, sexism etc.) (Chan and Chunn 2014) – all of which are disproportionately found among incarcerated populations – but where the interplay between these variables may exacerbate negative health outcomes for PHAs. Given the growth of mass incarceration and prison overcrowding, protecting the health of incarcerated citizens requires special consideration.

Deciding how to govern the health of incarcerated people engenders socio-political debate and prison reform efforts to improve the quality standards of conditions of confinement as a pathway to improve prisoner health. Reform efforts that aim to improve prisoner health by providing quality nutrition, medical care, more humane shelter conditions, and educational, rehabilitative, and treatment programming are often contested by those in favour of a more retributive approach to carceral governance. Criminologists describe this as a result of the "less eligibility principle" (Sim 2009), a shifting cultural reference point that intimates that prisoners should not experience state-supported conditions of confinement that exceed the quality standards of those experienced by impoverished members of society.

Although this flawed argument fails to consider the structural connections between poverty, marginality, and criminality (Chan and Chunn 2014; Wacquant 2009, 2010), it is often used to justify austerity measures to reduce prison costs. For example, in January 2015 the Harper government switched all federal prisons from fresh to powdered milk to save approximately three million dollars per year, a change that conservative MP Rob Anders described in the House of Commons as "not sit[ting] well with the hug-a-thug crowd in the NDP" (Quan 2015). Populist punitive discourses echo the less-eligibility principle by suggesting that criminalized people do not deserve carceral treatment that adheres to civic standards of decency, compassion, and, as this chapter discusses, health protection. The principle's legacy continues today and deeply contrasts the Ottawa Charter for Health Promotion (1986) "health for all" mantra and the fact that "the principle of equivalence is fundamental to the promotion of human rights and proper health care standards within prisons" (Lines 2007, 62).

To contextualize HIV prevention in carceral spaces, this chapter begins by identifying how neoliberalism affected Canada's evolving approach to public health and penality, which Wacquant (2010) describes as producing a kind of "daddy state" – where, in contrast to the "nanny state" provision of collective social welfare, the state acts as protector, authority figure, and source of security. These discussions segue into a closer examination of how the last decade of federal politics in Canada has engaged in legal moralism, legal paternalism, and the politics of blame when crafting criminal justice legislation and correctional policies on HIV prevention, which sets up the final section that explores the HIV risk environment specific to carceral spaces. I focus on the federal correctional system to exemplify the effects of neoliberal penality at the national level.

## Neoliberal Evolution of Health Discourses in Canada

Public health, as it was originally conceived, encompassed two key efforts – health promotion and health protection – and emphasized behavioural modifications and self-government as the mechanisms through which citizens are expected to achieve improved health. As such, "public health is bound up with moralistic notions of acceptable and unacceptable behaviours" (Orsini 2007, 348) that create a divide between healthy (good) and unhealthy (bad) people. Orsini (349) identifies a parallel emergence of a "shadow responsibilization paradigm" that emphasizes individual lifestyle changes to improve health and engages in victim-blaming for having developed certain illnesses. The increasing criminalization of HIV-positive people for not disclosing their HIV status to their sexual partners evidences the messiness of responsibilization discourses and the politics of blame at work.

As early incarnations of public health gave way to "the new public health," the role that "communities" play in improving health was accented (Orsini 2007; Robertson 1998). When public health efforts did not provide the cost-savings that health economists predicted, there was increased demand for evidence-based policy and medicine in future efforts to better the health of the population (Orsini 2007; Robertson 1998). The "population health" approach is widely considered an improvement on the public health framework, because it considers the social determinants of health as a way to identify health disparities between groups and to assess ways of effecting targeted change in the health of those who fare poorly on certain health and illness indicators. However, reflection on the social aspects of health is often "sloppy," stripped of context and "excessively reductionist and insensitive to the context in which health (and illness) is experienced by the individual as mediated through community and societal structures" (Orsini 2007, 353). For example, while demographic data demonstrate that individuals with lower socio-economic status have poorer overall health outcomes than those with higher incomes, this finding does not consider how political, socio-economic, and other macro structural forces create health disparities between the rich and the poor, or how to rectify this inequity through public health efforts. The population health approach certainly tips its hat to the social determinants of health, but it does not offer policy reforms or solutions to the structural forces at the root of health inequality.

This evolution of Canadian health discourses occurred as Western nation states began to adopt neoliberal approaches to governance in

earnest. Following Wacquant's (2009, 2010) argument for a sociological (rather than purely economic) specification of neoliberalism, I argue
that the trajectories of these two movements are not simply parallel, but
fused: the shift to the population health framework is itself an effect of
the neoliberalization of health care. Relatedly, the ascendancy of the conservative "get tough on crime" approach that drove Canada's criminal
justice policy agenda under Harper similarly engages responsibilization discourses that blame individual prisoners for their criminalization
without considering the social and structural forces that disadvantage
some groups more than others – most notably, Indigenous Canadians
and other racialized minorities, immigrants, and the poor (Chan and
Chunn 2014; Wacquant 2009). The next section considers the role neoliberal discourses play in Canadian penality.

### Lock 'em up style: Conceptualizing Neoliberal Penality

Whether described as a "punitive turn" or the less aggrandizing "penal
intensification" (Sim 2009), it is unquestionable that neoliberalism has
dramatically shaped the criminal justice policy and legislative landscape in most Western democracies. Canada is no exception. While it is
beyond the scope of this chapter to provide an in-depth review of the
emergence of neoliberal governance in Canada and the role the growing apparatus of penality played in this development, it is important to
outline the main contours of how I employ the concept of neoliberalism. Adopting Wacquant's (2009, 2010) thesis that neoliberalism does
not actually shrink the size and power of government, but rather creates what he calls a hierarchical and divisively classed "centaur state"
that has less governmental regulation at the top for the wealthy yet
strict control at the bottom for the poor, neoliberalism "entails not simply the reassertion of the prerogatives of capital and the promotion
of the marketplace, but the close articulation of four institutional log-
ics: (1) economic deregulation; (2) welfare state devolution, retraction
and recomposition; (3) an expansive, intrusive, and proactive penal
apparatus; and (4) the cultural trope of individual responsibility"
(Wacquant 2010, 213).

   To situate Wacquant's work in the Canadian context I focus on the
orientation of penal policy and criminal justice legislation created during the last decade of federal conservative rule under Prime Minister
Stephen Harper.[1] With historical commitment to correctional rehabilitation, Moore and Hannah-Moffat (2005) describe Canada's punishment

industry as donning a "liberal veil"; while falling short of the progressive nature of Scandinavian carceral exceptionalism (Pratt 2007, 2008), Canada has also avoided the negative repercussions flowing from American style mass incarceration (Webster and Doob 2007, 2015). One of the few Western democracies to maintain a relatively stable prison population over time – even during the 1980s–1990s upswing of neoliberal governance and global carceral expansion – Canada is often considered a global anomaly (Wacquant 2009, 2010).

However, during Harper's tenure as prime minister, the Conservatives introduced ninety new criminal justice bills, including two massive omnibus pieces of legislation that contained bills that were introduced separately while the party held a minority government but for various reasons, including prorogation, failed to receive approval in the House of Commons or royal assent. These include new mandatory minimum sentences for certain drug offences, gun crimes, and child exploitation offences; the abolition or tightening of parole review criteria; reduction of credit for time served in pretrial custody; more restricted use of conditional sentences; and the elimination of the faint hope clause (OCI 2012). Doob and Webster (2015) argue that the use of omnibus bills showcases a dramatic political shift away from Canada's traditional approach of securing parliamentary consensus on criminal justice legislation that is grounded in empirical research. This new strategy illustrates the rejection of social scientific evidence in favour of a distinctly neoliberal approach to governing crime that stresses individual choice and responsibility for criminality and supports retributive responses to law-breaking. Just as neoliberal health discourses underscore behavioural modification and self-government to improve health (Orsini 2007; Robertson 1998), this logic is mirrored in criminal justice legislation and correctional policy and practice (Harcourt 2010; Wacquant 2009, 2010).

Wacquant (2010, 201) argues that the neoliberal state governs social insecurity through an expanding penal apparatus that is "detectable in the reallocation of public budgets, personnel, and discursive precedence and the colonization of the welfare sector by the panoptic and punitive logic characteristic of the post-rehabilitation penal bureaucracy." Under Harper, the federal correctional system witnessed significant growth in fiscal cost and carceral population expansion. The Office of the Correctional Investigator (2012) reported that between 2010 and 2012, the federal prison population increased by 1,000 prisoners (6.8 per cent), "which is the equivalent of two large male medium security institutions." While the OCI (2012) maintains that "at a time of widespread budgetary restraint, it seems prudent to use prison sparingly, and as the last resort it was intended to be," the federal correctional budget expanded 43.9 per cent between 2005–6 and 2010–11 and is now over $3 billion.

The government also planned to add 2,700 new or renovated cells across thirty existing institutions "at a cost of more than $630M," expenditures that cover only "construction, not operation, staffing or ongoing maintenance" (OCI 2012). The OCI also found that more than 17 per cent of federal prisons are double-bunked (placing two prisoners in a cell designed for one), thus compromising prisoner, staff, and public safety. These legislative changes coincided with a surge in austerity, a component of the Conservative government's deficit-reduction action plan, that cut spending by eliminating innovative harm-reduction programs[2] like the pilot tattoo program created under the preceding Liberal government, while increasing costs to impoverished prisoners, for example through the new victim fine surcharge. The tattoo program allowed prisoners to earn work experience and build a portfolio that would help them find employment upon release, and reduced HIV risk by decreasing unsafe tattooing practices (e.g., sharing needles and handmade tattoo ink and gear) that are common in prison.

Larger budgetary allotments were also afforded to bolster the policing of carceral populations; for example, in 2008 the minister of public safety announced an additional $120-million investment in the Correctional Service Canada's (CSC) anti-drug strategy. The monies were specifically reserved for carceral law enforcement: "the expansion of drug-detector dog teams to all federal prisons; the hiring of new Security Intelligence Officers; purchase of new or advanced detection and interception technologies, such as ION scanners, x-ray machines and metal detectors, thermal imaging goggles and cellular phone detection systems; and more stringent search standards, augmented staff training and more robust deployment rosters at principal entrances and perimeters" (OCI 2012). At the same time that the government began scaling up funding for drug detection and correctional policing technologies, CSC's substance abuse programming budget fell from $11 million in 2008–9 to $9 million in 2010–11 despite the significant increase in the number of incarcerated citizens. These facts are in contradistinction to the national anti-drug strategy's stated emphasis on treatment and prevention.

Prison is more costly than community-based forms of treatment, social housing, and social assistance,[3] so we must question the economic sensibility of a government that defines itself as fiscally responsible and yet spends millions of dollars on more punitive crime control strategies when crime rates are declining (Doob and Webster 2015; Webster and Doob 2007, 2015). O'Malley (1999) suggests that this inconsistency is due to the twinning of neoliberal and neoconservative rationalities in a "new right penality" that creates "volatile and contradictory punishment," which Wacquant argues is a deliberate "exercise in state crafting" (2010, 210). The next section outlines how the philosophies of legal moralism and legal paternalism facilitate the new right's push to use law to control crime and morality, taking as examples the government's discursive reconstruction of harm-reduction technologies and efforts to eliminate evidence-based HIV prevention efforts.

**Legal Moralism, Legal Paternalism, and the Politics of Blame**

In his classic liberal conceptualization of the harm principle, Mill (1859) argued that the individual citizen is sovereign, and only when one's actions are known to cause harm to another person may the law impose a limit to autonomy. Contrary to Mill, many legal philosophers contend that the state may limit freedom in order to enforce particular standards of morality, including when protecting the individual from self-harm, what Mill called "self-regarding actions." Proponents of the principle of legal moralism maintain that the law may legitimately be used to prohibit behaviours that are in conflict with society's collective moral judgments, even when those behaviours do not cause harm to others (Devlin 1965; Dworkin 1972). This position implies that the state is permitted to use coercive power to enforce a sense of collective morality; it also suggests that state authorities have the power to determine what constitutes moral behaviour. For example, in response to the World Health Organization's (WHO) release of a new guide for HIV prevention at the XVII International AIDS Conference in Mexico City, Health Minister Tony Clement stated, "Allowing and/or encouraging people to inject heroin into their veins is not harm reduction, it is the opposite. We believe it is a form of harm addition" (Picard 2008).

Building on the effort to enforce a common morality, legal paternalism goes so far as to advocate "interference with a person's liberty of action justified by reasons referring exclusively to the welfare, good, happiness, needs, interests, or values of the person being coerced" (Dworkin 1972, 65). Accordingly, the state may legislate impositions on individual freedom, such as laws requiring that citizens wear bicycle helmets and seatbelts to protect individuals from harm. Wacquant describes the consequences of these legal philosophies in practice: "The new priority given to duties over rights, sanction over support, the stern rhetoric of the 'obligations of citizenship,' and the martial reaffirmation of the capacity of the state to lock [up] the trouble-making poor (welfare recipients and criminals) ... all these policy planks pronounce and promote the transition from the kindly 'nanny state' of the Fordist-Keynesian era to the strict 'daddy state' of neoliberalism" (Wacquant 2010, 201).

Legal moralist and paternalist discourses echo the neoliberal emphasis on self-government found in contemporary health and penal discourses. Over the past decade of conservative federal leadership, moral arguments about the dangers of drug use and unsafe sex became prominent in political debate, shaping public health strategies, criminal justice legislation, and correctional policies that were drafted or amended during this era. At this point, it is worth quoting Stephen Harper at length.

> Conservatives need to reassess our understanding of the modern Left. It has moved beyond old socialistic morality or even moral relativism to something much darker. It has become a moral nihilism – the rejection of any tradition or convention of morality, a post-Marxism with deep resentments, even hatreds, of the norms of free and democratic western civilization. This descent into nihilism should not be surprising because moral relativism simply cannot be sustained as a guiding philosophy. It leads to silliness such as moral neutrality on the use of marijuana or harder drugs mixed with its random moral crusades on tobacco. It explains the lack of moral censure on personal foibles of all kinds, extenuating even criminal behaviour with moral outrage at bourgeois society, which is then tangentially blamed for deviant behaviour. On the moral standing of the person, it leads to views ranging from radical, responsibility-free individualism, to tribalism in the form of group rights. (Harper 2003, 75)

Harper's position calls for a return to traditional morals, vaguely defined, and situates complex issues as black or white, moral or immoral. For Harper, there is no such thing as a moral person who uses drugs. Under his leadership, the conservative movement in Canada effectively attacked the civility and compassion of "the modern Left['s]" engagement with harm-reduction approaches as the cornerstone public health response to HIV and drug-use prevention by constructing moral relativism as a nihilistic "descent" into libertinism. In one decisive narrative turn, this passage rejects the fact that greater divisions of wealth between the rich and poor leads to increased social disorganization, health inequality, and criminality and espouses the Conservative Party of Canada's neoliberal emphasis upon individual responsibility and neoconservative moral censure that evokes the politics of blame for addiction, poverty, and criminality.

The Conservative view that drug use is a concern for criminal justice rather than for health was politically solidified in 2008, when leadership for Canada's drug strategy was relocated from Health Canada to the Department of Justice. While the Conservative party lost the federal election in October 2015 and now constitutes the official opposition, it remains to be seen whether or not the party will begin to accept empirical evidence in support of harm reduction practices. However, it is noteworthy that just four months prior to her election as the interim leader of the Conservative party, Health Minister Rona Ambrose reported being "outraged" by the Supreme Court of Canada's unanimous decision to expand the definition of marijuana for medicinal purposes to include oils and foodstuffs (Mulholland 2015), which suggests that Harper's narrative reflects the position of the broader conservative movement in Canada rather than his singular, isolated views.

Harcourt wrote that "the logic of neoliberal penality *facilitates* contemporary punishment practices by encouraging the belief that the legitimate space for government intervention is in the penal sphere – *there and there alone*" (2010, 80; emphasis in original). Harper's article similarly emphasizes free market solutions to social issues while advocating the strong arm of the law to facilitate Canada's return to traditional moral values. To illustrate the legal paternalism of the conservative neoliberal "daddy-state," I offer two broad examples related to harm reduction that contribute to constituting elevated HIV risk environments both in the community and specific to carceral spaces.

First, consider the shifting political discourse on harm reduction[4] as a component of state drug policy and HIV prevention. Internationally, harm reduction is widely accepted as the best practice for responding to drug use as a public health concern. It has not been linked with increased substance use and is a pathway to treatment for many (Beirness et al. 2008; Jürgens 2007a, 2007b; Rhodes 2009; Stöver and Nelles 2003), yet critics suggest that the concept of harm is too vaguely defined and there is disagreement over the degrees of harm associated with particular behaviours. The Conservative government stated explicitly that many drug-related harm-reduction strategies "*appear* to sanction or even enable substance use, and therefore may facilitate the "legalization" of illicit substances, or may send "the wrong message" (CCSA 2005, 11). When politicians engage moral arguments about the dangers of illicit substance use, they tend to follow with paternalist claims that a more punitive criminal justice response to drugs via increased state law enforcement is the only way to prevent addiction, a position that simultaneously undermines harm reduction by suggesting it encourages drug use – as per Clement's comment noted above.

Such was the case when for the first time since 1987 the term *harm reduction* were removed from Canada's National Drug Strategy, which in 2007 was renamed the National *Anti*-Drug Strategy (DeBeck et al. 2009). While this might appear to be a simple linguistic alteration to forcefully indicate that the Conservative government remains staunchly prohibitionist, the elimination of harm reduction as one of the four pillars of Canada's national drug strategy (in addition to law enforcement, treatment, and prevention) is a regressive step in Canadian social policy. As a public health initiative, harm reduction is an essential component of any strategy that aims to promote the health and safety of people who use drugs (CAMH 2008). Despite claims that the new anti-drug strategy would focus on treatment and prevention, and funding in these areas increased from 14 to 17 per cent and 3 to 4 per cent respectively, 70 per cent of base government funding remained earmarked for law enforcement, while harm-reduction initiatives decreased from 3 to 2 per cent of the budget (DeBeck et al. 2009). This trend shows no signs of slowing; for an example specific to the prison environment, the opioid substitution program (methadone maintenance) budget decreased by 10 per cent in 2013 (OCI 2014).

I offer a second and related example. After rejecting overwhelming empirical evidence in support of harm-reduction initiatives as methods to improve and protect public health, the Harper government undertook a dramatic and costly legal struggle to close down Vancouver's supervised injection facility, Insite, and to prevent the creation of similar facilities in other locations (Payton 2015). Since Insite opened in 2003, Vancouver's downtown eastside has shown a 35 per cent reduction in overdose mortality (Marshall et al. 2011), greater injection drug use cessation (DeBeck et al. 2011), and a 30 per cent increase in detoxification service use that was found to be associated with increased rates of long-term addiction treatment and reduced injecting at Insite (Wood et al. 2007). On 29 September 2011, the Supreme Court of Canada unanimously ruled that the decision to withdraw Insite's exemption under the Controlled Drugs and Substances Act (CDSA) was "arbitrary, undermining the very purposes of the CDSA, which include public health and safety. It is also grossly disproportionate: the potential denial of health services and the correlative increase in the risk of death and disease to injection drug users outweigh any benefit that might be derived from maintaining an absolute prohibition on possession of illegal drugs on Insite's premises" (Attorney General of Canada v PHS Community Services Society 2011).

Following this decision, the Conservatives tabled Bill C-65, The Respect for Communities Act, to create a federal regulatory framework for supervised injection sites with specific criteria for certification and inspection. The bill gives the federal minister of health sole authority for approving exemptions to the CDSA and requires support letters from provincial health and public safety ministers before a site may be licensed. While Bill C-65 died with prorogation, its nearly identical replacement, Bill C-2, received royal assent in June 2015. Subsequently, all applicants seeking an exemption for activities at supervised drug consumption sites must provide evidence of community and stakeholder support; once open, they must report on how the facility affects local crime rates, as well as both public and individual health. While requiring supervised injection sites to document the degree to which they affect local crime rates might provide correlative evidence that they reduce some forms of crime, it also ties a life-saving health-care practice to the penal sphere and thus to neoliberal penality's primary space of legitimate government intervention (Harcourt 2010).

In concluding this section it is important to return to Dworkin (1972), who identified three limits to legal paternalism: the state must demonstrate that (1) the proposed restriction that limits individual freedom is legitimate only if there is sufficient reason to believe that the harm the law aims to prevent is of the sort that a reasonable person would want to avoid; (2) the potential harm done by the restriction of autonomy outweighs the benefits of the restricted behaviour; and (3) the proposed control takes the least restrictive form possible. The removal of harm reduction from the national anti-drug strategy and the legal attempt to close down Insite and restrict the proliferation of new supervised consumption sites do not meet Dworkin's criteria. First, these restrictions do not prevent harm that law's "rational man" would want to avoid, but rather promote harm by blocking access to interventions that prevent HIV and other forms of communicable disease transmission. Second, these restrictions do not take the least restrictive form possible and instead promote punitive and harm-inflicting responses to drug use, namely an increased reliance on law enforcement and thus criminalization and incarceration.

While different harm-reduction strategies operate in communities across the country, after incarceration there are very few measures in place to prevent HIV transmission. The political move away from harm reduction towards criminalization is linked to the growing number of HIV-positive and other vulnerable people in Canadian prisons, where the legal moralism of the broader federal policy discourse takes specific forms in practices that elevate HIV risk. The final section of this chapter examines the specific HIV risk environment of carceral spaces.

### Carceral Spaces as Elevated HIV Risk Environments

To more accurately assess the risks and harms of drug use, Tim Rhodes (2002) argues that we must develop a broader understanding of the notion of the "risk environment," which requires examining the interplay of the physical, social, economic, and policy environments at both the micro and macro levels. Naturally, carceral spaces are physical environments, but as total institutions with their attendant characteristics (e.g., austere living conditions, physical barriers between groups of people, hierarchical authority structure, oppressive and authoritarian regime, excessive reliance on surveillance and dehumanizing forms of isolation, restraint, and punishment) (Goffman 1961), prisons, jails, and detention centres are some of the most difficult institutional spaces in which to engage in progressive and humane policy reform. As the CSC is legally responsible for protecting and promoting the health of prison populations, we must consider the HIV risk and prevention-enabling environments specific to carceral spaces.

A "risk environment" framework situates harm as an outcome of one's social structural environment and shifts responsibility for the reduction of those harms away from the individual "alone to include the social and political institutions" that together contribute to the production of harm (Rhodes 2002, 2009, 193; Small et al. 2007). "A shift in focus towards the 'risk environment' as a unit of analysis and change helps to overcome the limits of individualism, which characterizes most HIV prevention interventions as well as to appreciate how drug-related harm intersects with health and vulnerability more generally. This in turn raises the importance of 'non-drug' and 'non-health' interventions for harm reduction and the facilitation of alliances between harm reduction and other social movements oriented to tackling vulnerability as a means of promoting public health" (Rhodes 2002, 85).

A constellation of factors, notably the significantly higher rates of HIV and HCV infection in prison populations, neoliberal carceral expansion, and the inaccessibility of essential harm-reduction technologies in carceral settings, constitutes the prison as an elevated HIV risk environment. The 2007 National Inmate Infectious Diseases and Risk-Behaviours Survey conducted by CSC found that 4.6 per cent of federally sentenced prisoners (4.5 per cent of men and 7.9 per cent of women) reported being HIV-positive, and 31 per cent (30.8 per cent of men and 37.0 per cent of women) reported being HCV-positive (Zakaria, Thompson, and Borgatta 2010; Zakaria, Thompson, Jarvis et al. 2010; Thompson, Zakaria, and Grant 2011). Aboriginal women are a particularly high-risk group, reporting the highest rates of both HIV (11.7 per cent) and HCV infections (49.1 per cent) (Zakaria, Thompson, Jarvis et al.; Thompson, Zakaria, and Grant 2011). The OCI (2012) also reported that the rates of HCV infections in prison increased approximately 50 per cent between 2000 and 2008.

The survey also found that 17 per cent of men and 14 per cent of women (and 21 per cent of Aboriginal women) injected drugs while in prison, and nearly half shared injection equipment, including with prisoners they knew to be HIV- and/or HCV-positive or who had unknown infection statuses (Zakaria, Thompson, and Borgatta 2010; Zakaria, Thompson, Jarvis et al. 2010). In fact, the CSC estimates that 33 per cent of reported HCV infections since admission result from the use of shared injection equipment (Zakaria, Thompson, and Borgatta 2010, iii–iv). Moreover, 17 per cent of men and 31 per cent of women reported engaging in oral, vaginal, or anal sex while incarcerated (Thompson, Zakaria, and Grant 2011). While the majority of prisoners are aware that policy requires CSC to make available condoms, lubricant, dental dams, and bleach, only 57 per cent of sexually active prisoners reported that they attempted (successfully or unsuccessfully) to access these items, although the majority of those who injected drugs, received a tattoo, or were pierced used bleach to clean the equipment (Zakaria, Thompson, Jarvis et al. 2010).

While prisoners reported trying to access barrier protection and bleach, they also reported a number of obstacles in these efforts. Condoms, lubricant and dental dams were not always located in discreet locations that would facilitate anonymous retrieval, with some institutions requiring that prisoners request these items from nursing staff. When these items were available in discreet locations, dispensers were often empty or damaged. Prisoners must ask staff members for permission to access bleach, which is often diluted with water (Zakaria, Thompson, and Borgatta 2010; Zakaria, Thompson, Jarvis et al. 2010; Thompson, Zakaria, and Grant 2011), a practice that weakens its effectiveness as a disinfectant (Jürgens 2007a; Stöver and Nelles 2003).

Interestingly, the CSC reports that harm-reduction items are being used as intended by prisoners and that reducing access issues will help to optimize use (Zakaria, Thompson, and Borgatta 2010; Zakaria, Thompson, Jarvis et al. 2010). Despite this finding, and international evidence of successful syringe/needle exchange programs operating without incident in prison environments (Epele and Pecheny 2007; Stöver and Nelles 2003), the federal government continues to prohibit such programs in Canadian prisons out of fears that syringes will be used as weapons against other prisoners or staff members and that this practice encourages continued drug use. This illustrates the marginalization and inconsistency of correctional harm-reduction practices in favour of surveillance and punishment.

The absence of key harm-reduction practices in carceral environments coheres with the Harper government's removal of harm reduction as a pillar of the national anti-drug strategy,[5] but it fails to align with the guiding aims of the WHO's Health in Prison Project; in particular, the goals of reducing prisoners' exposure to communicable diseases so as to prevent prisons from being focal points of infection, and encouraging prison health services to provide care that is equivalent to what is accessible in the community (Gatherer, Moller, and Hayton 2005; Lines 2007). The totalizing features of the prison work to institutionalize certain harmful behaviours – such as unprotected sexual encounters, and shared drug injection, tattoo, and piercing equipment – demonstrating how the prison environment contributes to a carceral syndemic that may facilitate comorbid HIV and HCV infection and aggravate one or both illnesses. Goffman (1961) describes institutionalization as a structural and functional process that entrenches particular norms, social identity roles, values, and modes of behaviour within an organization, social system, or society as a whole. The failure to offer resources in prison settings that are known to reduce harm and promote health, especially when these resources are available in the community, effectively embeds harmful health behaviours into the routine practices of an already vulnerable and marginalized population. With the emergent trend of lengthier prison sentences and carceral expansion (Webster and Doob 2015), and evidence that the longer people are incarcerated, the more likely they are to be exposed to HIV and HCV through shared needles and drug injection equipment (Zakaria, Thompson, and Borgatta 2010; Zakaria, Thompson, Jarvis et al. 2010), prisons are actively facilitating the transmission of communicable diseases and institutionalizing HIV risk behaviours. Table 1 provides a more detailed sketch of the HIV risk and prevention-enabling environments specific to carceral spaces.

For carceral settings to become HIV-prevention-enabling environments, harm-reduction efforts must be scaled up and expanded to include syringe/needle exchanges, safer tattooing programs, easier access to low-threshold opioid substitution, and anonymous and confidential access to all forms of harm reduction. In addition to individual-level efforts to reduce harm, these enabling interventions should also include broader socio-political policy shifts, including augmented fiscal support for community social housing and welfare, and decriminalization and/ or legalization of drug use to diminish carceral expansion. This would require a significant paradigm shift in how the federal government conceptualizes drug use, from framing it as an immoral crime requiring punishment to instead responding to it as a public health concern. This would help to counter neoliberal penal efforts that are shored up by moralist discourse and paternalist legislation and would facilitate more fiscally responsible interventions that do not contribute to the hypermarginalization of already vulnerable citizens.

## Conclusion

While incarceration provides an opportunity to access consistent long-term health care for some individuals (Ginn 2013), the evidence presented here suggests that prisons are far from effective health-care institutions. In order to create an "enabling environment" for HIV-related harm/risk reduction in carceral settings, Canada's political positioning and subsequent policy environment must undergo a paradigm shift that prioritizes the health of prisoners as citizens with equal human rights in lieu of demonizing them as threats to society's moral fabric and our collective social welfare. Shifting away from the normative,

Table 1 The HIV Risk and Prevention-Enabling Environments Specific to Carceral Spaces

| Types of Environment | | Micro-Level Environment Influence | Macro-Level Environment Influence |
|---|---|---|---|
| *Physical* | | | |
| | Risk | Drug using, injecting, and sex locations | Carceral expansion (partially resulting from mandatory minimum sentences, criminalization of HIV nondisclosure, and other legislative and policy changes) |
| | | Drug injecting in surveilled space leads to "hurrying & worrying" (Small et al. 2007) | |
| | Intervention | Closed total institution | Decriminalization of drug possession for personal use |
| | | Overcrowding | Scaling up harm-reduction interventions including supervised injection/inhalation sites (SIS) and S/NEP |
| | | Harm-reduction interventions including syringe/needle exchange (S/NEP), opioid substitution | |
| *Social* | | | |
| | Risk | Social and peer "risk" norms (high rates of drug using and HIV+ prisoners) | Prisoners disproportionately come from socio-economically marginal communities that experience high levels of social disorganization, un/underemployment, homelessness, and precarious housing |
| | | Inter-prisoner and prisoner-staff violence | Disproportionately high rates of Indigenous and other racialized minorities |
| | | Random cell searches | High rates of gender-based violence and trauma |
| | | Sexual assault and coercion | Weak civil society and community advocacy |
| | | Geographic dislocation from family, friends, community | Stigmatization and marginalization |
| | Intervention | Peer support programs | Mass media and social marketing of harm reduction |
| | | Developing low threshold accessible harm-reduction services for people who use drugs, tattoo equipment, and safe sex practices | Fostering collective actions in combination with policy changes |
| | | Community health partnerships | Strengthening civil society infrastructure |

|  |  | | |
| --- | --- | --- | --- |
| *Economic* | | | |
| Risk | Federal prisoners earn a maximum pay of $6.90 per day | | Austerity measures leading to the elimination of programming (e.g., Lifeline, canine program, prison farms) |
| | Work programs are not available in all prisons | | Cuts to social housing and health spending |
| Intervention | Distribution of free prevention materials | | Increase investment in harm reduction relative to drug enforcement |
| | Elimination of "unfree labour" | | Increase investment in social housing |
| | | | National prescription care plan |
| | | | Increase use of compassionate release for individuals with chronic illnesses |
| *Policy* | | | |
| Risk | Prohibition of key harm-reduction practices (S/NEP and SIS) | | Public health policy governing harm reduction and drug treatment; shift from National Drug Strategy to National Anti-Drug Strategy and removing harm reduction as a pillar |
| | Availability of harm-reduction practices (i.e., bleach, condoms, conjugal visits) subject to discretionary implementation by staff; threatens confidentiality if prisoners must request to see a nurse to obtain items | | Laws governing drug possession |
| | No consultation or inclusion of prisoners or drug-users in the policy-setting agenda | | Laws governing protection of human and health rights |
| | Strip and body cavity searches | | Federal government going to Supreme Court of Canada to try to close Insite and restrict marijuana for medicinal purposes |
| | Inhumane segregation practices (e.g., segregating mentally ill prisoners and those who self-injure) | | No consultation or inclusion of prisoners or drug-users in the policy-setting agenda |
| | Threats to confidentiality for HIV testing and treatment when this information is in the prisoner's correctional file | | Mandatory minimum sentences leading to prison overcrowding |
| | Random cell searches and urinalysis | | Criminalization of HIV nondisclosure |
| | Failure to renew safer tattoo program | | |

Source: Adapted from Rhodes (2002, 2009). Note that this is not an exhaustive list of potential examples.

albeit empirically unsupported, neoliberal discourse that austere punishment provides the collective public safety would require a transformation of correctional policy towards a more inclusionary framework
that promotes "health for all" (Ottawa Charter for Health Promotion
1986), in line with the aims of the WHO's Health in Prison Program.

The risk-environment framework developed by Tim Rhodes (2002,
2009) can foster the creation of an HIV prevention-enabling approach
that combats the politics of blame that is a component of neoliberal
health (Orsini 2007) and penal discourses (Harcourt 2010; Wacquant
2009, 2010). As Rhodes (2009, 194) suggests, a risk environment framework counters the public health inclination to conceptualize harm
primarily as the outcome of individual behaviours and "shifts responsibility for harm to include the social and political-economic institutions
which have a role in harm production." Rhodes's risk environment
framework dovetails with the notion of the syndemic as they both examine how the interaction between disease(s), environment, and other
health disparities "elevate negative health outcomes" (Eisenberg and
Blank 2014, 1006). For example, individuals with serious mental illness,
which is disproportionately high among incarcerated populations (OCI
2012, 2014), are at "increased risk for both contracting and transmitting
HIV ... due to high rates of substance use including injection drug use
(IDU), risky sexual behaviour, sexual victimization, and prostitution"
(Eisenberg and Blank 2014, 1006). To examine the "carceral syndemic"
and thus the role that prisons play in promoting and reducing harm entails considering the ways in which risk is socially situated, which "offers impetus to understanding how risk environments are experienced
and embodied as part of everyday practices. This helps build ground-
up or 'emic' understandings of risk subjectivity and environment"
(Rhodes 2009, 194). As noted in table 1, facilitating the generation of
HIV-prevention interventions rooted in lived experience requires that
policymakers include the meaningful participation of those who use
drugs in policymaking and program development.

Problematically, being denied access to the full range of HIV prevention harm-reduction technologies can lead to the institutionalization of
harm-promoting behavioural practices, including unsafe sex and sharing drug injection, tattooing, and piercing equipment, that are empirically linked to the transmission of communicable illnesses. The absence
of key harm-reduction strategies in carceral settings is the direct result
of political gerrymandering, where embracing get-tough-on-crime rhetoric to shore up moral views on self-regarding actions (Mill 1859) enables

the political entrenchment of legally paternalist legislation that disproportionately affects the poor and visible minorities, including Canada's
Indigenous peoples. To conclude, it is worth returning to Wacquant
(2009, 2010, 218), who argues that legal paternalism arises from struggles "between the various sectors of the bureaucratic field, which vie
to gain 'ownership' of the social problem at hand and thus valorize
the specific forms of authority and expertise they anchor." Redefining
the "modalities of public action" with respect to HIV prevention neces-
sitates shifting away from conservative moralism and neoliberal penal
discourses and moving ownership of harm reduction back to the public
health sector. Without prioritizing health above punishment, the risks
of HIV exposure and transmission in prison will undoubtedly remain.

NOTES

1 This era also boasts economic deregulation in favour of corporate interests,
   in particular those that favour the oil and gas industry (Peters 2012), and
   massive cuts to social housing and welfare (e.g., cuts to the federal housing
   program, restricting access to employment insurance, and increasing the
   age before Canadians can receive old age security) that are linked to the
   criminalization of poverty (Chan and Chunn 2014).
2 Longstanding rehabilitative programs like Lifeline, the canine project,
   and the prison farm program were also cut to reduce costs.
3 "The annual average cost of keeping a federal inmate behind bars has
   increased from $88,000 in 2005–06 to over $113,000 in 2009–10. It costs
   $578 per day to incarcerate a federally sentenced woman inmate and just over
   $300 per day to maintain a male inmate. In contrast, the annual average
   cost to keep an offender in the community is about $29,500" (OCI 2012, np).
4 Harm reduction generally entails five key tenets: pragmatism; humane values
   (e.g., dignity, compassion, no moralistic judgment, and de-stigmatization);
   a focus on reducing the immediate harms of drug use at the individual,
   political, social, and environmental levels; balancing the costs and benefits
   of the intervention, drug-related harm, and community and societal concerns; and the priority of immediate goals (Beirness et al. 2008, 3–4).
5 Unlike CSC, provincial correctional systems do not make data on HIV
   rates and harm reduction technology usage public, if they are collected
   at all. Provincial prisons are more overcrowded than federal prisons and
   offer limited to no programming; many make condoms, dental dams,
   and lubricant available, but none provide syringe exchange.

REFERENCES

Beirness, Douglas J., et al. 2008. *Harm Reduction: What's in a Name*. Ottawa: Canadian Centre on Substance Abuse.

CAMH. 2008. *The National Anti-Drug Strategy: A CAMH Response*. Toronto: Centre for Addiction and Mental Health.

CCSA. 2005. *Substance Abuse in Canada: Current Challenges and Choices*. Ottawa: Canadian Centre on Substance Abuse.

Chan, Wendy, and Dorothy Chunn. 2014. *Racialization, Crime and Criminal Justice in Canada*. Toronto: University of Toronto Press.

DeBeck, Kora, et al. 2011. "Injection Drug Use Cessation and Use of North America's First Medically Supervised Safer Injecting Facility." *Drug and Alcohol Dependence* 113 (2–3): 172–6. https://doi.org/10.1016/j.drugalcdep .2010.07.023.

DeBeck, Kora, et al. 2009. "Canada's New Federal 'National Anti-Drug Strategy': An Informal Audit of Reported Funding Allocation." *International Journal on Drug Policy* 20 (2): 188–91. https://doi.org/10.1016/j.drugpo .2008.04.004.

Devlin, Patrick. 1965. *The Enforcement of Morals*. Oxford: Oxford University Press.

Doob, Anthony N., and Cheryl M. Webster. 2015. "The Harper Revolution in Criminal Justice Policy ... and What Comes Next." *Policy Options* (May–June). http://policyoptions.irpp.org/magazines/is-it-the-best-of-times-or-the-worst/doob-webster/.

Dworkin, Gerald. 1972. "Paternalism." *Monist* 56 (1): 64–84. https://doi.org/ 10.5840/monist197256119.

Eisenberg, Marlene M., and Michael B. Blank. 2014. "The Syndemic of the Triply Diagnosed: HIV Positives with Mental Illness and Substance Abuse or Dependence." *Clinical Research in HIV/AIDS* 1 (1): 1006. https://www .jscimedcentral.com/HIV-AIDS/HIV-AIDS-1-1006.php#citation.

Epele, M.E., and M. Pecheny. 2007. "Harm Reduction Policies in Argentina: A Critical View." *Global Public Health* 2:342–58.

Gatherer, Alex, Lars Moller, and Paul Hayton. 2005. "The World Health Organization European Health in Prisons Project after 10 Years: Persistent Barriers and Achievements." *American Journal of Public Health* 95 (10): 1696–700. https://doi.org/10.2105/AJPH.2003.057323.

Ginn, Stephen. 2013. "Promoting Health in Prison." *British Medical Journal* 346:1–6.

Goffman, Erving. 1961. *Asylums: Essays on the Social Situation of Mental Patients and Other Inmates*. New York: Doubleday.

Harcourt, Bernard E. 2010. "Neoliberal Penality: A Brief Genealogy." *Theoretical Criminology* 14 (1): 74–92. https://doi.org/10.1177/1362480609352785.

Harper, Stephen. 2003. "Rediscovering the Right Agenda: The Alliance Must Commit to Ideals and Ideas, Not Vague Decision-Making Processes: The Canadian Alliance Leader Outlines How Social and Economic Conservatism Must Unite." *Citizens Centre Report Magazine* 30:72–7.

Jürgens, Ralf. 2007a. *Interventions to Address HIV in Prisons: Needle and Syringe Programmes and Decontamination Strategies*. Geneva: World Health Organization.

– 2007b. *Interventions to Address HIV in Prisons: Prevention of Sexual Transmission*. Geneva: World Health Organization.

Lines, Rick. 2007. "HIV Infection and Human Rights in Prison." In *Health in Prison: A WHO Guide to the Essentials of Prison Gealth*, edited by L. Møller, H. Stöver, R. Jürgens, A. Gatherer, and H. Nikogosian, 61–72. Geneva: WHO.

Marshall, Brandon D.L., et al. 2011. "Reduction in Overdose Mortality after the Opening of North America's First Medically Supervised Safer Injecting Facility: A Retrospective Population-Based Study." *Lancet* 377 (9775): 1429–37. https://doi.org/10.1016/S0140-6736(10)62353-7.

Mill, John Stuart. 1859. *On Liberty*. London: John W. Parker and Son.

Moore, Dawn, and Kelly Hannah-Moffat. 2005. "The Liberal Veil: Revisiting Canadian Penality." In *The New Punitiveness: Trends, Theories, Perspectives*, edited by J. Pratt et al., 85–100. Cullompton, UK: Willan Publishing.

Mulholland, Angela. 2015. "Ambrose 'Outraged' by SCC Marijuana Ruling." CTV News, 11 June. http://www.ctvnews.ca/canada/ambrose-outraged-by-scc-s-marijuana-ruling-1.2417118.

OCI. 2012. *Annual Report of the Office of the Correctional Investigator 2011–2012*. Ottawa: Office of the Correctional Investigator. http://www.oci-bec.gc.ca/cnt/rpt/annrpt/annrpt20112012-eng.aspx.

– 2014. *Annual Report of the Office of the Correctional Investigator 2013–2014*. Ottawa: Office of the Correctional Investigator. http://www.oci-bec.gc.ca/cnt/rpt/annrpt/annrpt20132014-eng.aspx.

O'Malley, P. 1999. "Volatile and Contradictory Punishment." *Theoretical Criminology* 3 (2): 175–96. https://doi.org/10.1177/1362480699003002003.

Orsini, Michael. 2007. "Discourses in Distress: From 'Health Promotion' to 'Population Health' to 'You Are Responsible for Your Own Health.'" In *Critical Policy Studies*, edited by M. Orsini and M. Smith, 347–63. Vancouver: UBC Press.

Payton, Laura. 2015. "Conservatives Spent More Than $4.7 Million Fighting 15 Losing Court Cases." CBC News, 23 April 23. http://www.cbc.ca/

news/politics/conservatives-spent-more-than-4-7-million-fighting-15-losing-court-cases-1.3042725.

Peters, John. 2012. *Boom, Bust and Crisis: Labour, Corporate Power and Politics in Canada*. Halifax: Fernwood Publishing.

Picard, André. 2008. "Clement's Insite Attack Leaves WHO Red-Faced." *Globe and Mail*, 6 August. http://www.theglobeandmail.com/life/clements-insite-attack-leaves-who-red-faced/article1058485/.

Pratt, John. 2007. "Scandinavian Exceptionalism in an Era of Penal Excess: Part I: The Nature and Roots of Scandinavian Exceptionalism." *British Journal of Criminology* 48 (2): 119–37. https://doi.org/10.1093/bjc/azm072.

– 2008. "Scandinavian Exceptionalism in an Era of Penal Excess: Part II: Does Scandinavian Exceptionalism Have a Future?" *British Journal of Criminology* 48 (3): 275–93. https://doi.org/10.1093/bjc/azm073.

Quan, Douglas. 2015. "All of Canada's Federal Prisons Are Switching to Powdered Milk – Which Should Save $3.1M a Year." *National Post*, 30 January. http://news.nationalpost.com/news/canada/all-of-canadas-federal-prisons-are-switching-to-powdered-milk-which-should-save-3-1m-a-year.

Rhodes, Tim. 2002. "The 'Risk Environment': A Framework for Understanding and Reducing Drug-Related Harm." *International Journal on Drug Policy* 13 (2): 85–94. https://doi.org/10.1016/S0955-3959(02)00007-5.

– 2009. "Risk Environments and Drug Harms: A Social Science for Harm Reduction Approach." *International Journal on Drug Policy* 20 (3): 193–201. https://doi.org/10.1016/j.drugpo.2008.10.003.

Robertson, Ann. 1998. "Shifting Discourses on Health in Canada: From Health Promotion to Population Health." *Health Promotion International* 13 (2): 155–66. https://doi.org/10.1093/heapro/13.2.155.

Sim, Joe. 2009. *Punishment and Prisons: Power and the Carceral State*. Los Angeles: Sage Publications.

Small, Will, et al. 2007. "Public Injection Settings in Vancouver: Physical Environment, Social Context and Risk." *International Journal on Drug Policy* 18 (1): 27–36. https://doi.org/10.1016/j.drugpo.2006.11.019.

Stöver, Heino, and Joachim Nelles. 2003. "Ten Years of Experience with Needle and Syringe Exchange Programmes in European Prisons." *International Journal on Drug Policy* 14 (5–6): 437–44. https://doi.org/10.1016/j.drugpo.2003.08.001.

Thompson, Jennie, Dianne Zakaria, and Brian Grant. 2011. *National Inmate Infectious Diseases and Risk-Behaviours Survey for Women*. Ottawa: Correctional Services Canada.

Wacquant, Loïc. 2009. *Punishing the Poor: The Neoliberal Government of Social Insecurity*. Durham, NC: Duke University Press. https://doi.org/10.1215/9780822392255.

– 2010. "Crafting the Neoliberal State: Workfare, Prisonfare, and Social Insecurity." *Sociological Forum* 25 (2): 197–220. https://doi.org/10.1111/j.1573-7861.2010.01173.x.

Webster, Cheryl M., and Anthony N. Doob. 2007. "Punitive Trends and Stable Imprisonment Rates in Canada." *Crime and Justice* 36 (1): 297–369. https://doi.org/10.1086/592807.

– 2015. "US Punitiveness 'Canadian Style'? Cultural Values and Canadian Punishment Policy." *Punishment & Society* 17 (3): 299–321. https://doi.org/10.1177/1462474515590893.

Wood, Evan, Mark W. Tyndall, Ruth Zhang, Julio S.G. Montaner, and Thomas Kerr. 2007. "Rate of Detoxification Service Use and Its Impact among a Cohort of Supervised Injecting Facility Users." *Society for the Study of Addiction* 102 (6): 916–19. https://doi.org/10.1111/j.1360-0443.2007.01818.x.

Zakaria, Dianne, Jennie Mae Thompson, and Frederic Borgatta. 2010. *Rates of Reported HIV and HCV Infections since Admission to Canadian Federal Prison and Associated Incarceration Characteristics and Drug-Related Risk-Behaviours*. Ottawa: Correctional Services Canada.

Zakaria, Dianne, et al. 2010. *Summary of Emerging Findings from the 2007 National Inmate Infectious Diseases and Risk-Behaviours Survey*. Ottawa: Correctional Services Canada.

**Legal Cases**

*Canada (Attorney General) v PHS Community Services Society* [2011] 3 SCR 134, 2011 SCC 44.

# 4 Feeling Sick, Looking Cured!: The Iatrogenic Effects of HIV Public Health Policy on HIV-Positive Gay Men

FRANCISCO IBÁÑEZ-CARRASCO

*"I think the biggest problem with healthcare today is not its cost – which is a big problem – but for all that money, it's not an expression of our humanity."*
Jonathan Bush – CEO, athenahealth

This is a reflection on policy effects and not one of those routine "I-have-big-data-therefore-it-is-true" research cases so pervasive in the literature today. I point to the perpetuation of safer sex guidelines as business as usual in this millennium, and the painful denial and double bind of HIV as both normal and a disability, as two factors among many that maintain perceived and anticipated stigma and increase uncertainty among gay men, especially those living with HIV. My reflection presupposes that gay men continue to perceive HIV largely as a sexual illness one autonomously brings onto oneself – like guilt – and not as mutually reinforcing epidemics or syndemics (Singer and Clair 2003) provoked by a fatal combo of an outdated health system, pervasive erotophobia (Fisher et al. 1988), sexual/gender stigma and a gay culture of victimhood (Campbell and Manning 2014), misplaced notions of hetero and mono-normative romanticism (Bauer 2014) and the industrial production of fuck (of which porn is one vilified example). If the ultimate issue is "whether and to what extent should public health (government) get into the business of modifying human behaviour, even if it does so to improve health" (Bayer 1989, 79), in which the public good supersedes individual choice, we ought to consider what being HIV-positive means for gay men today, what the actual (not the expected) behaviours and cultural practices are, and the consequences for all, including new infections, continuing stigmatization, and uncertainty. To push the boundaries of this reflection as far as possible, I focus on gay men who are barebackers and meth users, as they represent the extreme in the public imaginary, even in the burgeoning presence of the Undetectable = Untransmittable campaign or "U = U" (Prevention Access Campaign 2017).

The invitation from the kind editors of this volume to write about HIV-related policy felt like a set-up. Why me? I'm a researcher in stuff other than public health policy. I am a teacher and educational theorist, a memoirist embroidering overly personal things in broad social fabrics. That is how I wrote *Giving It Raw*, my AIDS memoir (Ibáñez-Carrasco 2015). I write in a way that frees me from the shackles of academic papers, clinical reports, and policy. Was this an invitation to write about the ties that bind me?

Then I visited my friend Josh, who lives in that lovely Canadian city by the ocean. I had not seen him in years. I recalled him as strapping, assertive, sweet, and kinky as all hell. All decked in leather, we swore brotherhood love to each other at Dundas Square in Toronto during the special HIV vigil on the occasion of the XVI International AIDS Conference in 2006. Josh and I are both more than fifty now and alive. By all medical accounts, we are healthy and thriving. We checked each other out like old dogs and our sex was hurried and weird; two old fuck buddies trying to conjure a ghost that had long flown from their bodies. We barebacked and did drugs, of course; anything else would have signalled distrust. He lives in a small concrete box where patients have to leave their IDs at the entrance (not a concierge, more like a warden), and drug users come knocking at your door at odd times of the night to borrow lighters or money – a seeming accomplishment of housing policy for people with HIV.

In that factual manner that long-time patients develop – jarring to those not yet in constant contact with the medical system – Josh told me he sweats too much, hyperhidrosis, the silent handicap. He commented that he can't really get an erection without TriMix injected directly in his penis, and that his heart failed once as the result of HIV medications, which took away his joy of using electro-toys in sex and other fetish play. He told me that he works out a lot to calm his anxiety and fight long-set musculoskeletal morbidity. His body is inked and pierced to put together that aggressive and bulky exterior effect much needed to live in such environs. He has no vainglory about his weirdly shaped muscles, but they fit a helpful stereotype – "white trash" – that affords him far more "street cred" than having survived decades as

HIV-positive and certainly more than being a barebacker. He explains his muscles as side effects of long-term use of HIV medication, the way a geologist describes the tortured topography of a mountain. In his nearly thirty years living with HIV, Josh has been offered the entire pharmacopeia available to HIV-positive people. He should be grateful that he is alive. However, he is reminded of abstinence in polite terms, reminded of the shelter of monogamous relationships, and told that he faces *a new illness* now: aging with HIV. We laugh sarcastically: sex has become safer sex, getting old has become accelerated aging, and any deviation from clinically prescribed injection/digestion/inhalation of medical drugs is deemed recreational and a gateway to problematic use, abuse, and addiction. Nobody asks him about the aggregation of side effects, life experience, collective trauma, skilful trial and error, and epic joys of poz sexuality. Nobody would ever dare to ask him about kink and sexual health and how gay men his age still avoid him with fear and disgust and a new crop of pan-sexual, poly-amorous young-sters think Josh is really "cool" even if they do not understand his nos-talgia or believe HIV exists. And they are sweetly curious and carnal about his habits, his experience with sex and drugs and his values.

This un-holistic approach to reporting and circulating the medical his-tory of people living with HIV, especially queers that do not fit a main-stream cookie-cutter, is what I call an iatrogenic effect of HIV health policy. Its invisible but impactful repercussions ripple throughout the entire clinical and social experience of those of us surviving and those starting their journey as HIV positive persons.

I left Josh with the sad feeling I had visited him in prison but with the conviction that I had to write about this reality of gay men living with HIV.

## Iatrogenic Thinking

The notion of iatrogenesis, or "sickness produced by medical activity," was explored by philosopher Ivan Illich in his *Medical Nemesis* (1974) along with the term *medicalization*. My reflection borrows three features of iatrogenesis: the clinical, "the unwanted side-effects of medications and doctor ignorance, neglect, or malpractice, which poison, maim or even kill the patient"; the social, by which medical practice makes peo-ple hypochondriac and acquiescent; and the cultural, "by paralysing 'healthy responses to suffering, impairment and death'" (Scott 2014, 327).

It takes years to "manage" the physical, mental, and social aftermath of an HIV diagnosis (kids thinking of HIV as a common cold can't see this), but the paralysing and homogenizing effects of the *medicalization* of HIV continue to plague us (Conrad 2007). HIV positive scholar Kane Race (2009) describes how medicalization and self-governmentality of the body as a site of tragedy, deficit, or moral deviance has taken over from catechism or direct state control; Marty Fink (2015, 252) reminds us that HIV prevention, the staple of public health, remains "a hollow message if such materials fail to represent and affirm the identities of those dually excluded from queer and national movements ... [It] requires understanding desire and sexuality as linked to experiences of racism, migration, colonization, diaspora, cissexism, poverty and other complex facets of identity."

However, few doctors are trained to, are interested in, or have the administrative time or patience to pay attention to the complexity of our poz lives. Doctors have morphed from seemingly cultured and wise members of our communities to 9-to-5 highly paid technicians/ specialists with a prescription pad and too much power. Complexity is time-consuming and time is valuable currency; complexity is not as attractive as rudimentary medical suffering, adherence, and compliance. Public health makes regular salutations to protecting "priority populations." It contracts out key sexual health activities to small organizations (one could assume for political sanitization reasons) and remains focused on success measured as number of HIV tests taken, number of follow-ups to care, and number of people on treatment.

Josh sees plenty of young specialists who do not appear to consult with each other much or read each other's reports. While fighting the daily medical grind, there is another set of sickening effects, a combo of fear, uncertainty, and mental health problems brought about by the public health system, that is to say, *an effect induced by health-care policies*. Worse, it affects the way Josh and I and many others devalue our patient experience, disavow ourselves of power, and become helpless. Don't get me wrong, he complains and uses previous clinical hours to pursue complaints. However, the idea of diverse groups of HIV positive people gathering to protest the medical system died a slow death in the late 1990s. Iatrogenic thinking is lonely and confined.

One of the most insidious effects of iatrogenic thinking is that maintained by an obsolete but sacred safer sex code (a codex written on vellum, on our skins) that demands adherence on the basis of refuted medical evidence and disregarded social use, to integrate Thomas Szasz (1977) notions of theology in medicine. What is stopping us is the lack of nerve and red-tape of public health to reform the outdated codex, to integrate HIV as an episodic disability, and most recently to find ways to integrate the U = U messaging into the code thus sustaining a widely accepted fantasy of gay/queer liberation and implicitly a state of queer sexual apartheid. The iatrogenic thinking around HIV is ambivalent: it is cured and it is not, gay men are free of HIV and we are not, and this forms a double bind for gay men living with HIV.

## Resisting the Code: Boundary Play

How can the safe(r) sex code be an example of a policy that might have iatrogenic effects? Safer sex is a code that no queer I have ever met has ever really followed completely and constantly. Over time, safer sex has created an indelible cultural "effect": sex only seems to only come with negative consequences including emotional ones such as loneliness, envy, and jealousy and with only tenuous connections to desire and pleasure (Vicioso et al. 2005; O'Byrne and Holmes 2011a). Sex is often depicted as mechanical and bodies are machines at risk of terrorist attacks from others' bad intentions, neglect, or stupidity (Ibáñez-Carrasco 1997/1998). Queer sex in particular, guided by the old beacon of safer sex, and aided by a selection of research evidence that supports safer sex, has been consistently under colonizing attack as perilous, irrational and unproductive; hardly a positive contribution to queer sexual health.

To accept any iatrogenic effect, we must first appreciate that in the information age, audiovisual texts are powerful tools mediating between institutions, individuals, and their separate and collaborative motivations/policies and practices. Safer sex has been historically synergistic with an arsenal of medical tools to mostly measure illness and not wellness. In everyday practice, health-care professionals and HIV-positive "patients" are guided, some blindly, by viral loads and CD4 counts and/or psychometric tests (for those lucky enough to access mental health care) that measure, but do not explain, the state of being and mindset of a person living with HIV (or any other permanent un/manageable condition). The safer sex codex is the carnival spectre that leads the parade of accumulating fears about fluctuating numbers gaging the levels of enemies in the blood, the levels of anxiety and distress. The fanfare is funereal, in the much touted medical interview, fast and technical, commanded by the physician. There is little or no room for any counteractive medicine to the medical spectre of low counts or increasing depression.

The Public Health Agency of Canada's (PHAC) safer sex guidelines hint at risk[1] as a biomedical category, but the cultural and sexual practices of gay men include sophisticated and contradictory forms of risk and outcomes. In blatant denial, the government of Canada, in the last ten years, has not clearly endorsed "harm reduction" in sex. It is only a guess when or if PHAC will confront the game-changer messaging of U = U (which still relies heavily on medicalization of drug use). As far as public health policy is concerned, gay men remain either risky or safe, which in street parlance translates into clean and HIV-negative or dirty and HIV-positive. In our culture this has instigated a sexual apartheid that intersects with race and class (Wright 2008). This apartheid is sustained by the lateral violence of gay men themselves, ever submissive to safer sex and its heritage. Is "apartheid" too strong a word for you? Try living as an HIV positive person for 32 years, as I have, and encountering rejection, disdain, and accusations in private and in public all the time! The bottom line is that safer sex guidelines are ineffective medical guidelines. They lack necessary but cumbersome relativism: there should be a set of principles that must be interpreted differently in different settings for different purposes and by very different individuals.

In textual mediations, the "gay subjectivity" gets lost in translation. I refer here to that historical and multiplex homo-culture that suffers and seeks deliverance, that (over)acts and strives, and that preserves and reveres, even in the biting irony of camp, as queer theorist John Champagne explains on the basis of Nietzsche's historical modes (1995, 133). Historically, we have had to adapt to social, emotional, and sexual experimentation mediated by hide-and-seek technologies such as the Internet and drugs; this includes safer sex. If safer sex was really created by white gay men to protect the tribe, its usefulness as text became obsolete long ago.

Social science research often narrativizes our experience. For example, current research tells us that drugs and alcohol are "used intentionally to engage in unsafe sex, and then to justify this behavior after the fact" in a practice termed "boundary play": "a process during which individuals navigate a variety of edges, or 'play' with various boundaries including the limits between sanity and insanity, legality and illegality, safety and danger, chaos and order, and life and death. The boundary is the dividing line between two opposing states of existence, and playing with such boundaries is the act of approaching or treading on these lines" (O'Byrne and Holmes 2011b). Although used in an aseptic tone by the authors, I love the phrase and I invite us to think of, and reclaim, boundary (ludic) play as productive of a gay subjectivity, the way we are freed and subjugated at the same time, by others, by institutions, and by ourselves collectively and individually. The irony that, increasingly, queers are engaging in diverse forms of sexual "edging" should not be lost on us.

Barebackers are at the very epicentre of queer moral panic and at the same time displaced by supposedly valuable social/sexual/emotional practices/events such as marriage and the care of children. Whether this gay subjectivity is nurtured or natural merits a separate discussion. The point is that gay subjectivity and boundary play have no place in the safe(r) sex codex, and never did.

Since Douglas Crimp's (1988) seminal collection, cultural critics have often flagged safer sex, and specifically the odious second skin of latex, as a contention barrier for the complexity of queer sex. Barebackers and meth users are often bagged together. Some carefully staged empirical research shows clear connections between being high and having unprotected sex – this has been enough to convict us in the court of public opinion, the way that fetishists and sadomasochists were repudiated yesteryear. It is rare to see any research attention and funding being given to the potential linkages between "party drugs" and positive mental and physical health outcomes.[2] Greatheart and Birch (2015) explore the connections between meth and gay sex in the prologue of their inaugural issue of *Annals of Gay Sexuality: The Contemporary HIV Zeitgeist* (2015): "If we see ourselves as seminal to evolution rather than a biological aberration, our storyline gets far more interesting. In only four and a half decades we've run the proverbial gauntlet. From invisibility to disco ball frenzy, near annihilation to killing ourselves with meth to learning how to find intimacy with transmen" (17).

And what is the response of public health to this change in the zeitgeist? In this new millennial carnival of desire and pleasure, ambulance chasers follow behind a sexual pageantry of felons, ghouls, and monsters doling out their pills to everyone. They call it "treatment as prevention" or TasP, which seems to work for those gay men who are housed, well fed, and enjoying a modicum of socio-economic privilege. Clinicians are giving pills (pre-exposure prophylaxis or PrEP) to the innocent bystanders of sex to protect them from already aviremic pozzies and to those who slipped up last night or are the (often middle-class) "worried well," eager to consume anything in the health marketplace because it is an available product. For them, medics have post-exposure prophylaxis (PeP).

In the social sciences, the response of gay men is often veiled by the archaic and operant third-person narrative. Queers in the social sciences pass as "not too gay" while siding with veiled cultural/moral interpretations of gay sex closely dangerous to conventional public health guidelines and moral panic (Ibáñez-Carrasco 2012). This narrative seal is often unbreakable until one sees in-person the swish of the presenting authors/scientist toeing the line of neutral academia and public health. The researcher as openly queer and sexual and HIV-positive exists, and so does the danger of academic suicide.

Regardless of the disclosures or closets of queer academics regarding safer sex for queers, it is often an *othering* voice interpreting queer reality in this realm. For example, a report stemming from a 2006 study in New York on whether HIV-positive gay men are concerned about getting infected concludes, "The challenge still remains as to how these men could be engaged in using [serosorting and other] approaches more consistently and effectively" and how techniques that include "pre-contemplation" and "contemplation" are necessary (Balán et al. 2013, 11). Another report from the same study seems much more philosophical in its discussion of barebacking (Frasca, Dowsett, and Carballo-Diéguez 2013). For me, this and other narrativizations of barebacking signal something more than having different squeezes of qualitative data; these narratives evidence the very ambivalence of social science. Not unlike pornographers, social scientists writing about barebacking awkwardly jockey between positions as they try to occupy a middle ground between radicalism and acceptability.

I turn again to Kane Race's incisive analysis to highlight that the scientific narrative evidence infecting public health remains dead set on bodies, sexual technique, and outcomes; it focuses on complete and constant intentionality, compliance, adherence, and good lifestyle choices by sexual beings instead of focusing on erratic and even elusive bodies, desires, and pleasures. The former focus allows for technical expectations, creates a demonic "bad gay," and emphasizes "consumer beware" choices such as engaging in sex with those who use hard drugs. Gay sex and the use of licit and illicit drugs or even innovative emotional arrangements become antithetical to a health gay lifestyle, and cross the moral panic boundary from "medical" (e.g., erectile dysfunction drugs) to "recreational" that decent gays can access, to "problematic," which medicalize the morally at fault – any use of drugs for fun is wrong, especially among the disadvantaged.

The ghostwriters of AIDS in the social sciences are often complicit in maintaining the panic narrative of the barebacker (the endemic patient zero?) with all its trappings. The barebacker (individual) shows lack of concern, the result of childhood trauma, and his individualistic behaviour is incompatible with safer sex that "emphasises better access to information, services, and resources"(Garcia 2013, 1032). Barebacking is not accepted as collective sexual-cultural behaviour and, potentially, the result of Anglo-normative and hetero/homo-normative moral panic, the result of resistance, or even a form of "medicine" for panic and rejection.

This panic-based set of guidelines will continue to relegate to the periphery of current public health guidelines the fact that gay men (in fact all persons!) will bareback at one time, or many frequent or sporadic times in their sexual lifespan, in pursuit of individualistic or collective pleasure. The genre of public health text and social sciences tends to render barebacking as unspeakable in positive/productive terms, and render it invisible in their mediating texts, while, at the same time, exuberantly visible in the fantasy of porn as well as in many other versions of the gay collective imaginary.

While a sexual-cultural revolution has taken place, the public health sector has held steadfast to the safer sex code – the band played on and they sank with an obsolete Titanic of sexual health. However, the culturally obsolete ideas of disembodied, moralistic, purely reflective sexuality continue to be taught in schooling institutions from elementary to universities – albeit with refinements and salutations to sexual orientation, consent, and communication, but most often swatting aside the nebula of desire and pleasure as a foul fart odour.[3] Safer sex takes care of those who can be harmed by barebackers. But who takes care of *barebackers on meth*, the most villainous of the sexual offenders today? Rarely have we seen systematic efforts to help gay men with clinical, behavioural, and spiritual supports, and programs (harm reduction or not) for gay men using meth. I imagine that there may be organized/ institutionalized efforts to help men use meth efficiently or pleasurably, but could not find evidence at the time of this writing (this in contrast with a barrage of clinical work on the use of cannabis; not much of this focus seems to be on its use as pleasure).

After thirty years of hammering safer sex over the heads of LGTBQ communities, our few dedicated psychotherapists and psychiatrists, frontline workers, etc. are seeing an accumulation of shame, guilt, and anger for not having sex the (supposedly) right way (albeit having it good), for continuing to be a vector of infection, even more of a problem than drug users whose seroconversion rates have decreased over the last twenty years. Drug users learn to use their syringes; why can't gays just learn to use their dicks to inject semen safely?

Public health funds campaigns, programs, and tools to meet gay men where they are, to eroticize their messaging, and to discuss barriers such as pig (rough) sex, sex in public places and HIV-related stigma.[4] However, safer sex lives on, especially in the oral tradition of gay men, in our folklore mixed with our much-glorified spectacular escapades. Safer sex is theory, or faith, and there is the reality of what gay men do in their everyday lives.[5] Gay liberation has married safer sex and bare-backing forever in sickness and health. We cannot have one without the other. This is poorly understood in research and programming. In addition, the role of using hard substances (meth, ketamine, or GHB) is often researched in relation to safer sex and the individual, but not in relation to a community psyche, collective post-traumatic syndrome, and group identities.

If we accept that all audiovisual texts such as brochures, referral forms, informational videos, and clinical psychometric tests mediate between individual/collective practices and institutional/public policy, we must accept that we have dry and aseptic representations of safer sex for gay men on one hand, and self-recorded videos of barebackers self-injecting meth on the other; the chasm is too wide and too deep. There are a bunch of really confused "patients" and health-care providers caught in the middle.

## Denying Disability

In his novel *Amped*, Daniel H. Wilson predicts a world of amplified disabled people who become often more productive and energetic than those of us who deem ourselves fully able-bodied. However, Wilson also depicts shame and turmoil. An amplified person can be perceived as spectacular but dangerous, say a gay man who adheres to the technology of medications and doesn't practise safe sex. Although HIV-negative men are starting to feel amped by Truvada and other pre-exposure prophylactics, I doubt HIV-positive gay men have ever felt and acted "amped" and duly protected by taking HIV medications. In Canada, the gay cultural dialogue seems greatly influenced by "treatment as prevention" and PrEP. As a result, in social media and other fora, bare-backing and barebackers are not as vilified as they used to be. It feels like HIV-negative men are giving permission to their poz counterparts. And yet, if poz gay men avoided or hid the "disabled" designation before, now that the playing field seems to have levelled, it would seem foolish to want to reclaim the stigmatizing condition of HIV. The indulgence of the culture of victimhood doesn't extend that far. In contrast, clinical and social scientists keep on weaving psychometrics and grim scenarios of deficiencies, concerns, and accelerated inflammations.

There were timid and hurried policy changes to designate people living with HIV as disabled so they would be able to collect social as-sistance; these were hard to achieve in the 1990s. I recall activists from the (former) BC Persons with AIDS Society fighting hard for us to get provincial disability status. We were dying; it really wasn't a disability policy but enacting catastrophic rights. In spite of its benefits at times of crisis, this policy put and maintained a generation of HIV-positive gay men on welfare, unemployed and stigmatized. Western societies consider earning a salary as a key element in one's autonomy and ma-turity. Policies are cut and dried and in the area of HIV and disability, they tend to designate persons fully able or fully disabled.

Disability and rehabilitation in HIV have been influenced by the World Health Organization's International Classification of Function-ing, Disability and Health (2001) which includes disabilities, handicaps and impairments and, significantly, includes lack of social participa-tion and contextual barriers (Worthington et al. 2005). The invisibility of disability and lack of rehabilitation services connected to treatment permeate the lives of people living with HIV as we live longer and a whole generation ages living with HIV. I have pushed the agenda for HIV as episodic disability, even as I see it in daily opposition to queers wanting to be "healthy" and "safe." I want to try and explain this am-bivalence. Are AIDS patients trying to have two incompatible things when it is convenient? Normalcy and disability. No. Disabled people have the right to sexuality and are also impacted by the erroneous notions of sexuality supported by the safer sex codex.

Poz gay men I meet through research, work, teaching, and social life, like my friend Josh, were forced, and are still forced to decide to either stay on government or private issued disability and do nothing, which reduces their social participation and their social standing in the eyes of others; volunteer, sometimes almost as much or more than full-time paid work; or choose work and study under the table with ensuing stress, rejoining work life with fear, initial loss of benefits, and often keeping their status secret from employers. In many cases, poz gay men avoid claiming rights as a person living with an episodic disability. The result is a lost generation of poz gay men with varying levels of schooling and interrupted professional lives that we prefer not to account for.

Clearly the toll of disability, even as medications get more effective, has been much greater on those with less cultural and schooling capital, who have to work in low-paying menial industries. The iatrogenic effect of public policy is not battling the stigma of HIV as episodic disability and fuelling the fantasy that HIV is a chronic, long-term manageable condition with room to thrive. It is a weakening disability stigmatized inside and outside queer communities. *HIV should be a disability to be amped about; instead, it is filled with shame and feelings of inadequacy.*

I doubt any gay man, including my friend Josh, will hook up online and say, "Hey, I have an episodic disability but I am amped, better than normal, really!" The silent code is that it is better to keep quiet than claiming a dubious badge of personal politics, "patient" skills, and resilience. HIV stigma is one of the leading social problems in the epidemic, everywhere (Chambers et al. 2015). Lateral symbolic violence perpetrated by gay men against each other in the context of HIV is an enclave of HIV stigma (see https://www.thefactsite.org.uk The LGBT Fact Site, the home of health and life advice for LGBT people, published by HERO – The Health Equality and Rights Organisation). We have a long way to go before we understand and embrace "sluts" and "barebackers" as experts and "patient navigators" (not hired by public health). My mission and toll in public life – and that of many sibling queers in lust – reminds me of seeing Quentin Crisp in 1991 speak about the promiscuous gay man as "The Naked Civil Servant" (1968) who teaches gay men about being gay, and imparting the "wisdom of whores" that Elizabeth Pisani refers to in her 2008 book.

Weak public health policies on rehabilitation, especially as the lack of social participation detected in the World Health Organization definition (the lack of support services – a situation that many other disabled people endure – has resulted in a timorous, de-politicized poz gay group of long-term survivors who feel, and who are told, they have been well looked after because they get effective medications. However, we are rarely told we are triumphant or well-adjusted. The normalization of HIV has put the last nail on the coffin of oblivion of the 1980s and 1990s generation. We are still sick but we look cured. Disability is stigmatized. HIV is a double bind, stigmatizing you whether you keep it hidden or voice it. Public health has done nothing but cosset gay men into another gay fantasy of wellness.

## Interpreting Uncertainty

Continued implementation of public health programs with an ahistorical safer sex codex, in conjunction with the lack of clarity of HIV as an episodic disability, contributes to the stigmatization of HIV and the uncertainty that gay men living with HIV feel about the future of being HIV-positive (Solomon et al. 2013; Furlotte and Schwartz 2017). My view is that uncertainty is buttressed by an altered notion of time, an intergenerational disconnect between the young and the old in queer communities (brought about death and social reclusion of high numbers of infected queers), and emerging complications from HIV (such as HIV/AIDS associated neurocognitive disorders or HAND), we can maybe refer to it as "radical uncertainty" when patients don't know that they don't know (as opposed to knowing that they don't know). In a world that is, arguably, risky and uncertain for most, I suggest that the safer sex spectre especially contributes to the uncertainty of poz queers.

More than lack of access to rehabilitation services such as occupational therapy or physiotherapy, one of the preoccupations for aging queers (and those young aging with HIV) is having their altered notion of time, and ambivalence about planning for the future. We thought HIV medications and clinical certainty had resolved this! I interpret this "uncertainty" using a phenomenological lens. Thus, uncertainty is an epithelial tissue that covers one's motivations and interests. It is a distorted sense of one's circumstances and one's future – the opposite of that youthful sense of invincibility. In this respect, one can say that "uncertainty" captures the zeitgeist of Western societies. This fluid sense of uncertainty cannot be measured or even pinpointed as manifest. This renders it invisible to public health practitioners. It might not be a practical priority, a concrete action to take – racism, minority stress, transphobia, and other well-researched maladies were once invisible too, and we have come around to considering them and combating them in health systems – but it must be addressed as an underlying current in the lives of those living with HIV, especially those who have lived with HIV for a long time.

Gay men living with HIV do have an altered sense of time. Those from the "old guard" who were expected to die are still amazed we are here. Those getting infected today also see their corporeal time out of synch with their sense of time. Young or old, in spite of the biomedical normalization of HIV, this paradigm shift is not bringing about "a parallel shift in the embodied experiences of being HIV-positive" (Persson 2013 abstract).

Here I reclaim uncertainty among HIV-positive men who are confused and ambivalent about *what will please others*, because they are expected to toe the line of good, decent, gay (married with children) and be the last bastion of cultural and sexual resistance, *the sexual radicals who know what gay men really want*: communing physically with others, marking each other's bodies with clinically glorified DNA, seeding, breeding, or augmenting one's sense of belonging to a proscribed group. As a clinical tool and a teaching tool for clinicians and non-clinicians, safer sex guidelines fail miserably to examine a broad Western uncertainty of what Adam calls "the neoliberal sexual actor," that is to say, the "rational, adult, contract-making individual in a free market of options" (Adam 2005, 344).

However, our technocratic quest is to quantify complex motivations, actions, and outcomes – to translate the untranslatable. It has been said that "something similar is happening when health economists use measures like the QALY to evaluate the costs of disease or the benefits of treatments: it is an imperfect yet seemingly necessary technology to enable tragic choices, translating impossible moral judgments about suffering into a technical and calculable form" (Rose 2008, 38). In the case of many "isms," "phobias," and "stressors," we measure to eliminate, as if that were possible. We rarely reflect and work with these ailments to consider the function they have in society. I am the first one to condemn homophobia and the last one to reflect on what possible role it can have in society – that would be heretical.

### Fighting back the Bio-morality of Safer Sex!

At the root of "uncertainty" we find (HIV) stigma, lucidly defined by Erving Goffman in 1963, refined over time to distinguish between enacted, anticipated, and internalized stigma (Gray 2002) and greatly buttressed by the bio-morality of health (Parhizgar, Parhizgar, and Parhizgar 2006).[6] Bio-morality is the expectation that each *individual* has enough space and tools for healthy decision-making; that healthy choices (e.g., no salt, sugar, meth, or raw semen) are not only desirable but (financially) valuable; they contribute to the public good and they are good in themselves. The idea of wellness and mindfulness

– "lifestyle medicine" they call it – are now packed with morality (Holloway 2015). Say it is expected that my friend Josh should be planning for his (uncertain) future instead of smoking too much weed and spending his welfare money on booze and drugs and extreme sex. That he keeps away from HIV-negative men, especially the young ones. This is a function of "uncertainty": keeping patients neutralized and adherent. This is close to what thinker Ivan Illich proposed in *The Limits to Medicine*.

Some of our adaptive individual and group reactions to "uncertainty" are "resilience" and "empowerment" – we applaud them. Stigma is also an epithelial skin that envelops everything but seems invisible, hard to pinpoint, to say, "See? Here it is!" Stigma makes us look paranoid, and the result is deep uncertainty of ourselves. I go as far as suggesting that the "spoiled identity" (Goffman) of HIV gay pozzies is that of never being fully normal men. This insidiously reaffirms the historical (not defunct) idea that gay men were never fully masculine with responsibilities and families and lasting relationships.

We have faith in the bio-moral public health imperative of preventing harm (Murphy 2015). This guides our beliefs on abortion, stem cell implants, euthanasia, and many other significant aspects of our health lives. This faith still permeates our concerns with HIV, those who carry it and what they do with "it." Most often than not, the belief is that nothing good may come from giving and getting HIV, no sense of relief at having finally become infected and not having to be so scared, no character growth, no post-traumatic growth, and no sense of meaning. Indeed, research in the area of HIV and aging is showing that pozzies have great coping mechanisms (Brennan et al. 2013). Gay pozzies may possess a degree of "cultural capital" (some might call it "wisdom") that makes us defiant and resilient; by the same token, it is in the interest of the status quo to keep us neutralized and stigmatized and uncertain. The alternative would be to have aviremic pozzies having sex with everyone and openly. It certainly doesn't seem that pozzies feel "distinct" and poz proud when public health, conventional schooling, and the legal system help little in this respect.

How do many gay men fight uncertainty when there are no *generative redemptive narratives* (McAdams and Guo 2015) for the likes of my sexual friend Josh? We resort to well-proven sheltering practices such as living in a closet, albeit of a different kind. In this case, our closet is managing our HIV status information with all people and at all times. Lützén and Ewalds-Kvist (2013) theorize that one of the most important strategies of resilience is making meaning of one's historical and individual situation, and "despair is suffering without meaning." Understanding the effects of colonization on our health is one of the central de-colonizing projects in Indigenous movements (Linda Tuhiwai Te Rina Smith 1999). What is the queer option? Or is it even possible to compare these two historical processes?

To fight the iatrogenic effects of public health and the safer sex code seems like an insurmountable battle. How? The work of AIDS Action Now! in Toronto is very local but exemplar (http://www.aidsaction now.org). They have called for the decriminalization of HIV, the re-establishment of a formal and effective National HIV Strategy in Canada, and the building of a National Pharmacare Program. They have also engaged in some representational work reminiscent of ACT UP (AIDS Coalition to Unleash Power) in 1988 and the work of Gran Fury, the AIDS activist artist collective from New York City.

A great deal of contemporary political work may never have the teeth of early AIDS activism, because most queers do not care and HIV is medically managed. The work that individuals living with HIV have to make visible what we have to live everyday seems piecemeal and Sisyphean. In its most technical version, it is important to access inter-professional programs for health-care providers and medical students. The number of hours that (mostly young) health-care students get to understand the complexity of AIDS is negligible. However, the newer generations, diverse and politically correct and differently savvy (functioning in an intensely mediated context) tend to exhibit an open attitude to considering the complexity of sexual health, the fragmentation of the medical system, the need to continue redrawing the archaic forms of communication and decision-making between the ill and the healers, and the significance of understanding the breadth of disability (including HIV as an episodic nearly invisible disability).

In my corner of the world, where education and training still matter, the maintenance of pre-clerkship programs, the creation of small-scale research courses for students to work collaboratively with people living with HIV, the creation and support of patient councils (Bertelsen, Kanstrup, and Olsson 2015), patient-assisted training (Towle and Godolphin 2015; Lenton and Storr 2015), and the engagement of patients in health research (following a long-held tradition in HIV community-based research in Canada) and other consultative and collaborative modalities may go a long way in fighting the iatrogenesis of public health. I acknowledge the extent of my contradiction here by suggesting that we continue to invest in the human cogs of the very machinery that produces barebackers, the medical system and public health; I don't see any better, feasible, systematic, and sustainable strategies today.

## Conclusion

The bio-moral quality of public health policy in the context of HIV is manifest in outdated safer sex guidelines, in the inability to conceptualize HIV as an episodic disability, in its inability to keep up with the sexual/cultural conversation and practices of gay men, its timid response to the criminalization of the non-disclosure of HIV, and its inability to connect physical spaces (much less the Internet) with public health policies. Uncertainty is one of the greatest iatrogenic effects of public health policy on gay men living with HIV, and by extension on entire sexual-cultural networks. Nothing will change unless we value in concrete ways our HIV positivity, its wisdom and enactments. In this reflection on the possible iatrogenic effects of public policy, I have given a special salutation to barebackers and hard drug–users as resilient sexual and cultural pioneers that effect cultural resistance, take on the uncertainty of life and the ambiguity of public spaces, and perform radical disability.

NOTES

1  See Government of Canada (2015).
2  In this regard, it is hopeful and helpful that Evan Wood, renowned HIV researcher, has recently reinvigorated the dialogue on the use of "psychedelic medicine" by publishing a review that includes detail on the use of MDMA-assisted psychotherapy (a psychedelic "party drug" to relieve post-traumatic stress disorder) and foreshadows the study of MDMA-assisted therapy as a treatment for social anxiety in adults with autism. See K. Tupper et al., "Psychedelic Medicine: A Re-emerging Therapeutic Paradigm," *Canadian Medical Association Journal* 187, no. 14 (2015): 1054–9.
3  See the 2015 controversy surrounding the Ontario's new sexual education curriculum, "Sex Education in Ontario" (2016).
4  For TowelTalk see http://www.catie.ca/en/pc/program/towel-talk; for "Sex Pigs," see http://img.thebody.com/confs/aids2008/pdfs/

THPE0347_kathy_triffitt.pdf; and for the Canadian HIV Stigma campaign in 2008, see http://www.hivstigma.com.

5  In contrast to the lack of cultural production on these issues in Canada, HIV-positive media collectives are fruitful in other countries, such as Three Flying Piglets in the United Kingdom, http://threeflyingpiglets.co.uk/, part of the Gay Men's Health Collective, http://gaymenshealthcollective .co.uk/, who tackle chemsex, bareback sex, and other issues.

6  HIV stigma is being widely explored by researchers, and most significantly, it has been documented by persons living with HIV using a global community–based research approach: "The People Living with HIV Stigma Index provides a tool that measures and detects changing trends in relation to stigma and discrimination experienced by people living with HIV. In the initiative, the process is just as important as the product. It aims to address stigma relating to HIV while also advocating on the key barriers and issues perpetuating stigma – a key obstacle to HIV treatment, prevention, care and support." People Living with HIV Stigma Index, "Home" (2017), www.stigmaindex.org.

## REFERENCES

Adam, B.D. 2005. "Constructing the Neoliberal Sexual Actor: Responsibility and Care of the Self in the Discourse of Barebackers." *Culture, Health & Sexuality* 7 (4): 333–46. https://doi.org/10.1080/13691050500100773.

Balán, Ivan, et al. 2013. "Are HIV-Negative Men Who Have Sex with Men and Who Bareback Concerned about HIV Infection? Implications for HIV Risk Reduction Interventions." *Archives of Sexual Behavior* 42 (2): 279–89. https://doi.org/10.1007/s10508-011-9886-2.

Bauer, Robin. 2014. *Queer BDSM Intimacies: Critical Consent and Pushing Boundaries*. New York: Palgrave Macmillan.

Bayer, R. 1989. "AIDS, Privacy, and Responsibility." *Daedalus* 118 (3): 79–99.

Bertelsen, P., A.M. Kanstrup, and S. Olsson. 2015. "Patient Perspectives on Patient Participation: Results from a Workshop with a Patient Council in a General Practice." *Studies in Health Technology and Informatics* 208:72–7.

Brennan, D.J., et al. 2013. "Socio-demographic Profile of Older Adults with HIV/AIDS: Gender and Sexual Orientation Differences." *Canadian Journal on Aging / La Revue canadienne du vieillissement* 32 (1): 31–43. https://journals.scholarsportal.info/details?uri=/17101107/v32i0001/31_spooawhgasod.

Campbell, Bradley, and Jason Manning. 2014. "Microaggression and Moral Cultures." *Comparative Sociology* 13 (6): 692–726. https://doi.org/10.1163/15691330-12341332.

Chambers, Lori A., et al. 2015. "Stigma, HIV and Health: A Qualitative Synthesis." *BMC Public Health* 15:848. https://bmcpublichealth .biomedcentral.com/articles/10.1186/s12889-015-2197-0.

Champagne, John. 1995. *The Ethics of Marginality: A New Approach to Gay Studies*. Minneapolis: University of Minnesota Press.

Conrad, Peter. 2007. *The Medicalization of Society: On the Transformation of Human Conditions into Treatable Disorders*. Baltimore, MD: Johns Hopkins University Press.

Crimp, Douglas, ed. 1988. *AIDS: Cultural Analysis, Cultural Activism*. Cambridge, MA: MIT Press.

Crisp, Quentin. 1968. *The Naked Civil Servant*. HarperCollins.

Fink, Marty. 2015. "Don't Be a Stranger Now: Queer Exclusions, Decarceration and HIV/AIDS." In *Disrupting Queer Inclusion, Canadian Homonationalism and the Politics of Belonging*, edited by H. Dryden OmiSoore and Suzanne Lenon, 150–68. Vancouver: University of British Columbia Press.

Fisher, W.A., et al. 1988. "Erotophobia-Erotophilia as a Dimension of Personality." *Journal of Sex Research* 25 (1): 123–51.

Frasca, Timothy, Gary W. Dowsett, and Alex Carballo-Diéguez. 2013. "The Ethics of Barebacking: Implications of Gay Men's Concepts of Right and Wrong in the Context of HIV." *International Journal of Sexual Health* 25 (3): 198–211.

Furlotte, C., and K. Schwartz. 2017. "Mental Health Experiences of Older Adults Living with HIV: Uncertainty, Stigma, and Approaches to Resilience." *Canadian Journal on Aging / La Revue canadienne du vieillissement* 36 (2): 125–40.

Garcia, Christien. 2013. "Limited Intimacy: Barebacking and the Imaginary." *Textual Practice* 27 (6): 1031–51. https://doi.org/10.1080/0950236X.2013 .830828.

Government of Canada. 2015. "Prevention of HIV and AIDS." https://www .canada.ca/en/public-health/services/diseases/hiv-aids/prevention-hiv-aids.html.

Government of Ontario. 2016. "Sex Education in Ontario." https://www .ontario.ca/page/sex-education-ontario.

Gray, A.J. 2002. "Stigma in Psychiatry." *Journal of the Royal Society of Medicine* 95 (2): 72–6. https://doi.org/10.1258/jrsm.95.2.72.

Greatheart, M., and R. Birch, eds. 2015. *Annals of Gay Sexuality: The Contemporary HIV Zeitgeist*, with art direction by Pan. Toronto, Ethica.

Holloway, Kali. 2015. "'Wellness' Is Making Us Sick: How Corporate America's Favourite Mantra Leaves Us All Feeling Inadequate. Mindfulness Has Become a Tool to Distract Us from Societal Ills and Further Enrich

Our Corporate Overlords." Salon, 14 August. http://www.salon.com/
    2015/08/14/wellness_is_making_us_sick_how_corporate_americas_
    favorite_mantra_leaves_us_all_feeling_inadequate_partner.
Ibáñez-Carrasco, J. Francisco. 1997/1998. "Explorations and Border-Crossings:
    The Risks of Safer Sex Discourse." Trans/forms: Insurgent Voices in Education
    3 (4).
– 2012. "Making the AIDS Ghostwriters Visible." In Sexualities in Education:
    A Reader, edited by Therese Quinn and Erica R. Meiners, 309–20. New York:
    Peter Lang.
– 2015. Giving It Raw: Nearly Thirty Years with AIDS. Oakland: Transgress.
Illich, Ivan. 1974. Medical Nemesis: The Expropriation of Health. London: Calder
    & Boyars.
Lenton, Carrie, and Emma Storr. 2015. "Patients as Teachers for Under-
    graduates: Real-Life Experiences of Long-term Conditions." Education
    for Primary Care 26 (2): 109–12.
Lützén, K., and B. Ewalds-Kvist. 2013. "Moral Distress and Its Interconnection
    with Moral Sensitivity and Moral Resilience: Viewed from the Philosophy
    of Viktor E. Frankl." Journal of Bioethical Inquiry 10 (3): 317–24. https://doi
    .org/10.1007/s11673-013-9469-0.
McAdams, D., and J. Guo. 2015. "Narrating the Generative Life." Psychological
    Science 26 (4): 475–83. https://doi.org/10.1177/0956797614568318.
Murphy, Timothy F. 2015. "Preventing Ultimate Harm as the Justification
    for Biomoral Modification." Bioethics 29 (5): 369–77. http://ssrn.com/
    abstract=2604588.
O'Byrne, P., and D. Holmes. 2011a. "Desire, Drug Use and Unsafe Sex:
    A Qualitative Examination of Gay Men Who Attend Gay Circuit Parties."
    Culture, Health & Sexuality 13 (1): 1–13. doi:10.1080/13691058.2010.510610.
– 2011b. "Drug Use as Boundary Play: A Qualitative Exploration of Gay
    Circuit Parties." Substance Use & Misuse 46 (12): 1510–22. http://doi.org/
    10.3109/10826084.2011.572329.
Parhizgar, Kamal Dean, Suzan Parhizgar, and Fuzhan Parhizgar. 2006.
    "Bioethical Analysis of the Promethean and Biophilia Global Biobusiness."
    Competitiveness Review 16 (2): 170–84. http://www.emeraldinsight.com/
    doi/pdfplus/10.1108/cr.2006.16.2.170.
Persson, A. 2013. "Non/infectious Corporealities: Tensions in the Biomedical
    Era of 'HIV Normalisation.'" Sociology of Health & Illness 35 (7): 1065–79.
    https://doi.org/10.1111/1467-9566.12023.
Pisani, Elizabeth. 2008. The Wisdom of Whores: Bureaucrats, Brothels, and the
    Business of AIDS. Don Mills, ON: Penguin, Canada.

Prevention Access Campaign. 2017, 3 July. https://www.preventionaccess.org.

Race, K. 2009. *Pleasure Consuming Medicine: The Queer Politics of Drugs*. Durham, NC: Duke University Press.

Rose, N. 2008. "The Value of Life: Somatic Ethics & the Spirit of Biocapital." *Daedalus* 137 (1): 36–48. https://doi.org/10.1162/daed.2008.137.1.36.

Scott, J. 2014. *A Dictionary of Sociology*. 4th ed. Oxford: Oxford University Press.

Singer, Merrill, and Scott Clair. 2003. "Syndemics and Public Health: Reconceptualizing Disease in Bio-Social Context." *Medical Anthropology Quarterly* 17 (4): 423–41. https://doi.org/10.1525/maq.2003.17.4.423.

Solomon, P., et al. 2013. "Aging with HIV and Disability: The Role of Uncertainty." *AIDS Care* 26 (2): 240–5.

Szasz, Thomas. 1977. *The Theology of Medicine: The Political-Philosophical Foundations of Medical Ethics*. Syracuse, NY: Syracuse University Press.

Towle, A., and W. Godolphin. 2015. "Patients as Teachers: Promoting Their Authentic and Autonomous Voices." *Clinical Teacher* 12 (3): 149–54. https://doi.org/10.1111/tct.12400.

Tuhiwai Te Rina Smith, Linda. 1999. *Decolonizing Methodologies*. New York: Zed Books and University of Otago Press.

Vicioso, Kalil J., et al. 2005. "Experiencing Release: Sex Environments and Escapism for HIV-Positive Men Who Have Sex with Men." *Journal of Sex Research* 42 (1): 13–19, doi: 10.1080/00224490509552252.

World Health Organization. 2001. *International Classification of Functioning, Disability and Health*. http://www.who.int/classifications/icf/en/.

Worthington, Catherine, et al. 2005. "Rehabilitation in HIV/AIDS: Development of an Expanded Conceptual Framework." *AIDS Patient Care and STDs* 19 (4): 258–71.

Wright, Kai. 2008. "America's AIDS Apartheid." *American Prospect*, 20 June. http://prospect.org/article/americas-aids-apartheid.

# PART TWO

Services

# 5 Aging without a Net: Policy Barriers Facing Older Adults Living with HIV in Canada

KATE MURZIN AND CHARLES FURLOTTE

The first cohorts of people living with HIV (PHAs) in Canada are now reaching middle and older adulthood; these older adults are now navigating a complex aging process. The absence of coordinated, comprehensive, equitable social policy, especially at the federal level, means that many of these people are aging "without a net." As in all age cohorts, women, racialized people, and Indigenous people often experience forms of marginalization that can limit their ability to access care, resulting in poorer health outcomes (Cescon et al. 2015; Moore, Keruly, and Bartlett 2012; Patterson et al. 2015).

The furthest-reaching intervention with the greatest potential for population-level improvement in the well-being of older PHAs is a renewed commitment to healthy public policy. In the context of HIV and aging, this would include integrated health strategies for aging, HIV and chronic disease management, and fiscal and social policy that includes citizens who are aging, living with chronic illness, or otherwise marginalized.

Individuals, networks, and organizations working to support older PHAs are cobbling together a response without guidance from pan-Canadian HIV, aging/seniors, or chronic-disease-management strategies, and within benefits and health systems rife with barriers.

In this chapter, we explore some of the health and social challenges facing older PHAs, first discussing how they compare with the lived experiences of HIV-negative older people, and the applicability of "healthy aging" frameworks. We then critique existing public policies that significantly affect older PHAs, arguing that problematic features of these policies include HIV exceptionalism; lack of integration across HIV, chronic disease, and aging sectors; downstream approaches to disease management; suboptimal care delivery and physician payment models; inadequate attention to the importance of work (employment) and income security; lack of support for aging in place; and barriers to health service access. We conclude with recommendations to improve policies affecting older PHAs.

## Older PHAs in Canada

Some older PHAs have been living with HIV for years, and older adults also represent an increasing proportion of people newly diagnosed with HIV (PHAC 2014, 22). The population of people aging with HIV is therefore growing. But recent findings indicate that PHAs with low viral load and well-functioning immune systems are not at increased risk of death, compared to their same-aged HIV-negative counterparts (Rodger et al. 2013). So is aging with HIV just like aging without it?

In some ways, yes. The prevalence of heart disease, kidney disease, diabetes, high blood pressure, and high cholesterol increase with age among North Americans, regardless of HIV status (Arora et al. 2013, e420; CIHI 2011, 5; Statistics Canada 2013; Vance et al. 2011, 22). Older adults who are financially reliant on federal benefits receive the same income, whether they are HIV-positive or not. It is common for people living with HIV, like most older adults, to have experienced the death of peers, and to grieve these losses.

However, PHAs have a higher prevalence of age-associated non-communicable comorbidities than their HIV-negative counterparts (Schouten et al. 2014). PHAs are also at increased risk of pulmonary disease, heart attacks, end-stage renal disease, non-AIDS-defining cancers, and early-onset frailty (Althoff et al. 2014; Crothers et al. 2011; Desquilbet et al. 2007). Both HIV itself and long-term exposure to anti-retroviral therapies contribute to these health outcomes.

PHAs may also be more likely to experience mental health challenges: almost one sixth of people with HIV report experiencing depression, and one third report experiencing anxiety (Robertson et al. 2014, 1557). In older adults, depression is often linked to loneliness and/or HIV-related stigma (Grov et al. 2010, 637). Uncertainty is also common and centres on prognosis, ambiguity around causes of symptoms (e.g., HIV-related or age-related), and practical questions of where people will live and who will care for them as they grow older with HIV (Furlotte and Schwartz 2017; Rosenfeld et al. 2014; Solomon et al. 2014).

Post-traumatic stress disorder (PTSD) is also common among PHAs (Beckerman and Auerbach 2010; Sherr et al. 2011). It may result in part from events predating a person's HIV diagnosis, but can be exacerbated by this diagnosis (Gangbar and Globerman 2014; Halkitis 2014). In the case of many long-term survivors, prolonged exposure to intersecting forms of stigma, including the social marginalization and exclusion of gay men and substance users, and political reluctance to acknowledge the devastating effects of HIV in the early days of the epidemic, may be the root cause of trauma.

Health in the context of aging is significantly socially determined. The same social and financial factors contributing to HIV vulnerability (e.g., underemployment, social exclusion) can limit well-being after diagnosis. A person's financial status before or after HIV infection, in combination with the health issues and stigma that an HIV diagnosis may bring, may explain why PHAs are often financially disadvantaged. For long-term survivors, economic disadvantage can also be exacerbated by structural barriers: some PHAs have had no choice but to remain on social assistance or disability benefits since their diagnosis, as this was the only way they could maintain coverage for expensive HIV medications. PHAs in the workforce may often be engaged in precarious labour (LCO 2012), including holding part-time, temporary, or non-standard jobs, which provide flexibility to "work around" HIV-related episodic illnesses. Poor pay, job insecurity, and lack of pension, all characteristics of precarious employment, contribute to immediate poverty and limit the ability to save for retirement; it has also been linked to poor mental health among PHAs (Rueda et al. 2015).

When aging and HIV intersect, engagement in the workforce and income decline further. In one Canadian study, 60 per cent of older adults living with HIV reported being retired, unemployed, or otherwise disengaged from the labour force on account of disability (Brennan et al. 2013, 37). Almost 40 per cent of participants reported having a yearly income of less than $20,000.

It is important to understand how older PHAs experience aging and older adulthood. The relationship between "healthy aging" frameworks (that are now prominent in the study of aging) and the everyday lived experiences of older adults living with HIV is complex and can be somewhat unclear (Gahagan et al. 2012, 17). One way that healthy aging frameworks can be applied to HIV is through studies that examine successful aging (Rowe and Kahn 2015). The idea of successful aging is still in early stages of being applied to older adults living with HIV. While some successful aging paradigms define healthy aging as absence of infirmity in older adulthood, some authors have modified this definition, suggesting that for PHAs, the absolute absence of disease is not an appropriate criterion for healthy aging (Romo et al. 2013). Some studies have therefore asked PHAs to define "healthy" or "successful" aging for themselves (Emlet et al. 2016; Kahana and Kahana 2001; Moore et al. 2013; Vance, Struzick, and Masten 2008).

While self-reported successful aging has been found to be lower in older PHAs than their HIV-negative counterparts, despite poorer physical and mental health and greater stress, successful *psychosocial* aging with HIV is possible (Moore et al. 2013, e417). Older PHAs attribute aging well to both intrinsic coping strategies and social support (Emlet et al. 2016; Kahana and Kahana 2001). This emerging body of work suggests that resilience (hardiness), mastery, and optimism can contribute to successful aging with HIV.

## Public Policy Concerns for Older Adults Living with HIV in Canada

Some public policy features affect all older adults in Canada, including PHAs. These include an uncoordinated health-care system, including regional inconsistencies in product and service accessibility; lack of a national seniors' strategy; a shortage of geriatric experts and inadequate clinician training in gerontology; insufficient income supports for older adults and inflexible eligibility criteria for these supports; and fewer resources than needed allocated to aging in place, including underfunding of the social housing, home care, and long-term care sectors.

This section will touch on some of these aging-related public policy concerns, critically appraising them through the lens of HIV and aging. We will also explore policies that have few implications for older adults in general, but have the potential to significantly affect the well-being of older adults living with or vulnerable to HIV.

### Lack of Cross-Sectoral Integration

An overarching policy issue is lack of federal leadership on health. People often refer to the Canadian health-care system, when in fact there are fifteen distinct systems operating here: one system in each of the provinces and territories; a federal system governing the health care of

First Nations and Inuit people, military personnel and veterans, some refugees, and people in federal penitentiaries (Government of Canada 2012); as well as a growing private sector. The services and products that are publicly funded in each of these jurisdictions are determined separately, save for "medically necessary" care provided by physicians and in hospitals.

Like health-care services, access to subsidized prescription medication and medical devices differs from province to province. Even with federal guidance in the form of policy and strategy, as long as the responsibility for health is shared between the federal and provincial governments, there will be a piecemeal approach to health care across the nation.

Differences in what is covered from system to system result in inequitable access to critical health resources for older PHAs across Canada, and even within provinces (e.g., prisoners, Aboriginal people living on-reserve, and community-dwelling older adults within the same province access three different public health insurance systems). Older PHAs should not be expected to relocate in order to access comprehensive publicly funded care, and even if they were inclined to move, frailty, transportation costs, and the loss of social support and subsidized housing that may result would make migration especially challenging for this population.

In the absence of shared plans that shape expectations of support for people living with HIV and seniors across levels and silos of government, service providers and policymakers must cobble together provincial HIV, chronic illness, and aging policies to address HIV and aging in Canada. Unfortunately, disconnects between the sectors at the policy and health systems levels are often mirrored at the service provision level and interrupt continuity of care. With no common understanding of the constellation of policies and programs that contribute to good health outcomes for this population, the true complexity of aging with HIV remains invisible to decision-makers, and the multidimensional needs of this population are likely to remain unmet.

THE SPACE BETWEEN COMMUNICABLE AND CHRONIC ILLNESSES

HIV exists in a unique space between infectious and chronic illness and, as such, has been labelled "exceptional" until recently. There is now pressure to integrate HIV into one or the other of these policy areas, and either choice could alienate older adults living with HIV, specifically those living with the virus over the long term.

Given its trajectory, it is easy to see how HIV could be constructed as a chronic illness, for policy reasons. In theory, this characterization would normalize HIV, making screening, diagnosis, and treatment routine practice, as they are for other chronic, manageable conditions.

But two indicators within current chronic disease prevention and management policies suggest that integration may not be working. First, instead of using an obvious opportunity to draw a parallel between life with HIV and other chronic illnesses, many chronic disease prevention and management strategies reproduce the notion that HIV, and by extension people living with HIV, are different. References to the transmissibility of HIV within the health-care context unnecessarily evoke fear and reinforce negative attitudes towards HIV sometimes held by service providers outside the HIV sector.

Eleven provinces and territories in Canada have chronic disease prevention and/or management (CDPM) strategies, and/or prioritize CDPM within their primary care, community care, or health services strategies. Several policy documents describe chronic illness with the same terms used to characterize life with HIV such as long-lasting, incurable, requiring special treatment and coordinated care over time, and detrimental to functioning and quality of life (Government of New Brunswick 2010, 3; Government of Newfoundland and Labrador 2011, 2; Health PEI 2013, 7; Government of Ontario 2007, 3; Office of the Auditor General of Alberta 2014, 9; Saskatchewan Ministry of Health 2012, 13). However, only three make explicit mention of HIV, and these draw attention to its "infectiousness" to differentiate it from other chronic diseases (Government of New Brunswick 2010, 3; Government of Newfoundland and Labrador 2011, 2; Saskatchewan Ministry of Health 2012, 32). Another proclaims that chronic illnesses are, by definition, "not contagious" (Gouvernement du Québec 2010, 3).

The second issue, of particular importance to older adults living with HIV over the long term, who require formal social support, is that this approach to integration could ultimately lead to a reduction in earmarked funding for HIV/AIDS programming while simultaneously making less visible the unique challenges of living with HIV, such as enduring social stigma (Squire 2013). Expecting PHAs to participate in generalized chronic illness or aging-sector services that may not be welcoming or relevant to their needs could cause an already marginalized community to withdraw from service altogether.

The unique needs of PHAs are also likely to be lost if HIV is constructed as an infectious illness for policy purposes. While HIV shares common routes of transmission with other communicable diseases, it is among a handful that are incurable. Public health responses to infectious illnesses are often highly medicalized – including the UNAIDS 90-90-90 treatment targets[1] – and rely on a "test and treat" paradigm, which focuses primarily on the early stages of the care cascade. This approach is sufficient if treatment equals cure, as it can for tuberculosis, chlamydia, and even hepatitis C, but it fails to acknowledge the quality-of-life needs of people living with a life-long illness such as HIV after medical treatment is initiated. Lack of attention to post-treatment outcomes is a significant problem for older PHAs, since they are more likely to have complex needs related to their physical, mental, financial, and social well-being. Community-based HIV organizations have been safe havens of support for many long-term survivors, especially gay men. Some are wary that an integrated approach to infectious disease will stretch the already limited resources of the HIV sector too far by expanding the populace they are expected to serve. People living with HIV over the long term, mostly older adults, may particularly feel that they are being pushed aside when their need for support is highest.

HIV STRATEGIES

The Canadian HIV/AIDS Strategy, *Leading Together: Canada Takes Action on HIV/AIDS*, expired in 2010, leaving Canada without an official, federal HIV strategy (CPHA 2005). In 2013, a refreshed version was released, but this renewed report was not officially taken up as policy, and stakeholders were invited to consult this document "voluntarily" (LTCC 2013, 3). Most provinces and territories, as well as cultural groups within these jurisdictions, have created their own HIV strategies. Several acknowledge age as a determinant of HIV vulnerability. Few make the connection between HIV and chronic illness; however, Nova Scotia was a leader in this regard in 2003. Its HIV strategy explicitly recommends that actions taken to prevent and treat HIV should align with those outlined in other provincial strategies; it urges "intersectoral collaboration with other chronic disease groups" (Provincial HIV/AIDS Strategy Steering Committee 2003, 12). It also champions equitable implementation of disability policy, stating that people with HIV "should be able to avail themselves of rights and benefits similar to those available to persons with disabilities and/or other chronic diseases" (25). In a 2014 review of the strategy, the Nova Scotia Advisory Commission on AIDS acknowledges the aging-related health conditions experienced by PHAs and recommends public and health-provider education on

HIV and aging (NSACA 2014). Following suit over a decade later, policy frameworks introduced by Manitoba and Ontario in 2015 and 2017, respectively, integrate the management of chronic conditions into HIV care planning (Government of Manitoba 2015; Ontario Advisory Committee on HIV/AIDS 2017).

Over the last ten years, the HIV community has witnessed the rise and fall of a national HIV strategy for Canada. The fact that the strategy was not renewed may be interpreted by some as a symbol that HIV is no longer a priority for policymakers. In particular, people living over the long term with HIV may feel abandoned or invisible at a time when they are uncertain about their future needs.

AGING AND SENIORS' STRATEGIES

At all levels of government, consideration of the specific needs of older adults is sorely lacking in public policy. At the time of writing, there is no pan-Canadian seniors' or aging strategy. To fill this federal policy void, nearly all Canadian provinces and territories have developed their own seniors' strategies, but only about half are up-to-date (Gouvernement du Québec 2012; Government of British Columbia 2012; Government of Northwest Territories 2014; Government of Ontario 2013; Government of New Brunswick 2012; Government of Nunavut 2017). This results in regional disparities, such that older adults in some regions are more recognized in policy and have, in principle, better access to services than those in other regions.

Service access issues could be more significant for older adults living with HIV, but among eleven provincial and territorial aging strategies, only one framework mentions HIV (Government of Nova Scotia 2005). Three other aging strategies reference the sexual health of older adults (Gouvernement du Québec 2012; Government of Newfoundland and Labrador 2007; Government of Ontario 2013). Policymakers appear reluctant to acknowledge that sexual health is an important part of overall well-being for seniors; older adults living with HIV remain, for the most part, invisible within the aging sector. This lack of attention in policy translates into lack of education and support in practice, leaving older adults more vulnerable to HIV infection and less able to access aging-related services.

## Models of Care and Clinician Remuneration

Despite the proliferation of community-based, inter-professional health-care teams, dominant approaches to health-care provider remuneration still limit access to holistic care for people aging with HIV. For example, fee-for-service payments for physicians can encourage the implementation of "one problem per visit" policies, since shorter appointment times mean more appointments and therefore more compensation for the practitioner (Fullerton 2008, 623). This practice is especially problematic for older PHAs who are trying to manage a life-long illness, deal with comorbidity, cope with aging-related physical and mental health changes, and, in some cases, overcome significant social issues such as addiction and poverty.

The concept of singular focus is problematic not just for older PHAs in the context of a patient appointment. When combined antiretroviral therapy was first introduced, it was thought that specialist physicians were best positioned to manage the complexity of these medication regimens. As a result, PHAs were referred to HIV specialists who provided the major portion of their care. However, given the comorbidity that often accompanies aging with HIV, primary care physicians now have a more important role to play in the care of people living with HIV (Kendall et al. 2015). It is widely acknowledged that chronic disease prevention does not receive the attention it deserves within our healthcare system (Romanow 2002, 119), and HIV specialists may not have the time or training to provide preventive care. The lack of integration between HIV care and primary care, as well as the tendency to prioritize immediate health concerns over chronic issues, may lead to poorer health outcomes for older PHAs. More attention paid to secondary and tertiary prevention could lower the elevated prevalence of comorbidity within this population.

RETIREMENT BENEFITS

The impending transition from working-age income to retirement income can be a significant point of stress for older PHAs, who (especially those from minority groups) may have fewer financial resources, as compared to older adults in the general population (Joyce et al. 2005). The insufficiency of public pensions has been reported to have a substantial impact on PHAs' income security (Emlet et al. 2016).

Public retirement benefit programs do not take into account the heterogeneity among older adults in the population. Age-based benefit programs cater to people who are able to work until the designated retirement age of sixty-five. This may be an unrealistic goal for PHAs, since the burden of multi-morbidity may hasten functional decline. As the Law Commission of Ontario writes, "The common use of essentially arbitrary markers of old age, such as retirement from the work force or the attainment of age 65, while providing clarity and simplicity, do not accord with the realities of ageing, or the important role of attitudes, social expectations and specific context in how aging is experienced" (2008, 13–14).

The insufficiency and restrictive eligibility criteria for income supports across the life course are problematic for individuals and families, but the disconnect between benefits systems run by different government payers also drives financial inequity among PHAs across jurisdictions. For example, PHAs who cannot work into their mid-sixties may look to provincial disability income supports as a stopgap between work and retirement income. The amount of support they receive will then depend on the province they live in.

## CUMULATIVE IMPOVERISHMENT

Older adults' experiences and negative health risks accumulate across the life course and lead to social inequalities in morbidity and mortality later in life (Bartley, Blane, and Davey Smith 1998, 10). In addition, older adults living with HIV may experience cumulative impoverishment as they age. The concept of cumulative advantage and disadvantage, or "the systemic tendency for inter-individual divergence in a given characteristic (e.g., money, health, or status) with the passage of time" (Dannefer 2003, S327) helps us to construct an understanding of how financial precariousness and hardship experienced earlier in life can result in health inequalities in later life for people aging with HIV.

Part of the present cohort of people living for many years with HIV – sometimes referred to as long-term survivors – experienced a profound loss of social-connectedness, as well as income security, during the first wave of the AIDS epidemic (Rosenfeld, Bartlam, and Smith 2012). As described previously, the inability of many people living with HIV to work, or to work consistently, earlier in their lives may have limited personal saving and pension contributions, access to collective investments, and purchasing power for affordable housing.

Some older PHAs who did not hold jobs that provided access to long-term disability benefits have spent their entire life savings, and even cashed in their life insurance policies. This was most common among people diagnosed with HIV in the 1980s and early 1990s, who were faced with immediate financial pressures at a time when neither PHAs nor service providers thought they would live long enough to feel the repercussions of these financial decisions (Owen and Catalan 2012).

Policymakers seeking to foster income security among older PHAs must, therefore, consider the timing of an individual's diagnosis, not just chronological age. In addition, historical pre- and post-antiretroviral eras should be critically examined for how they affect the well-being of older people living with HIV today.

*Lack of Support for Aging in Place*

SOCIAL HOUSING

Housing is a key social determinant of health, and low-income populations, including many seniors and people living with disabilities, rely on social housing to address their need for shelter. Unfortunately, social housing remains poorly addressed in public policy (Raphael 2004). Canada is the only industrialized nation in the world without a national housing strategy, though one is expected in 2017, and fragmentation has been the norm for the last two decades (TSSHA 2013). This deficiency has resulted in demand that exceeds availability, and circumstances that limit secure access to social housing for people aging with HIV.

Older adults can face discrimination when renting market-rent units because they cannot provide employer letters of support to show that they can afford the rent, they are presumed to lack capacity for unit maintenance, or they may request costly accommodations from landlords (OHRC 2008, 18). PHAs may also face discriminatory housing practices (PSHP Research Team 2006). A recent study of people living with HIV found that approximately half experienced housing instability (OHTN and PSHP Research Team 2015). The study concluded that "housing instability, including inappropriate and unsafe housing, is significantly associated with poorer mental and physical health among people living with HIV" (7). An older PHA may experience the intersectional effects of both ageism and HIV stigma leading to housing instability.

HOME CARE

The possibility of aging at home is an important consideration for some older PHAs. Home care includes a variety of both publicly and privately funded medical and non-medical support services – that can enable older PHAs to continue to live independently in their own homes. Home care continues to be in a precarious condition across Canada, characterized by shifting budget allocations, and increasing demand. The adoption of a competitive market structure has produced an increased burden on informal caregivers, with questionable client satisfaction (CHCA 2013). Historically there has been tremendous advocacy in this area by seniors' groups, who fought hard for health and social care policies that would allow older adults to age in place (Finkel 2006, 163).

Of concern to older PHAs is the availability of kin and informal care-giver support, particularly given the decimated social networks some communities have experienced due to AIDS deaths and the social stigma that has often accompanied HIV. The U.S. Research on Older Adults with HIV study found that older PHAs do not have access to sufficient social support networks, and often must rely on formal care services, which can often be "ill prepared" for them (Karpiak, Shippy, and Cantor 2006, 5). Canadian research is limited in this area, but it can be reasonably assumed that some older adults living with HIV in Canada face similar challenges as they age with HIV (Wallach et al. 2013).

RETIREMENT HOMES AND LONG-TERM CARE FACILITIES

Admission to long-term care may evoke feelings of loss, anxiety, and fear (Saskatoon Health Region 2015, 15). In some cases, these negative feelings are reinforced by the poor living conditions in long-term care facilities. Poor investment in quality of care within the sector results in inadequate staffing, as well as low wages and limited opportunities for professional development for service providers (Armstrong 2009; Petch, Tierney, and Cummings 2013).

Access to retirement homes and to long-term care (LTC) facilities remains a major concern for many older PHAs (Furlotte et al. 2012, 38). It remains unclear whether retirement homes and LTC facilities are prepared to provide appropriate care for an influx of older PHAs, or whether community-based alternatives exist. Older PHAs may present unique care considerations for retirement homes and LTC facilities, including care and treatment needs (e.g., medications, services), intimate relationships and sexual identity, and the risk of social stigma (Foebel et al. 2015). HIV organizations are leading work across sectors to bring education about HIV and resources into these care environments (Murzin and Furlotte 2015).

*Health Service Accessibility Barriers*

Older PHAs are disproportionately affected by health service access barriers; two of the most significant are cost and stigma. With respect to cost, between 1995 and 2005, public funding for community-based rehabilitation services was decreased or discontinued entirely in most provinces (Gordon et al. 2007; Stabile and Ward 2007). Furthermore, many Canadians are still denied private health insurance on the basis of their HIV status. These policies contribute to community-dwelling older PHAs not being able to afford rehabilitation services (e.g., physiotherapy) that could vastly enhance their quality of life by reducing the negative impacts of HIV, treatment, and comorbidity.

The second barrier is stigma, which may be linked to age, HIV status, or both. HIV-related stigma is defined as prejudice, discounting, discrediting, and discrimination directed at people perceived to have HIV or AIDS (Herek et al. 1998). Stigmatizing encounters with service providers can limit engagement in care for older PHAs. Emlet et al. (2015) found that older PHAs reported significantly less stigma than younger PHAs, but that they tend to experience stigma via rejection, stereotyping, fear of contagion, violations of confidentiality, and internalized ageism (Emlet 2006). Anti-oppression policies and human rights policies help safeguard access to needed services for older PHAs who might otherwise face discrimination on the basis of age, HIV status, or both.

### Policy Coordination from Below: Community Responses to Policy Barriers

There are many barriers to optimal health for older PHAs, and these barriers are often reinforced by public policy. However, there is also a significant commitment to challenge the status quo, led by champions within the HIV community, including the National Coordinating Committee on HIV and Aging (NCC). Established in 2011, the NCC is a group of diverse stakeholders from across Canada (e.g., front-line service providers, researchers, academics, older adults living with HIV) who share an interest in HIV and aging. Members meet quarterly to exchange information on regional interventions that show promising potential for adaptation in other contexts, and to collaborate on joint awareness-raising, capacity-building, and policy-change initiatives that will improve the lives of older PHAs in Canada. For example, the NCC has been pushing government epidemiologists to manipulate data differently in order to give a better sense of the socio-demographic profile of older PHAs. The importance of this network is recognized by federal funders who provide financial support to Realize (formerly the Canadian Working Group on HIV and Rehabilitation), the secretariat for the NCC.

There is also work being done at the local and regional levels to improve support for older PHAs. A recent community-driven environmental scan that collected input from ninety-two service organizations across Canada confirmed that program planners are managing to creatively circumvent some of the organizational and social policies that restrict equitable access to health resources for older PHAs (Murzin and Furlotte 2015). While the majority of organizations surveyed did not offer specialized programming for older adults living with HIV, the research revealed twenty-one unique programs that were either tailor-made for or adapted to meet the needs of this population. These programs fell into four categories – health, home care, and practical support; support/peer groups; educational/informational programs; and national coordination.

Most of the policy recommendations stemming from this scan were operational: HIV organizations positioning themselves as leaders in a cross-sectoral response to HIV and aging; engaging in cross-sectoral dialogue on organizational values to ensure safer environments across the continuum of care; advocating for HIV prevention, support, and housing-related resources for older adults; and combating all forms of stigma. These recommendations are well supported by the contents of this chapter.

### Conclusion: Recommendations for Policy Action

On the basis of this analysis, we urge policymakers to take additional action at the provincial/territorial and federal government levels. First, age-based eligibility criteria for publicly funded benefits like Old Age Security and rehabilitation services should be reconsidered. These programs favour chronological age over functional capacity and are therefore inequitable. It is critical that we prevent the development and worsening of HIV and aging-related comorbidity and disability by minimizing poverty and maximizing access to health services. The elevated prevalence of mental health issues among PHAs underscores the importance of increasing the affordability and accessibility of mental health supports for this population.

Second, a cross-sectoral approach to policymaking is needed. Strategies focused on different but often overlapping populations should complement, rather than be implemented parallel to one another. An HIV strategy should explicitly mention the prevention, treatment, care, and support needs of older adults and should reference recommendations found in seniors' and chronic disease–management strategies within the same jurisdiction. A less siloed approach will ensure holistic support for PHAs and foster the creation of inclusive environments across health and social systems.

To this end, there is growing momentum behind the idea of a National Seniors' Strategy. It is vital that the HIV sector support policy change that has the potential to affect all older adults. Income supports, pensions, and housing are social determinants of health with substantial impact. Any future changes to "seniors" policy should be informed by, and relevant to, older PHAs. One way to do this is to ensure that new policies address complex and intersecting forms of exclusion.

And third, older PHAs are a relatively "new" aging population and so investment in both research and advocacy is needed if we are to fully understand and respond effectively to their needs. It is important that we rekindle the community spirit that was harnessed to tackle policy challenges in the early days of the HIV epidemic in Canada. Many older PHAs successfully struggled against the system in the early days and should be given the resources and support they need to make change again.

In many instances, public policy change could vastly improve the lives of older adults in Canada. A sustained effort is needed to change the status quo. Decision-makers must prioritize equitable outcomes, not equal investment, to improve the health and social lives of older adults living with HIV, a growing but underserved aging population in Canada.

NOTE

1 The 90-90-90 treatment target is part of a broader set of strategies proposed by UNAIDS to "end the AIDS epidemic by 2030" (Joint United Nations Programme on HIV/AIDS [UNAIDS] 2014). Widespread adoption of this target worldwide is based on shared recognition of cART as a highly effective tool for health promotion among people living with HIV as well as HIV prevention. To meet the targets, 90 per cent of people living with HIV will have been diagnosed, 90 per cent of those who have tested HIV-positive will be taking antiretroviral medication, and 90 per cent of those on treatment will have an undetectable viral load. The care cascade depicts a parallel engagement in the health-care system in which individuals are screened for HIV and are linked to, and subsequently retained in, HIV care, should they test positive.

REFERENCES

Althoff, K.N., et al. 2014. "Comparison of Risk and Age at Diagnosis of Myocardial Infarction, End-Stage Renal Disease, and Non-AIDS-Defining Cancer in HIV-Infected versus Uninfected Adults." *Clinical Infectious Diseases* 60 (4): 627–38. https://doi.org/10.1093/cid/ciu869.

Armstrong, Pat. 2009. "Long-term Care Problems: Both Residents and Care Providers Denied Fair Treatment: More, Better-Paid Staff Key to Improved Long-Term Care." *Monitor*, 1 May. https://www.policyalternatives.ca/publications/monitor/long-term-care-problems.

Arora, Paul, et al. 2013. "Prevalence Estimates of Chronic Kidney Disease in Canada: Results of a Nationally Representative Survey." *Canadian Medical Association Journal* 185 (9): E417–23. https://doi.org/10.1503/cmaj.120833.

Bartley, Mel, David Blane, and George Davey Smith, eds. 1998. *The Sociology of Health Inequalities*. Maldan, MA: Blackwell Publishers.

Beckerman, N.L., and C. Auerbach. 2010. "Post-traumatic Stress Disorder and HIV: A Snapshot of Co-Occurrence." *Social Work in Health Care* 49 (8): 687–702. https://doi.org/10.1080/00981389.2010.485089.

Brennan, David J., et al. 2013. "Socio-demographic Profile of Older Adults with HIV/AIDS: Gender and Sexual Orientation Differences." *Canadian Journal on Aging* 32 (1): 31–43. https://doi.org/10.1017/S0714980813000068.

Canadian Home Care Association (CHCA). 2013. *Portraits of Home Care in Canada*. http://www.cdnhomecare.ca/media.php?mid=3394.

Canadian Institute for Health Information (CIHI). 2011. "Seniors and the Health Care System: What Is the Impact of Multiple Chronic Conditions?" https://secure.cihi.ca/free_products/air-chronic_disease_aib_en.pdf.

Canadian Public Health Association (CPHA). 2005. *Leading Together: Canada Takes Action on HIV/AIDS (2005–2010)*. http://www.leadingtogether.ca/pdf/Leading_Together.pdf.

Cescon, Angela, et al. 2015. "Late Initiation of Combination Antiretroviral Therapy in Canada: A Call for a National Public Health Strategy to Improve Engagement in HIV Care." *Journal of the International AIDS Society* 18 (1). https://doi.org/10.7448/IAS.18.1.20024.

Crothers, Kristina, et al. 2011. "HIV Infection and Risk for Incident Pulmonary Diseases in the Combination Antiretroviral Therapy Era." *American Journal of Respiratory and Critical Care Medicine* 183 (3): 388–95. https://doi.org/10.1164/rccm.201006-0836OC.

Dannefer, Dale. 2003. "Cumulative Advantage/Disadvantage and the Life Course: Cross-Fertilizing Age and Social Science Theory." *Journals of Gerontology* 58 (6): S327–37. https://doi.org/10.1093/geronb/58.6.S327.

Desquilbet, Loic, et al. 2007. "HIV-1 Infection Is Associated with an Earlier Occurrence of a Phenotype Related to Frailty." *Journals of Gerontology* 62A (11): 1279–86. https://doi.org/10.1093/gerona/62.11.1279.

Emlet, Charles A. 2006. "'You're Awfully Old to Have *This* Disease': Experiences of Stigma and Ageism in Adults 50 Years and Older Living with HIV/AIDS." *Gerontologist* 46 (6): 781–90. https://doi.org/10.1093/geront/46.6.781.

Emlet, Charles A., et al. 2015. "The Impact of HIV-Related Stigma on Older and Younger Adults Living with HIV Disease: Does Age Matter?" *AIDS Care* 27 (4): 520–8. https://doi.org/10.1080/09540121.2014.978734.

Emlet, Charles A., et al. 2016. "'I'm happy in my life now, I'm a positive person': Approaches to Successful Ageing in Older Ddults Living with HIV." *Ageing and Society*, 1–24. https://doi.org/10.1017/S0144686X16000878.

Finkel, Alvin. 2006. "Social Policy and the Elderly, 1950–80." In *Social Policy and Practice in Canada: A History*, ed. Alvin Finkel, 151–68. Waterloo, ON: Wilfrid Laurier University Press.

Foebel, Andrea, et al. 2015. "Comparing the Characteristics of People Living with and without HIV in Long-term Care and Home Care in Ontario, Canada." *AIDS Care* 27 (10): 1343–53. https://doi.org/10.1080/09540121.2015.1058893.

Fullerton, Merrilee. 2008. "Understanding and Improving on 1 Problem per Visit." *Canadian Medical Association Journal* 179 (7): 623. https://doi.org/10.1503/cmaj.081239.

Furlotte, Charles, et al. 2012. "Got a room for me?' Housing Experiences of Older Adults Living with HIV/AIDS in Ottawa." *Canadian Journal on Aging* 31 (1): 37–48. https://doi.org/10.1017/S0714980811000584.

Furlotte, Charles, and Karen Schwartz. 2017. "Mental Health Experiences of Older Adults Living with HIV: Uncertainty, Stigma and Approaches to Resilience." *Canadian Journal on Aging* 36 (2): 125–40.

Gahagan, Jacqueline, et al. 2012. *HIV and Rehabilitation: Bridging Policy and Practice: A Scan of Policies Related to Access to Rehabilitation in Canada and the United Kingdom*. Halifax: Department of Health Promotion, Dalhousie University.

Gangbar, Kira, and Jason Globerman. 2014. *Rapid Response: Posttraumatic Stress Disorders among People Living with HIV/AIDS*. Toronto: Ontario HIV Treatment Network.

Gordon, Melanie, et al. 2007. "The Consequences of Delisting Publicly Funded, Community-Based Physical Therapy Services in Ontario: A Health Policy Analysis." *Physiotherapy Canada / Physiotherapie Canada* 59 (1): 58–69. https://doi.org/10.3138/ptc.59.1.58.

Gouvernement du Québec, Commissaire à la santé et au bien-être. 2010. *Appraisal Report on the Performance of the Health and Social Services System: Adopting an Integrated Approach to Chronic Disease Prevention and Management: Recommendation, Issues and Implications.* http://www.csbe.gouv.qc.ca/fileadmin/www/2010/MaladiesChroniques/CSBE_T4_Recommandations2010.pdf.

Gouvernement du Québec, Ministère de la Famille et des Aînés et Ministère de la Santé et des Services sociaux. 2012. *Vieillir et vivre ensemble: Chez soi, dans sa communauté, au Québec.* https://www.mfa.gouv.qc.ca/fr/publication/Documents/politique-vieillir-et-vivre-ensemble.pdf.

Government of British Columbia. 2012. "Improving Care for B.C. Seniors: An Action Plan." http://www2.gov.bc.ca/assets/gov/people/seniors/about-seniorsbc/pdf/seniorsactionplan.pdf.

Government of Canada. 2012. "Canada's Health Care System." https://www.canada.ca/en/health-canada/services/health-care-system/reports-publications/health-care-system/canada.html#a5.

Government of Manitoba. 2015. "Manitoba Sexually Transmitted and Blood-Borne Infections Strategy 2015–2019." http://www.gov.mb.ca/health/publichealth/cdc/sti/strategy.html.

Government of New Brunswick, Department of Health, Primary Health Care Branch, Addiction, Mental Health and Primary Care Division. 2010. "A Chronic Disease Prevention and Management Framework for New Brunswick." https://www.gnb.ca/0051/pub/pdf/2010/6960e-final.pdf.

Government of New Brunswick, Premier's Panel on Seniors. 2012. "Living Healthy, Aging Well." http://www2.gnb.ca/content/dam/gnb/Corporate/pdf/LivingHealthyAgingWell.pdf.

Government of Newfoundland and Labrador, Department of Health and Community Services. 2007. "Provincial Healthy Aging Policy Framework." http://www.cssd.gov.nl.ca/seniors/phapf/.

– 2011. "Improving Health Together: A Policy Framework for Chronic Disease Prevention and Management in Newfoundland and Labrador." http://www.health.gov.nl.ca/health/chronicdisease/cdcontrol.html#improv.

Government of Northwest Territories, Health and Social Services. 2014. "Our Elders: Our Communities." http://www.assembly.gov.nt.ca/tabled-documents/our-elders-our-communities.

Government of Nova Scotia Seniors' Secretariat. 2005. "Strategy for Positive Aging in Nova Scotia." https://novascotia.ca/seniors/pub/2005_StrategyPositiveAging.pdf.

Government of Nunavut. 2017. "Strategic Framework: Addressing the Needs of Nunavut Seniors." http://assembly.nu.ca/sites/default/files/

TD-285-4(3)-EN-Strategic-Freamework-Addressing-the-Needs-of-Nunavut-Seniors.pdf.

Government of Ontario, Ministry of Health and Long-Term Care. 2007. "Preventing and Managing Chronic Disease: Ontario's Framework." http://www.health.gov.on.ca/en/pro/programs/cdpm/pdf/framework_full.pdf.

Government of Ontario, Seniors' Secretariat. 2013. "Independence, Activity and Good Health: Ontario's Action Plan for Seniors." http://www.oacao.org/images/ontarioseniorsactionplan-en.pdf.

Grov, Christian, et al. 2010. "Loneliness and HIV-Related Stigma Explain Depression among Older HIV-Positive Adults." *AIDS Care* 22 (5): 630–9. https://doi.org/10.1080/09540120903280901.

Halkitis, Perry N. 2014. *The AIDS Generation: Stories of Survival and Resilience.* New York: Oxford University Press.

Health PEI, Community Hospitals and Primary Health Care Division. 2013. "Stemming the Tide: Health PEI Chronic Disease Prevention and Management Framework 2013–2018." http://www.gov.pe.ca/publications/getpublication.php3?number=2124.

Herek, Gregory M., et al. 1998. "Workshop Report: AIDS and Stigma; A Conceptual Framework and Research Agenda." *AIDS & Public Policy Journal* 13 (1): 36–47

Joint United Nations Programme on HIV/AIDS (UNAIDS). 2014. *Fast Track: Ending the AIDS Epidemic by 2030.* http://www.unaids.org/sites/default/files/media_asset/JC2686_WAD2014report_en.pdf.

Joyce, Geoffrey, et al. 2005. "A Socioeconomic Profile of Older Adults with HIV." *Journal of Health Care for the Poor and Underserved* 16 (1): 19–28. https://doi.org/10.1353/hpu.2005.0013.

Kahana, E., and B. Kahana. 2001. "Successful Aging among People with HIV/AIDS." *Journal of Clinical Epidemiology* 54 (12): S53–6. https://doi.org/10.1016/S0895-4356(01)00447-4.

Karpiak, Stephen E., R. Andrew Shippy, and Marjorie Cantor. 2006. *Research on Older Adults with HIV.* New York: AIDS Community Research Initiative of America.

Kendall, Claire, et al. 2015. "A Population-Based Study Comparing Patterns of Care Delivery on the Quality of Care for Persons Living with HIV in Ontario." *BMJ Open.* http://bmjopen.bmj.com/content/5/5/e007428.

Law Commission of Ontario (LCO). 2008. "The Law as It Affects Older Adults: Moving the Project Forward; Report on the Preliminary Consultation." https://www.lco-cdo.org/wp-content/uploads/2010/10/older-adults_Older%20Adults%20Consultation%20Paper%20-%20January%202009.pdf.

– 2012. "Vulnerable Workers and Precarious Work." http://www.lco-cdo
.org/wp-content/uploads/2013/03/vulnerable-workers-final-report.pdf.

Leading Together Championing Committee (LTCC). 2013. "Leading Together:
Canada Takes Action on HIV/AIDS." http://www.catie.ca/sites/default/
files/Leading%20Together_Final%20EN%20November%202013.pdf.

Moore, Raeanne C., et al. 2013. "A Case-Controlled Study of Successful Aging
in Older HIV-Infected Adults." *Journal of Clinical Psychiatry* 74 (5): e417–23.
https://doi.org/10.4088/JCP.12m08100.

Moore, Richard D., Jeanne C. Keruly, and John G. Bartlett. 2012.
"Improvement in the Health of HIV-Infected Persons in Care: Reducing
Disparities." *Clinical Infectious Diseases* 55 (9): 1242–51. https://doi
.org/10.1093/cid/cis654.

Murzin, Kate, and Charles Furlotte. 2015. "HIV & Aging: A 2013
Environmental Scan of Programs and Services in Canada – Community
Report." http://realizecanada.org/wp-content/uploads/Community-
Report-EN-Web-Ready-Low-Resolution.pdf.

Nova Scotia Advisory Commission on AIDS (NSACA). 2014. "Review of
Nova Scotia's Strategy on HIV/AIDS: Looking Back & Moving Forward."
http://novascotia.ca/aids/documents/Review-of-Nova-Scotia-Strategy-
on-HIV-AIDS-Executive-Summary.pdf.

Office of the Auditor General of Alberta. 2014. "Report of the Auditor General
of Alberta: Health – Chronic Disease Management." https://www.oag
.ab.ca/webfiles/reports/OAGSept2014Report.pdf.

Ontario Advisory Committee on HIV/AIDS. 2017. "Focusing Our Efforts:
Changing the Course of the HIV Prevention, Engagement and Care
Cascade in Ontario – HIV/AIDS Strategy to 2026." http://www.health
.gov.on.ca/en/pro/programs/hivaids/docs/oach_strategy_2026.pdf.

Ontario HIV Treatment Network (OHTN) and the Positive Spaces Healthy
Places (PSHP) Research Team. 2015. "HIV, Housing and Health: Research
in Action." http://www.ohtn.on.ca/wp-content/uploads/reports/
positive-spaces-healthy-places-pshp-report.pdf.

Ontario Human Rights Commission (OHRC). 2008. "Right at Home: Report
on the Consultation on Human Rights and Rental Housing in Ontario."
http://www.ohrc.on.ca/sites/default/files/attachments/Right_at_
home%3A_Report_on_the_consultation_on_human_rights_and_rental_
housing_in_Ontario.pdf.

Owen, Garath, and Jose Catalan. 2012. "'We never expected this to happen':
Narratives of Ageing with HIV among Gay Men Living in London, UK."
*Culture, Health and Sexuality* 14 (1): 59–72. https://doi.org/10.1080/1369105
8.2011.621449.

Patterson, Sophie, et al. 2015. "Life Expectancy of HIV-Positive Individuals on Combination Antiretroviral Therapy in Canada." *BMC Infectious Diseases* 15 (1). https://doi.org/10.1186/s12879-015-0969-x.

Petch, Jeremy, Mike Tierney, and Greta Cummings. 2013. "Improving Quality in Canada's Nursing Homes Requires 'More Staff, More Training.'" Healthy Debate, 20 June. http://healthydebate.ca/2013/06/topic/quality/improving-quality-in-canadas-nursing-homes-requires-more-staff-more-training.

Positive Spaces Healthy Places (PSHP) Research Team. 2006. "Fact Sheet #2: Stigma and Discrimination in Housing." Accessed 25 November 2015. http://www.pshp.ca/documents/fact-sheets/2006-PSHP-Fact-Sheet-Stigma.pdf.

Provincial HIV/AIDS Strategy Steering Committee. 2003. *Nova Scotia's Strategy on HIV/AIDS.* http://novascotia.ca/aids/documents/HIV-AIDS%20Stratgy-Full%20Report.pdf.

Public Health Agency of Canada (PHAC). 2014. *HIV and AIDS in Canada: Surveillance Report to December 31, 2013.* http://www.phac-aspc.gc.ca/aids-sida/publication/survreport/2013/dec/assets/pdf/hiv-aids-surveillence-eng.pdf.

Raphael, Dennis, ed. 2004. *Social Determinants of Health: Canadian Perspectives.* Toronto: Canadian Scholars' Press.

Robertson, Kevin, et al. 2014. "Screening for Neurocognitive Impairment, Depression, and Anxiety in HIV-Infected Patients in Western Europe and Canada." *AIDS Care* 26 (12): 1555–61. https://doi.org/10.1080/09540121.2014.936813.

Rodger, Alison J., et al. 2013. "Mortality in Well Controlled HIV in the Continuous Antiretroviral Therapy Arms of the SMART and ESPRIT Trials Compared with the General Population." *AIDS (London, England)* 27 (6): 973–9.

Romanow, Roy J. 2002. *Building on Values: The Future of Health Care in Canada.* Commission on the Future of Health Care in Canada. http://publications.gc.ca/collections/Collection/CP32-85-2002E.pdf.

Romo, Rafael D., et al. 2013. "Perceptions of Successful Aging among Diverse Elders with Late-Life Disability." *Gerontologist* 53 (6): 939–49. https://doi.org/10.1093/geront/gns160.

Rosenfeld, Dana, Bernadette Bartlam, and Ruth D. Smith. 2012. "Out of the Closet and into the Trenches: Gay Male Baby Boomers, Aging, and HIV/AIDS." *Gerontologist* 52 (2): 255–64. https://doi.org/10.1093/geront/gnr138.

Rosenfeld, Dana, et al. 2014. "Vital Scientific Puzzle or Lived Uncertainty? Professional and Lived Approaches to Uncertainties of Ageing with HIV."

*Health Sociology Review* 23 (1): 20–32. https://doi.org/10.5172/hesr
.2014.23.1.20.

Rowe, John W., and Robert L. Kahn. 2015. "Successful Aging 2.0: Conceptual
Expansions for the 21st Century." *Journals of Gerontology. Series B, Psychological
Sciences and Social Sciences* 70 (4): 593–6. https://doi.org/10.1093/geronb/
gbv025.

Rueda, Sergio, et al. 2015. "Is Any Job Better Than No Job? Labor Market
Experiences and Depressive Symptoms in People Living with HIV." *AIDS
Care* 27 (7): 907–15. https://doi.org/10.1080/09540121.2015.1015479.

Saskatchewan Ministry of Health. 2012. "Patient Centred, Community
Designed, Team Delivered: A Framework for Achieving a High Performing
Primary Health Care System in Saskatchewan." https://www.saskatchewan
.ca/~/media/files/health/additional%20reports/other%20ministry%
20plans%20and%20reports/primary%20health%20care.pdf.

Saskatoon Health Region. 2015. *Welcome Guide to Long Term Care Communities.*
https://www.saskatoonhealthregion.ca/locations_services/Services/
Senior-Health/Documents/ResidentFamilyResourcesPage/LTC%
20Welcome%20Guide%20Final%20June%209%20Optimized.pdf.

Schouten, Judith, et al. 2014. "Cross-sectional Comparison of the Prevalence
of Age-Associated Comorbidities and Their Risk Factors between HIV-
Infected and Uninfected Individuals: The AGEhIV Cohort Study." *Clinical
Infectious Diseases* 59 (12): 1787–97. https://doi.org/10.1093/cid/ciu701.

Sherr, L., et al. 2011. "HIV Infection Associated Post-traumatic Stress
Disorder and Post-traumatic Growth: A Systematic Review." *Psychology
Health and Medicine* 16 (5): 612–29. https://doi.org/10.1080/13548506
.2011.579991.

Solomon, Patricia, et al. 2014. "Aging with HIV and Disability: The Role of
Uncertainty." *AIDS Care* 26 (2): 240–5. https://doi.org/10.1080/09540121
.2013.811209.

Squire, Corinne. 2013. "From HIV's Exceptionalism to HIV's Particularity." In
*Living with HIV and ARVs: Three Letter Lives*, ed. C. Squire, 12–50. London:
Palgrave. https://doi.org/10.1057/9781137313676_2.

Stabile, Mark, and Courtney Ward. 2007. "The Effects of De-listing Publicly
Funded Health Care Services." In *Restructuring in Canada: New Evidence and
New Directions*, ed. Charles M. Beach, Richard P. Chaykowski, Sam Shortt,
France St-Hilaire, and Arthur Sweetman, 83–110. Montreal and Kingston:
McGill-Queen's University Press.

Statistics Canada. 2013. "Cholesterol Levels of Canadians, 2009 to 2011."
http://www.statcan.gc.ca/pub/82-625-x/2012001/article/11732-eng.htm.

Toronto Shelter, Support & Housing Administration (TSSHA). 2013. "2014–2019 Housing Stability Service Planning Framework." http://www.toronto.ca/legdocs/mmis/2013/cd/bgrd/backgroundfile-64008.pdf.

Vance, David E., et al. 2011. "Aging with HIV: A Cross-Sectional Study of Comorbidity Prevalence and Clinical Characteristics across Decades of Life." *Journal of the Association of Nurses in AIDS Care* 22 (1): 17–25. https://doi.org/10.1016/j.jana.2010.04.002.

Vance, D.E., T.C. Struzick, and J. Masten. 2008. "Hardiness, Successful Aging, and HIV: Implications for Social Work." *Journal of Gerontological Social Work* 51 (3–4): 260–83. https://doi.org/10.1080/01634370802039544.

Wallach, I., et al. 2013. "Le VIH et le vieillissement au Québec: Une recherché qualitative sur les expériences, les difficultés et les besoins des personnes vivant avec le VIH de 50 ans et plus." http://www.realizecanada.org/wp-content/uploads/Wallachetal_2013_RapportVIHvieillissement1.pdf.

# 6 Evaluation Policy at AIDS Service Organizations: Managing Multiple Accountabilities

NICOLE R. GREENSPAN

Community-based HIV prevention programs have been key in the response to HIV for the past thirty years. However, quantitatively capturing the effectiveness of the HIV prevention work carried out by these organizations, in a manner that might direct funding or programmatic decisions, has remained elusive. This has been a challenge in the context of increases in rates of new infections across several jurisdictions and populations in Canada, including men who have sex with men in Ontario, and various communities in Saskatchewan. For example, quantitative data on the impact of HIV prevention work have not been able to illuminate which programs are most needed among these communities. There have been calls to assess how HIV prevention might be more effective (Adam et al. 2007). In addition, over the past decade there has been an increase in the amount of monitoring and evaluation required by governments who provide funding for community-based organizations. Both are part of a social shift towards an "audit society," where previously trusted professionals and institutions are subject to more scrutiny, regulation, and monitoring (Power 2005). How this social shift has affected the practice of community-based HIV prevention is not well understood.

This chapter examines the impacts of this social shift on the practice of community-based HIV prevention. It provides insight into how community-based AIDS service organizations (ASOs) understand and evaluate their HIV prevention work, and how changes in evaluation policy have affected these organizations. It then highlights the role that tacit knowledge plays in evaluating HIV prevention, drawing on the lived experience of people living with and most affected by HIV. Tacit knowledge is important, not only for the insight it provides to challenging questions, but how it illuminates information derived from other sources and makes it meaningful to communities most affected by HIV. This chapter also provides recommendations for evaluation policymakers and practitioners, which can contribute to a more effective and responsive HIV movement in Canada. This chapter focuses on the kind of knowledge that ASOs draw on to make decisions about HIV prevention programs. While important questions remain about assessing the effectiveness of these programs, they are beyond the scope of this chapter.

In the first section, I discuss the key role community-based organizations have played, and continue to play, in Canada's HIV response; I also describe the intensification of monitoring and evaluation in the community sector, in order to set the stage for understanding the current state of evaluation practice at ASOs. The next section describes some of the results from empirical research I conducted with ASOs in Ontario, which show that evaluation practices are complex and assist in a collective "sense-making" of HIV prevention work within and across diverse communities (Greenspan 2015). The final section addresses ideal evaluation practice and policy and provides recommendations to harness the potential of evaluation to help enhance the responsiveness of HIV prevention work.

## ASOs as a Response to the HIV Epidemic

Community-based HIV prevention has been influenced by a number of international, national, and local factors, including Canada's distinctive organization and delivery of health services, which are funded by both federal and provincial sources, but delivered provincially and locally. Specific Canadian institutions and actors have developed over time in order to respond to local issues and contexts related to HIV, such as national not-for-profit groups, provincial governmental departments, and local AIDS organizations. Community-based ASOs have been, and continue to be, an important piece of the Canadian national response to HIV. Their key role has been acknowledged in federal initiatives to address HIV, including the National AIDS Strategy (1990), and the Federal Initiative to Address HIV/AIDS in Canada (2004), which is a partnership of the Public Health Agency of Canada (PHAC), Health Canada, the Canadian Institutes of Health Research (CIHR) and Correctional Service Canada, and the main source of federal funding for HIV in Canada (Government of Canada 2004). ASOs are expected to use government funds to help reach communities most affected by HIV, to serve the needs of these communities, and provide them with tailored responses in order to address the epidemic in a responsive, timely, and effective way (ibid.). While ASOs are diverse, they share a history of emerging as a response to HIV with the intention of reflecting and responding to community concerns about the epidemic, which are often made up of people from socially marginalized groups that have been neglected or served poorly by traditional health care and social service providers (Altman 1994; Miller and Greene 2005). Early in the AIDS epidemic in Canada, government inaction prompted community groups to form in several major urban centres, in order to provide needed support, services, and education, and to promote policy change (Rayside and Lindquist 1992). Changes occurred when the AIDS movement secured government funds to support AIDS work, but this also changed the nature of the work carried out and shaped community-based AIDS organizations' agendas (Kinsman 1997). As Cain described (1993, 1995), ASOs in Ontario became more formalized and bureaucratic in the early to mid-1990s, and the political nature of their work changed, along with the strategies they employed. This was related to these organizations' reliance on state funding, rather than building organizations that relied solely on community membership and financial support (Cain 1995). While initially tied to larger social movements and political agendas (e.g., addressing poverty, homophobia, and other drivers of inequality), many of these goals were more ambitious and ambiguous than could be carried out once ASOs' relationships with government funders became routinized and integrated (ibid.).

ASOs still face pressures on the scope of their HIV work (Miller and Greene 2005). The mandate of most ASOs includes providing social support for people living with HIV and education for those who are not HIV-positive, as well as promoting social change (ibid.). The kinds of expertise that are required to carry out these functions may differ, and resources at ASOs are often limited. Some of these resource limitations have promoted a push to increase the evidence base of HIV prevention programs and services, and to use this research to inform and evaluate community-based HIV prevention practice in Canada. For example, CIHR and the Ontario HIV Treatment Network (OHTN) actively promote the use and production of research in community-based HIV programming (Flicker et al. 2009). In addition, federal Treasury Board rules require that all government programs (including the Federal Initiative to Address HIV/AIDS in Canada) evaluate their success and demonstrate their return on investment using a results-based management and accountability framework. The Federal Initiative to Address HIV/AIDS in Canada funds the HIV prevention work of community-based organizations. Reports on this program have identified the need for increasing evaluation capacity at community-based organizations (Natalie Kishchuk Research and Evaluation 2010), and emphasized the importance of tracking and monitoring government-funded HIV programs (Evaluation Directorate 2014). These pressures – to increase the use of research in community-based HIV prevention work, and to monitor and evaluate the work carried out by ASOs – are some of the tensions that characterize the relationship among ASOs, government funders, and the communities they serve, and are part of a broader shift towards evidence-based policy and practice noted in social services sectors in Canada and elsewhere.

HIV prevention is, admittedly, a complex undertaking (Auerbach, Parkhurst, and Cáceres 2011; Piot et al. 2008). Early prevention efforts involved providing basic information about HIV transmission, but this is not sufficient to reduce HIV transmission rates (Adam et al. 2007). Current common HIV prevention interventions include condom distribution, social marketing, and other interventions aimed at reducing HIV risk behaviours. Some of these are community-level interventions aimed at communities at higher risk of HIV (e.g., social marketing media campaigns aimed at men who have sex with men). While it is recommended that a variety of interventions be used to best reach target populations, the lack of consistent definitions or classifications can make it difficult to use standardized monitoring and evaluation techniques. This can contribute to the tensions that ASOs and their funders face in decision-making about which work to fund and carry out, given their limited resources.

Although the relationships between people from HIV-affected communities and ASOs are complex, these organizations play a significant role in providing HIV prevention and support programs, delivering HIV-specific strategies, and providing HIV-related education or leadership. People who work for ASOs often represent a collective social identity (e.g., gay men, people who use drugs, etc.) or form one in response to being similarly affected by HIV (Altman 1994; Miller and Greene 2005). Many people who work and volunteer at ASOs are from the communities that are strongly affected by HIV. The knowledge acquired by people who work or volunteer at ASOs, accumulated through their lived experience of HIV, thus contributes significantly to the work carried out by these organizations. ASO prevention workers in Ontario have reported bringing "their skills, past experience, passions, politics, and perseverance to the work" (Guenter et al. 2001, 45). While these workers reported perceiving their work as contributing to social change, the ways in which they drew on their lived experience and other knowledge they held has been unexplored; however, it is important to understand for evaluation practice. Moreover, the ways in which monitoring and evaluation practice in the community sector as a whole have developed are important in order to understand the organizational environment. This will be explored in the next section.

## The Rise of the "Audit Society"

The rise of the "audit society" has been characterized by the intensification of accountability, monitoring, and evaluation across sectors (including the community-based sector). Michael Power has been a prolific author in this area. He contends that Canada, like New Zealand and the United Kingdom, experienced an explosion in monitoring, beginning in the late 1980s and the 1990s, as a response to "political demands for greater accountability of public service providers [which were] tightly coupled to a neo-liberal preference for exercising economic control at a distance through the 'managerialist' instruments of accounting, budgetary control, auditing and quality assurance" (Power 2003, 191). Power (2000, 2005) showed that monitoring intensified without a critical understanding of these practices and their consequences, and suggested that this may be, fundamentally, an ideologically driven system for disciplining and controlling professionals in the public sector that were once regarded as experts and, therefore, not an instrument of genuine accountability. To Power (2000), making organizations and the work they carry out "auditable" has had "much to do with agendas for control of these organizations" (114). Performance measurement systems "create and support a window on organizational life, one which is often demanded by outside agencies, and which makes various kinds of internal and external intervention possible" (114). Given the tensions in the community-based response to HIV about who are the real "experts," and the complicated relationships between ASOs, governments, and the communities they intend to serve, these issues about "auditability" and power are particularly relevant.

There has been an intensification of monitoring and evaluation in health, social services, and the community sector for many years (Patton

2008; Freeman 2002; Feller 2002; Bowerman, Raby, and Humphrey 2000; Price et al. 2016). In particular, there has been a move towards monitoring for results; some even suggest that the current political environment is one of "outcomes mania" (Patton 2008, 248). "Results-based management" – a facet of New Public Management where managerial decision-making is based on outcomes – is said to increase accountability and improve programs and managerial decision-making (ibid.). However, there have been reports of the symbolic and ceremonial use of performance measurement systems, and their failure to improve performance valued by managers across jurisdictions (Feller 2002).

There is limited understanding about what the intensification of monitoring and evaluating looks like in practice, and what consequences it has had on community-based practice. Research has showed that public sector organizations (health care, police, and schools) in the United Kingdom have been subject to intensified monitoring, but the connections between these activities, external verification, and public accountability are a struggle (Bowerman, Raby, and Humphrey 2000), leading some to suggest that there is more of an "audit mess" than a coherent "audit society."

## Accountability

One driver of the intensification of monitoring and evaluation is the need to show accountability (Alkin 2013). Accountability is not a static concept, however. Aucoin and Jarvis (2005) described how within government, virtually everyone to whom an account is due is also accountable to someone else at a higher level, with the ultimate authority resting on the electorate. This has been described as the problem of "many eyes" in accountability, where there is a long list of potential stakeholders (who value a multitude of norms) that demand answers about programs (Bemelmans-Videc 2007). Many authors have called for careful consideration of issues such as who is being held accountable, to whom, for what, how, and with what consequences (Rogers 2005; Bemelmans-Videc, Lonsdale, and Perrin 2007).

Traditionally, accountability has focused on deriving information about the process or impact of government-funded work on external audiences, to confer credibility and legitimacy on the work and the distribution of government funds to service providers who undertake this work. Some question whether or not the goals of this traditional view of accountability are actually being achieved, citing that although there is increasing monitoring and evaluation, there is greater distrust from the general public towards government institutions (Bemelmans-Videc, Lonsdale, and Perrin 2007; Feller 2002; Freeman 2002). There has been a push to incorporate learning and practice improvement as a necessary part of the monitoring and evaluation practices that create accountability and confer legitimacy and credibility (Mayne 2007; Auditor General of Canada 2002; Perrin 2007). Some have questioned the meaningfulness of evaluation that solely meets the traditional demand for accountability: "Demand for evaluation ... may be motivated by a genuine desire to learn from experience, or merely to meet a bureaucratic requirement with no intention of using the gathered information. If the demand is genuine, evaluation information will potentially be used to help improve projects and programs ... However, if information is merely being collected as a bureaucratic ritual, there is little reason to expect any quality in the data, any motivation on the part of those generating the data to ensure accuracy or any substantial trust in the enterprise" (Rist quoted in Owen 2007, 191).

However, evaluation for the purpose of accountability differs from evaluation for facilitating improvements (or generating knowledge) in terms of modes of inquiry, suggested methods, and audiences (Mark, Henry, and Julnes 2000; Patton 2008). For example, critical literature about the "explosion" of performance measurement in social programs has highlighted the differences in indicators and practices that are intended to provide accountability, compared to those that are intended for learning and improvement (Freeman 2002; Power 2000; Price et al. 2016). Conflicts and complications can arise when evaluation tries to achieve too much, or serve too many audiences, ultimately fulfilling none of its objectives particularly well (Mark, Henry, and Julnes 2000; Lehtonen 2005).

These tensions about what is needed to be accountable, and whether learning or program improvement is required to confer legitimacy and maintain relationships with government funders matters when exploring what influences evaluation practice at ASOs; these helped frame my research into what influences evaluation practice, described in the next section.

## Evaluation Practice at ASOs

From 2011 to 2014, I conducted a qualitative case study of two ASOs in Ontario: a large ASO with relatively significant resources for HIV prevention programming and evaluation that serves multiple populations, and a smaller ASO with fewer resources for HIV prevention programming and evaluation that targets a specific racialized population. In this study, I employed some of the principles of community-based research, and used ethnographic methods to study the ASOs, including in-depth interviews with service providers and their funders, reviewing documents that related to program planning and evaluation, and I attended some meetings as a participant observer.

I interviewed eighteen service providers and five funders with a range of experience in the response to HIV. I reviewed roughly 100 documents related to HIV prevention programming and evaluation, and I attended meetings about monitoring and evaluation. To analyse the data, I employed interpretive description (Thorne 2008), and verified my findings in an iterative process with a community advisory committee.

I employed a broad, inclusive definition of evaluation. *Evaluation practice* was defined as "a set of practices that involve developing an action-oriented understanding that assists in the practical reasoning and reflection about a program or activity"; this definition draws on literature that understands evaluation as "assisted sense-making" (Julnes and Mark 1998; Mark, Henry, and Julnes 1999, 2000). Evaluation practice was understood as aiming to capture, make sense of, and assess programs for multiple purposes (such as assessing merit or worth, for oversight and compliance, for program improvement, or knowledge development) (Mark, Henry, and Julnes 2000), as well as other purposes that emerge in practice, such as to increase critical reflection, or to "tell the story" of a program.

The promotion of programmatic decision-making based on research, monitoring, and evaluation is influenced by a movement towards "evidence-based" and/or "evidence-informed practice" seen in many health and social service fields (Fink 2013; Brownson, Fielding, and Maylahn 2009; Armstrong et al. 2007; Roberts and Yeager 2006) in the United States and internationally (Korda 2013).

Locally, there have been a number of efforts to support community-based organizations with research and evaluation related to HIV programming in Ontario. These have occurred within the dense network of institutional actors that influence programming and evaluation practice at ASOs in Ontario. The largest provincial funder, the Ontario Ministry of Health and Long-Term Care's AIDS Bureau (AIDS Bureau) funded the Community-Linked Evaluation AIDS Resource (CLEAR) Unit at McMaster University from 1999 to 2007 to carry out research, evaluation, and capacity-building with community-based organizations receiving AIDS Bureau funding throughout the province (see fhs.mcmaster.ca/slru/clear/home.htm). Since 2008, the OHTN has offered a Rapid Response Service to ASOs in Ontario, to increase their access to research evidence and support evidence-informed programs, service delivery, and advocacy (see http://www.ohtn.on.ca/services-for-asos/rapid-response-service/). In addition, the OHTN Evidence-Based Practice Unit (EBPU) provides assistance with evaluation, creates guidelines for services at ASOs, and helps develop "a culture of accountability and continuous quality improvement" (OHTN 2013, 2). The EBPU brings together two monitoring and evaluation initiatives funded by the AIDS Bureau: the Ontario Community-Based Agency Services Evaluation (OCASE) and the Ontario Community-Based HIV and AIDS Reporting Tool (OCHART). OCHART is a collaborative project of the Ontario Regional Office of PHAC and the AIDS Bureau; it is a system that these two funders use to monitor the work carried out at organizations they fund. It includes a website (www.ochart.ca) where funded organizations complete and submit monitoring reports. The data that these organizations submit are analysed and summarized in a yearly report called *View from the Frontlines*. The funders also host an annual Knowledge Translation & Exchange (KTE) Day to review and discuss the report with organizations that receive funding. I examined this dense network of actors in detail in my qualitative case study.

Overall, my study found that despite differences in size of the organizations, there were common practices: discrete one-time evaluations, routine monitoring, and tacit assessments, which informed each other in complex ways. In addition, relationships were an important theme: they indicated programmatic success; and monitoring and evaluation practices helped maintain relationships between organizations and their funders. Accountability to government funders required monitoring and evaluation that was different from what was needed to maintain relationships with the communities these organizations served. Community-based discernment strategies that helped these organizations build knowledge merged their tacit knowledge and experiences with formal research were an important part of practice. The rest of this chapter will focus on the important role of tacit knowledge in ASO work. Government funders require explicit information derived from standardized monitoring and evaluation, and tacit knowledge is relied upon to make that information meaningful.

## The Many Faces of Evaluation

My study identified evaluation practices in HIV prevention programs employed by ASOs, and explored what influences those practices. Such practices are complex because it is difficult to classify HIV programs (Akers and Hervey 2003) – the size and scope of what is considered a "program" varied considerably, therefore assessing or comparing them in a standardized way was very difficult. Complexity was also introduced because multiple kinds of evaluation were being undertaken at these organizations concurrently, such as discrete one-time evaluations, formal routine monitoring, and tacit assessment. Some were intended to be connected to each other, but in practice they did not connect or inform each other well, so they increased the complexity of evaluation practice. An example of this is how routine monitoring for funders and tacit assessments informed each other.

Routine monitoring for funders was the most explicit evaluation practice carried out by this community of practice. Government monitoring requirements were complicated and detailed. Each reporting tool had its own format and internal logic that organized the data that agencies were required to submit, and agencies usually had several government grants with distinct reporting systems to manage. Even funders themselves recognized that filling out all these monitoring forms was a burden. As one funder described it,

> There is this constant tension ... between this incessant demand for very specific indicators and very specific evidence of particular types of change, and at the same time, there was a Blue Ribbon panel, probably close to seven years ago ... that recommended that we should be reducing the reporting burden of our funded projects and that we should just be collecting a couple of really key indicators and not overburdening them with ... big twenty-page reports. So we keep hearing that, and that's direction that we also hear from senior management, but we also hear, "But you need to collect all this really specific information."

The most developed and routinized monitoring system was OCHART, which required more effort to learn and maintain, compared to other monitoring and reporting systems. However, it also allowed funders to provide more information back to ASOs. For OCHART, reports on all agency activities were submitted semi-annually using a complex online system, which consisted of multiple linked pages where agency staff entered quantitative and qualitative data about their agency characteristics and all programming activities carried out during a reporting period. Data from each agency were amalgamated by government funders and published in a yearly report. Negotiations between agencies and funders over OCHART were evident. OCHART played a role in building shared meanings and repertoires within this community of practice – it assisted collective "sense-making" of complex HIV prevention work between the funders and service providers. Whether or not OCHART was a good source of information for programmatic or agency decision-making was disputed; however, there was agreement on OCHART's role in monitoring for accountability. When added to other reporting requirements, the OCHART system contributed to the complexity of monitoring and evaluation practices at the case organizations. At the ASOs under study, OCHART was considered an insufficient source of information for programmatic decisions or assessment of the impact of the programs they carried out, and had to be supplemented by other routine monitoring, as well as tacit assessment.

Tacit assessment of prevention programs was a preponderant evaluation practice. It involved informal (often non-recorded) appraisals of merit or other information, and was based on embodied, intuitive, or experiential knowledge. Professional and social interaction between program implementers and program participants, non-participants, other program implementers, funders, etc., was important in formulating tacit assessments. Tacit assessment was used to judge the process as well as the impacts of program activities, and could also be applied to other issues in decision-making, such as developing greater understanding of clients' needs, or assessing individual or organizational performance. It helped evaluate programs in a way that informed future programmatic decisions. The ways in which it was used in combination with more formal evaluation methods were complex: while some elements of programs were only assessed tacitly, often tacit assessments were combined with other evaluation processes when formally sharing information about a program. Tacit assessment was regarded as a meaningful and responsive form of evidence building, and contributed to the overall complexity of evaluation practice. The ability to tacitly assess a program and make changes was linked to the idea of program implementers having embodied and intuitive knowledge as a result of being members of the community that the programs sought to reach. As one manager described it,

The concept of just "the gut" I think is really important. And kind of that sense of automatic feedback ... we recruit people based on that sense of knowing ... we recruited [name of staff] because she was a young woman who ... [lived and] operated in some of those communities and came up through our programs ... She knows what's best. You know, the [funder name] doesn't know what's best. I don't know what's best, in terms of those populations. She knows what's best ... evaluation can take place in a number of ways, and sometimes, it's "You know what? This workshop isn't going so well, and I'm going to turn it this way." It's as simple as that.

This is important to highlight because traditional notions of monitoring and evaluation seldom acknowledge the role of tacit knowledge. Tacit assessment and knowledge building contributed to the extensive information that members of this community of practice held in their minds and memories about programs and their impacts, and provided valuable information for decision-making about future programming. Tacit assessments combined in complex ways with other evaluation practices. Staff and managers often drew on tacit knowledge when writing narrative reports to funders. Tacit knowledge was also used to evaluate or explain explicit information that was captured by other evaluation methods, which made the information more meaningful. For example, tacit knowledge was crucial in explaining trends in participant numbers. It was also relied upon to make sense of OCHART data; it informed the analysis of the data presented in the yearly report, and it was drawn upon during discussions at OCHART KTE Day to interpret the meaning of data and derive plans for future action. It provided an infrastructure through which new information was made sense of and turned into information that could inform future plans. In contrast, traditional evaluation practice seldom values the role of tacit knowledge in evaluation.

Evaluation practice could also be characterized as being plural – evaluation measures and practices contained multiple dimensions, including an appeal to different stakeholders. According to Greene (2005), different stakeholder groups require different evaluative information; using this framework, we can contrast how the intended beneficiaries of the program (and their communities) valued different evaluation criteria compared to the general public. This relates to the "many eyes" of accountability, where there are multiple potential stakeholders, who value a multitude of norms (Bemelmans-Videc 2007).

Both case organizations had members; people from communities served by the organization paid a small annual fee to attend and vote at AGMs. At these meetings, and within annual reports and newsletters distributed to members, organizations used some standard monitoring and evaluation results to capture and describe their work and its success to members. However, this information was not presented and discussed as it was in OCHART KTE Days or reports. For example, the number of program participants, services provided to clients, and volunteer hours contributed over the past year were important indicators of success, but were stated only briefly. Stories of the personal impact of the organization on individuals were lauded, as was the ability of organization leaders to dialogue about and respond to issues that were affecting the community they served.

This approach can be contrasted to evaluations that address the concerns of people who were not part of this sector or linked to community-based organizations. For example, an ASO manager described the experience of reviewing an analysis in a yearly report that estimated the number of averted HIV infections and cost savings to Ontario's healthcare system due to HIV prevention programs. This information was not useful for the manager or the agency in making decisions about programs or activities. But stakeholders who were not part of the organization or the community sector, and who might not see the value of providing HIV prevention programming to communities most affected by HIV might find such information convincing; this is important, as taxpayer support for all community services, including HIV prevention, is under increasing scrutiny and threat of termination. From this, we see that the accountabilities of ASOs to the communities they serve, the government bodies that fund them, and the general public vary considerably. This creates great pressure on ASOs – which must function with limited resources – to maintain good relationships with all stakeholders by managing their multiple accountabilities.

### Recommendations

Ideal evaluation practice at ASOs would balance the need to maintain accountability to multiple stakeholders, and provide information to help ASOs learn from their work and make decisions about it. It would combine the tacit knowledge of people with lived experience of HIV, with explicit knowledge gathered through monitoring, evaluation, and research. It would shed light on the complexity of capturing the effectiveness of HIV prevention programs that that often involve addressing people's sexual and drug use behaviours that are resistant to change, and other important principles in community-based health promotion practice and the social determinants of health. However, current evaluation policy emphasizes standardized monitoring, often motivated by meeting increasing demands for accountability to the general public. There are challenges in meeting this ideal, including that much of the tacit knowledge held is not well suited to standardized monitoring and issues about managing accountability to different audiences. Evaluation policymakers need to consider the limitations of standardized monitoring procedures in capturing tacit knowledge and in capturing effectiveness, and the burden they place on community-based organizations. The following section addresses these challenges and provides recommendations for more effective and useful evaluation policy.

*Acknowledging and Strengthening the Role of Tacit Knowledge*

Current HIV prevention evaluation practice involves several approaches. However, the pressure to monitor for accountability to government funders was dominant at the ASOs I studied, and was growing. In particular, there was pressure to demonstrate program improvement based on explicit knowledge derived from monitoring practices, which was conceived of as linear, sequential, or, at best, iterative. If pressure to monitor or demonstrate a certain kind of learning moves this sector away from the concerns of the communities they hope to serve and towards making decisions based on limited and limiting information that standard monitoring practice amasses, it is unlikely that the response to HIV will find relevant and timely ways to address the epidemic in communities most affected by HIV. As one manager explained,

> "Is it an art or is it a science?" And it's really, in so many ways, both. And it has to be, to be ... truly responsive. And if [a program is] peer based, and if it's led by community members, and if ... it's coming from a place of knowing the community that you're working with ... Nor do we need to be collecting humongous amounts of data to tell us that the programs are going well ... [We need to show] people are coming to the program and they're engaged and they're staying and they're learning ... We [need to be] epidemiologically [informed], and in terms of transmission, that has to be accurate, absolutely. We need to have the science down. But when it

comes to kind of the human side of it, the art-based side of it, they [program staff and volunteers] know what they know.

Another way to respond to this pressure may be to become more adept at articulating the experiential knowledge gained in delivering programs or interacting with the communities they serve, and relying on this knowledge when asked to explain program planning and improvement. Nonaka and von Krogh (2009) suggest that a degree of tacit knowledge can be articulated. Patton (2004) suggests that to "be useful and insightful ... evaluation ... need[s] to match the nature of ... HIV ... which is best understood as a dynamic, complex systems phenomenon" (169). This framing of the HIV epidemic could allow for more diverse kinds of knowledge to be valued in the response to HIV. This would have important impacts on monitoring and evaluation practice, and it could also allow for more diversity in addressing the complexity of capturing the effectiveness of community-based HIV prevention programs.

## Attending to the Burden of Evaluation for Accountability

Managers and staff at ASOs who reported to government funders agreed with funders that monitoring for accountability was necessary. However, what constituted appropriate monitoring continued to be negotiated. These negotiations were based on the impacts that increased monitoring requirements had on practice, especially when they burdened community-based agencies with further data collection and reporting. They were also based on ideas and rationalizations about how increased monitoring for accountability might provide benefits. According to funders, more monitoring information was needed, even if the benefits of increased reporting were not explicit. Some respondents expressed the hope that increased monitoring would produce information that could "prove" the important impact of community-based HIV prevention work to the public, which may not be well attuned to the issues faced by communities at high risk for HIV. However, converting reporting on outputs to information about outcomes can be difficult (or impossible); and knowing more about different outputs does not necessarily result in knowing more about impacts. In addition, it is hard to persuasively quantify the impact of community-based work, especially for stakeholders who may hold social or political views that are opposed to government-funded social health and welfare programs. These are examples of complications that arise when there is a desire to know about effectiveness, but it is difficult to assess, and there are multiple evaluation stakeholders. It seems unlikely that more monitoring can resolve these complications. Another proposed benefit – that organizational learning and program improvement would result from more monitoring – also seems unlikely. As discussed above, it was not evident that program planning or improvement at the ASOs studied occurred as a result of OCHART data. Overall, negotiations about what is appropriate monitoring for accountability would benefit from closer examination of the proposed benefits, in order to balance them thoughtfully against the additional burdens that are created by increased monitoring.

## Supporting Capacity-Building in Evaluation

The need for community-based organizations to monitor and evaluate their HIV prevention programs for several reasons, including providing information to a variety of stakeholders, is clear. However, how they fulfil this requirement is less clear. There is a need to support this sector's capacity in formal monitoring and evaluation, as well as recognize the value of tacit knowledge. ASOs depend on the skills and capacities of individuals, usually staff (and sometimes volunteers), to monitor and evaluate. Few have had training. In addition, a funder also talked about her incapacity to make recommendations on the evaluation plans of organizations who were applying for funding. Support for formal monitoring and evaluation capacity-building in the entire sector seems warranted. This would likely be better if it fostered formal monitoring and evaluation capacity along with building strategies that recognize tacit knowledge.

The impact of community-based HIV prevention programs on participants is difficult to capture. For example, a program that successfully engages participants might not change their behaviour in ways that make them less likely to contract HIV, but it could increase other health-promoting behaviours (like HIV testing) or build social relationships that will have a positive effect no matter what their HIV status. Capacity building in ways to identify, assess, adopt, or create tools and measures that are reasonable and appropriate for ASOs to use to better capture their work is recommended. For example, better tools and measures could be developed to capture and understand how programs enhance relationships that support health and well-being in communities at high risk for HIV.

While ASOs have been part of the community-based response to HIV since the beginning of the epidemic, the response to HIV has always involved tensions between scientists, government officials, and affected communities as to who are seen as "experts" (Altman 1994; Miller and Greene 2005). Given the need to understand divergent perspectives, constructivist, collaborative, and participatory approaches to evaluation make a particularly good fit. In this study, I noted that this community of practice tended to use participatory monitoring and evaluation approaches, as described by Jackson (2005), for instrumental (rather than transformative) reasons. This seems to be an appropriate response to the possible threat of more "top-down" approaches, in which outcomes and ways to measure them are established by people who do not work in the field of community-based HIV prevention. This echoes Knaapen's (2014) description of how the medical profession has repositioned the tools for evidence-based medicine as a "defensive strategy to avoid externally controlled regulation" (830). This maintains the collective autonomy of the profession (albeit at the cost of individual practitioners' autonomy) and introduces a new kind of hierarchical intra-professional regulation, where instead of third parties outside the sector, it is the "knowledge and administrative" elite of the profession that employs standards to order, assess, and direct the work of the rank-and-file professions, and wards off external control. The hierarchies among practitioners who deliver community-based HIV programs may be less visible and formalized. Participatory approaches to monitoring and evaluation that build capacity and give voice to more marginalized individuals and groups will likely be the most useful in furthering monitoring and evaluation practice that can meaningfully inform a relevant response to the HIV epidemic.

*Preparing for the Future*

Attending to the diversity and complexity of programming, and capacity building in evaluation approaches that give voice to more marginalized groups, should be considered in future evaluation policy and practice in this sector, given that there is a move to integration of services related to HIV, hepatitis C, and other sexually transmitted and bloodborne infections (CATIE 2015). While it is difficult to predict the effects that this move will have on individual ASOs, it could require significant organizational changes, including expanding the range of services provided or communities served. For example, an ASO could evaluate its level of community engagement using tools to measure the ways in which people living with HIV are meaningfully involved in organizational decision-making; this is referred to as the greater involvement and meaningful engagement of people living with HIV/AIDS (GIPA/ MIPA) (OAN 2011). However, an integrated approach may require an organization to consider the needs of people living with hepatitis C, and how they can meaningfully engage people from this community in their organizational decision-making. There may be a need to adapt existing tools, and develop new ones to appropriately evaluate the aims and work carried out by these organizations.

## Conclusion

Many challenges remain in addressing HIV and the social determinants of health that underlie inequities in health and well-being among Canadians. Monitoring and evaluation have the potential to enhance this work. ASOs must maintain relationships with stakeholders that value different aspects of their work, and how they evaluate it. Supporting ASOs to balance their multiple accountabilities requires creating evaluation policies that support tacit knowledge development, and allow for learning in ways that address and respond to the needs of people from communities most affected by HIV and other inequities in health. Responsive monitoring and evaluation will prevent these practices from becoming bureaucratic rituals, and instead harness their potential to meaningfully contribute to innovative progress in the response to HIV.

REFERENCES

Adam, B.D., et al. 2007. *Risk Management in Circuits of Gay and Bisexual Men: Results from the Toronto Pride Survey.* Toronto: AIDS Committee of Toronto.
Akers, T.A., and W.G. Hervey. 2003. "Why Classification for HIV/AIDS Prevention Interventions?" *JANAC: Journal of the Association of Nurses in AIDS Care* 14 (4): 17–20. https://doi.org/10.1177/1055329003254853.
Alkin, M., ed. 2013. *Evaluation Roots: A Wider Perspective of Theorists' Views and Influences.* 2nd ed. Thousand Oaks: Sage.
Altman, Dennis. 1994. *Power and Community: Organizational and Cultural Responses to AIDS.* Bristol, PA: Taylor & Francis.
Armstrong, Rebecca, et al. 2007. "The Nature of Evidence Resources and Knowledge Translation for Health Promotion Practitioners." *Health*

*Promotion International* 22 (3): 254–60. https://doi.org/10.1093/heapro/dam017.

Aucoin, Peter, and Mark D. Jarvis. 2005. *Modernizing Government Accountability: A Framework for Reform*. Toronto: Canada School of Public Service Canada.

Auditor General of Canada. 2002. *Modernizing Accountability in the Public Sector*. Ottawa: Queen's Printer.

Auerbach, J.D., Justin O. Parkhurst, and Carlos F. Cáceres. 2011. "Addressing Social Drivers of HIV/AIDS for the Long-term Response: Conceptual and Methodological Considerations." In "Social Drivers of HIV and AIDS," supplement, *Global Public Health: An International Journal for Research, Policy and Practice* 6 (s3): S293–309. https://doi.org/10.1080/17441692.2011.594451.

Bemelmans-Videc, Marie-Louise. 2007. "Accountability, a Classic Concept in Modern Contexts: Implications for Evaluation and for Auditing Roles." In Bemelmans-Videc, Lonsdale, and Perrin, 21–39.

Bemelmans-Videc, Marie-Louise, Jeremy Lonsdale, and Burt Perrin, eds. 2007. *Making Accountability Work: Dilemmas for Evaluation and for Audit*. New Brunswick: Transaction Publishers.

Bowerman, M., H. Raby, and C. Humphrey. 2000. "In Search of the Audit Society: Some Evidence from Health Care, Police and Schools." *International Journal of Auditing* 4 (1): 71–100. https://doi.org/10.1111/1099-1123.00304.

Brownson, Ross C., Jonathan E. Fielding, and Christopher M. Maylahn. 2009. "Evidence-Based Public Health: A Fundamental Concept for Public Health Practice." *Annual Review of Public Health* 30 (1): 175–201. https://doi.org/10.1146/annurev.publhealth.031308.100134.

Cain, R. 1993. "Community-Based AIDS Services: Formalization and Depoliticization." *International Journal of Health Services* 23 (4): 665–84.

Cain, R. 1995. "Community-Based AIDS Organizations and the State: Dilemmas of Dependence." *AIDS & Public Policy Journal* 10 (2): 83–93.

CATIE. 2015. "Integrated Approaches to Sexually Transmitted and Blood-Borne Infections and Tuberculosis." http://www.catie.ca/en/hiv-canada/8/8-3.

Evaluation Directorate. 2014. "Evaluation of the Federal Initiative to Address HIV/AIDS in Canada 2008–09 to 2012–13."

Feller, Irwin. 2002. "Performance Measurement Redux." *American Journal of Evaluation* 23 (4): 435–52. https://doi.org/10.1177/109821400202300405.

Fink, A. 2013. *Evidence-Based Public Health Practice*. Thousand Oaks, CA: Sage. https://doi.org/10.4135/9781506335100.

Flicker, S., et al. 2009. "Community-Based Research in AIDS-Service Organizations: What Helps and What Doesn't?" *AIDS Care* 21 (1): 94–102. https://doi.org/10.1080/09540120802032650.

Freeman, Tim. 2002. "Using Performance Indicators to Improve Health Care Quality in the Public Sector: A Review of the Literature." *Health Services Management Research* 15 (2): 126–37. https://doi.org/10.1258/0951484021912897.

Government of Canada. 2004. "The Federal Initiative to Address HIV/AIDS in Canada."

Greene, J.C. 2005. "Stakeholders." In *Encyclopedia of Evaluation*, edited by S. Mathison, 398. Thousand Oaks, CA: Sage.

Greenspan, N.R. 2015. "Frontline Measures: Evaluating HIV Prevention at AIDS Service Organizations." Toronto: Health Policy, Management and Evaluation, University of Toronto.

Guenter, D., et al. 2001. "Doing HIV Prevention Work in Ontario's AIDS Service Organizations." CLEAR Working Paper Series. Hamilton, ON: McMaster CLEAR Unit.

Jackson, E.T. 2005. "Participatory Monitoring and Evaluation." In *Encyclopedia of Evaluation*, edited by S. Mathison, 296–7. Thousand Oaks, CA: Sage.

Julnes, George, and M. Mark. 1998. "Evaluation as Sensemaking: Knowledge Construction in a Realist World." *New Directions for Evaluation* 1998 (78): 33–52. https://doi.org/10.1002/ev.1099.

Kinsman, G. 1997. "Managing AIDS Organizing: 'Consultation,' 'Partnership,' and 'Responsibility' as Strategies of Regulation." In *Organizing Dissent: Contemporary Social Movements in Theory and Practice*, edited by W.K. Carroll, 213–39. Toronto: Garamond.

Knaapen, Loes. 2014. "Evidence-Based Medicine or Cookbook Medicine? Addressing Concerns over the Standardization of Care." *Sociology Compass* 8 (6): 823–36. https://doi.org/10.1111/soc4.12184.

Korda, Holly. 2013. "Bringing Evidence-Based Interventions to the Field: The Fidelity Challenge." *Journal of Public Health Management and Practice* 19 (1): 1–3. https://www.ncbi.nlm.nih.gov/pubmed/23169396.

Lehtonen, Markku. 2005. "OECD Environmental Performance Review Programme: Accountability (f)or Learning?" *Evaluation* 11 (2): 169–88. https://doi.org/10.1177/1356389005055536.

Mark, M., Gary Henry, and George Julnes. 1999. "Toward an Integrative Framework for Evaluation Practice." *American Journal of Evaluation* 20 (2): 177–98. https://doi.org/10.1177/109821409902000202.

– 2000. *Evaluation: An Integrated Framework for Understanding, Guiding, and Improving Policies and Programs*. San Francisco: Jossey-Bass.

Mayne, John. 2007. "Evaluation for Accountability: Myth or Reality?" In Bemelmans-Videc, Lonsdale, and Perrin, 63–84.

Miller, R.L., and G.J. Greene. 2005. "Transferring HIV Prevention Technology to Community-Based Organization: How Can HIV Prevention Scientists Play an Effective Role in Practice?" In *Community Interventions and AIDS*, edited by Edison J. Trickett and Willo Pequegnat, 196–221. New York: Oxford University Press.

Natalie Kishchuk Research and Evaluation. 2010. "AIDS Community Action Program (ACAP) Evaluation Summary Report 2007–09."

Nonaka, Ikujiro, and Georg von Krogh. 2009. "Tacit Knowledge and Knowledge Conversion: Controversy and Advancement in Organizational Knowledge Creation Theory." *Organization Science* 20 (3): 635–52. https://doi.org/10.1287/orsc.1080.0412.

Ontario AIDS Network (OAN). 2011. *Living and Serving 3: GIPA Engagement Guide and Framework for Ontario ASOs*. Toronto: OAN.

Ontario HIV Treatment Network (OHTN). 2013. *OHTN Report to the Board July–September 2013*. Toronto: OHTN.

Owen, J.M. 2007. "Making Policy Interventions More Effective: The Case for Accountability up and Accountability Down." In Bemelmans-Videc, Lonsdale, and Perrin, 181–92.

Patton, M.Q. 2004. "A Microcosm of the Global Challenges Facing the Field: Commentary on HIV/AIDS Monitoring and Evaluation." *New Directions for Evaluation* 2004 (103): 163–71. https://doi.org/10.1002/ev.130.

– 2008. *Utilization-Focused Evaluation*. 4th ed. Thousand Oaks, CA: Sage.

Perrin, Burt. 2007. "Towards a New View of Accountability." In Bemelmans-Videc, Lonsdale, and Perrin, 41–84.

Piot, Peter, et al. 2008. "Coming to Terms with Complexity: A Call to Action for HIV Prevention." *Lancet* 372 (9641): 845–59. https://doi.org/10.1016/S0140-6736(08)60888-0.

Power, M. 2000. "The Audit Society: Second Thoughts." *International Journal of Auditing* 4 (1): 111–19. https://doi.org/10.1111/1099-1123.00306.

– 2003. "Evaluating the Audit Explosion." *Law & Policy* 25 (3): 185–202. https://doi.org/10.1111/j.1467-9930.2003.00147.x.

– 2005. "The Theory of the Audit Explosion." In *The Oxford Handbook of Public Management*, edited by E. Ferlie, L.E. Lynn, and C. Pollitt, 326–44. Oxford: Oxford University Press.

Price, A., et al. 2016. "Pursuing Performance and Maintaining Compliance: Balancing Performance Improvement and Accountability in Ontario's Public Health System." *Canadian Public Administration* 59 (2): 245–66. https://doi.org/10.1111/capa.12151.

Rayside, David M., and Evert A. Lindquist. 1992. "AIDS Activism and the State in Canada." *Studies in Political Economy* 39 (1): 37–76. http://dx.doi .org/10.1080/19187033.1992.11675417

Roberts, A., and K. Yeager, eds. 2006. *Foundations of Evidence-Based Social Work Practice.* New York: Oxford University Press.

Rogers, Patricia J. 2005. "Accountability." In *Encyclopedia of Evaluation,* edited by S. Mathison. Thousand Oaks, CA: Sage.

Thorne, Sally. 2008. *Interpretive Description.* Walnut Creek, CA: Left Coast.

# 7 Living and Aging with HIV: Tiptoeing through a Pan-Canadian Policy Maze

RON ROSENES

## The Personal Is Political

As a long-time activist and advocate living and aging with HIV, I often ponder the factors that have enabled me to reach the seventh decade of my life, while so many friends and colleagues, still in their prime, were lost along the way. For half of those decades, some thirty-five years, HIV has been my constant companion, at times whispering in my ear, at other times crying out to be heard, always there to remind me of my limitations – and on good days, of my personal potential and the potential we share collectively to ensure that everyone has an equal opportunity to lead a productive and healthy life. In this chapter, I reflect on the challenges of living and aging with HIV, and some of the ways in which we could improve on the maze of public policies that affects Canadians of all ages living with HIV and other chronic diseases, including the disease of poverty.

Research into options to improve access to essential medicines and provide income security are just two examples of growing evidence to suggest there is a better way to use public policy to level the playing field. People with HIV may be among the whistle-blowers who point out the inequities of the current tangle of policies, but our lived experience can inform a better and fairer way forward for all Canadians facing unexpected or chronic illness.

I agree to talk about myself, but on the condition that it serves as a way to talk about others. If I have enjoyed relatively good health and longevity, it may be due to "luck and genes." Genetically, I am favoured with a single delta32 gene that makes it more difficult for HIV to attach to the CD4 cells, which it normally prefers. This is well documented in the literature and is thought to have occurred among Northern European people at the time of the bubonic plague. One copy of this delta32 gene seems to lessen the severity of infection and may be found in up to 20 per cent of Caucasians. There is a lesson here, a reminder that while some aspects of health can be controlled, such as diet and exercise, individual health is variable and unpredictable. Income plays an obvious and important role as well.

There are other aspects of good fortune that have nothing to do with genetics – being born, for example, into a loving and stable middle-class family in Ottawa with parents who made it possible for me to receive a good education. I taught French and Russian language and literature at CEGEP in Montreal through the 1970s. I left teaching and moved to Toronto, where I had a successful business and relationship with a wonderful man that ended in 1991 when he succumbed to opportunistic infections related to HIV that could not be controlled by the few medications available at the time. Losing my life partner and my mother in the space of a year was devastating for me. Shortly after, on the advice of a sympathetic counsellor at the AIDS Committee of Toronto, I activated a private long-term disability (LTD) policy that I had purchased while still working – and prior to receiving a confirmatory diagnosis of HIV. This insurance policy provided a monthly income that placed me well above the poverty line for the next twenty-one years, although it did not cover the cost of drugs. To pay for my antiretroviral treatments, as they became available, I turned to Trillium, the Ontario catastrophic drug program, which came about as a result of pressure from the HIV community at the time. We fought for and succeeded in getting the Trillium Drug Program established in Ontario, not just for people with HIV but to assist everyone in the province facing excessively high drug costs with little or no private insurance. It's far from perfect, requiring an income-based deductible, but we will get to that.

Upon reaching sixty-five, I was unceremoniously handed off to the Canada Pension Plan – welcome to old age and not much security. My personal response was a decision to take the past twenty-five years of experience working as a volunteer, activist, and advocate in the HIV sector, and become a paid consultant specializing in organizational development for non-profits. The work is extremely gratifying but precarious. I am unsure how long I will be able to work and whether there will be sufficient funds to enjoy a future I did not anticipate.

My personal journey has evolved from *survivor*, to *witness*, and now unexpectedly to *pioneer*. It has been clear to me for many years now that my destiny and responsibility as a long-term survivor is to act as a witness, not only to the loss of so many friends and colleagues, but also to the remarkable advances in treatment and understanding of the underlying social conditions that drive HIV infection. Born in 1947, I am at the leading edge of those baby boomers who are among the first to face the challenges of aging with HIV.

Others in this book are writing about certain aspects of aging with HIV, but here is a primer on what has been learned so far about the biomedical, social, and economic aspects of the challenges we now face. Until a few years ago, we thought our chances of aging with a minimum of complications were good if HIV was well controlled, particularly for those on newer medications with lower pill burden and fewer side effects. Despite data showing we are nudging closer in high-income countries to a lifespan equal to that found in the general population, we are not there yet (Lohse et al. 2009).

In the 1980s and 1990s, having AIDS meant succumbing to opportunistic infections that we no longer hear about since the advent of triple antiretroviral therapy in 1996. We are no longer dying of diseases that arose from weakened immune systems, with names that terrified: toxoplasmosis, cytomegalovirus, PCP pneumonia, *Mycobacterium avium* complex or Kaposi sarcoma. Today, we are more likely to die from a cancer that is unrelated to HIV, from cardiovascular disease, bone disease, or organ failure – end-stage kidney or liver disease. We no longer see the type of fulsome dementia that occurred in untreated HIV, but we are seeing an increase in asymptomatic and milder forms of cognitive impairment, which can be challenging to diagnose but can still affect daily function. Memory decline and confusion, along with frailty and bone disease, appear to be "accelerated" in HIV – that is, these conditions are occurring at a younger age when compared to the general population. Other chronic conditions, such as cardiovascular disease and type 2 diabetes, appear to be accentuated – they are found in greater prevalence than in the general population, although they may not be occurring sooner.

In their attempts to explain causality, researchers present compelling data to suggest that low levels of ongoing viral activity exacerbate the inflammatory processes associated with the cellular damage of "normal" aging. This may also be due to the virus's ability to lie in wait in places such as the lymphatic system, leading the body to believe it must mount a non-stop defence. Some researchers refer to this process as "inflammaging" (see, for example, Guaraldi et al. 2014). It seems to occur despite the success of ARV therapies in reducing viral load to the so-called holy grail of "undetectable," and the re-establishment of CD4 marker cells that indicate substantially restored immune function. Drugs to treat HIV today may have fewer unwanted side effects, but that does not mean they are free of toxicities.

In addition, a growing epidemic of type 2 diabetes (in the general and HIV-positive populations), and co-infection with hepatitis C, further complicate matters. With death due to so many possible causes, one has to wonder if HIV is being captured at all on death certificates today.

Biomedical issues are not the only comorbidities. Intersecting layers of social and structural comorbidities, or syndemics, each add weight and oppression to a delicate house of cards that risks collapse with each new assault. These may include: stigma and discrimination, childhood trauma from sexual abuse or the effects of colonization, intimate partner violence, addictions, mental health issues including depression, unstable housing, and last, but far from least, poverty – poverty that is due to life circumstance or poverty that results from illness. Simply put, poverty can drive HIV and HIV often leads to poverty.

The effect is both additive and cumulative. The ability of an individual to maintain and manage her or his health is in direct relationship to the number of negative contributing factors each may experience, be they medical, social, or economic. Despite the fact that medications to treat HIV are generally thought of as accessible for most people living with HIV (PHAs) in Canada, many are forced onto restrictive social programs in order to obtain those medications along with other drugs they need to treat a host of additional acute and chronic conditions. As one friend wryly pointed out, "I am taking about forty pills a day but only three of them are for HIV."

The Canadian Working Group on HIV and Rehabilitation (rebranded as Realize) has done much to raise awareness of HIV as an episodic disability: an ongoing illness where periods of good health may be interrupted by periods of illness or disability. It can be difficult to predict when these episodes will occur or how long they will last. They can occur at any age and cause significant employment and income support challenges. These issues are not unique to HIV and are faced by growing numbers of Canadians with lifelong episodic disabilities including multiple sclerosis, cancer, diabetes, lupus, and mental health and mood disorders. For this reason, sound public health policy must reflect the entire lifespan and have the flexibility to provide a safety net that does not force an individual out of the workplace or onto social assistance when disease or disability causes a temporary setback.

## The Role of Public Health Policy
## in Increasing Access to Essential Medicines

During our fourteen years together at the helm of the Canadian Treatment Action Council (CTAC), Louise Binder and I developed a good understanding of the medical, social, and economic complexities of living with HIV. Nonetheless, we founded the organization to focus on "narrow and deep" work on the issue of access to essential medicines. We spent endless hours debating what would be required from a policy perspective to improve access to medicines across the country, and in particular for those who can least afford them – at any stage of life.

Take the example of Glen (not his real name) who had to stop working when he was diagnosed with HIV in his early thirties. He was on his own, working in the service sector, with a typically low-paying job as a waiter in a mid-price restaurant in downtown Toronto. Unfortunately, he learned his HIV status after becoming ill with an opportunistic infection, and needed to both rest and to start treatment urgently. With no insurance, and forced to stop working, the only way to get on treatment was to apply for social assistance. That way, he would get a drug card, minimal dental benefits, and the princely sum of $554 basic needs allowance plus a shelter allowance of $445 each month. That's a total of $999 for rent and food in downtown Toronto. In 2015.

Adisa (not her real name) came to Canada in her fifties as a refugee from an African country in the 1990s. She and her daughter (who is HIV-negative) have successfully settled in Atlantic Canada, but settlement services are few and ill-equipped to deal with the double stigma of having HIV and being a refugee. Getting access to the health-care system took over a year, and confidentiality is not well understood or protected at the clinic she attends. The challenges of accessing medications, not just for HIV, but for other age-related conditions, with trying to work and raise a child, are enormous. She also finds it difficult to access mental health services, both because they are lacking in her community and she does not feel they would be culturally safe for her.

Thus began a quest for answers: What is the best way to ensure a choice of options for people with HIV, and others who need essential medicines, within the Canadian health-care system? What would efficiencies in the system look like if they could improve access to the optimal range of essential medicines, regardless of age, address, or ability to pay? Who decides what the list or formulary of essential medicines covers? Can we provide for all without lowering the bar in what the public system is able to cover? Finally, how can we maintain the principles of affordability, comprehensiveness, and universality throughout the lifespan?

Through the history and evolution of the Canadian federation, considerable power has become vested in the provinces and territories, allowing them to manage their own affairs, particularly in the area of health and social programs. The result is the patchwork of public policies, which regulate access to essential medicines and income supports across the country. We can begin to fix this with a Universal Public Drug Plan (UPDP) or Pharmacare that builds on what we currently have and creates a safety net that fills the gaps in the current system. It can be done incrementally. It doesn't require a "big bang" approach.

The plan we envisaged at CTAC would require contributions from every stakeholder in the system, including governments (60 per cent), employers (30 per cent), and individuals and families (10 per cent). Funding would essentially come through the progressive taxation system, which would be a fair way to ensure equity. The plan would in effect be pre-funded by all contributors, including younger healthy individuals. The plan would address the fact that public drug benefit programs in Canada evolved in ways that historically resulted in coverage for select populations only, including people with specific illnesses such as HIV/AIDS, cancer, MS, cystic fibrosis, and diabetes. All provinces offer public drug coverage at little or no cost to seniors and people on social assistance. The plan we envisaged would not apply to select populations or illnesses, it would cover everyone's needs, regardless of age. For people at all ages and stages of HIV, it would also cover the myriad essential medicines required to treat concomitant conditions. The keys to access should be financial need and failure to qualify for existing drug plans.

The provinces and territories have already begun to take the lead in achieving efficiencies related to price of drugs, with a focus on the classes required to treat chronic health conditions such as diabetes and cardiovascular disease. They have formed the pan-Canadian Pharmaceutical Alliance (pCPA) to take the lead in collectively negotiating lower drug prices with pharmaceutical manufacturers of patent and generic drugs. According to the pCPA, as of March 2015, collaboration had resulted in approximately $490 million in combined annual savings

(Council of the Federation 2016). Morgan et al. (2015) further suggest that universal public drug coverage would save taxpayer money in the long term. It is clear that greater economies can be achieved, but they are not going to result in "Pharmacare" without a new policy framework to support them.

If we are serious about achieving efficiencies in the delivery of health care, then we should not consider lower drug costs in isolation. Thirty per cent of Canada's health-care expenditures are on hospitals ($63.5 billion), 16 per cent on drugs ($33.9 billion), and 15 per cent on physicians ($33.3 billion). Interestingly, the share of public-sector health dollars spent on Canadian seniors has not changed significantly over the past decade, rising only one-half of a percentage point between 2002 and 2012 (from 44.6 to 45.2 per cent). Many of the cost increases to the system lie in the hospital sector and in the pay structure for physicians (all data from the Canadian Institute for Health Information 2014). The point is, we must continue to innovate and seek efficiencies throughout the system as a whole, bearing in mind that drugs in many cases keep people, including seniors, out of hospital, where costly acute care is delivered.

Inevitably, the provinces will continue to take the lead in providing public drug coverage for eligible people in Canada who need it, either because they do not qualify for private insurance or because that coverage is inadequate. But the federal government also needs to play its part in leadership, coordination, and helping to set national standards and guidelines. And as health-care consumers, or patients, our lived experience has value and we should be consulted in a meaningful way by both levels of government.

There will also likely be a continuing role for employers and their various private plans, either to cover high-income individuals or as a competitive benefit of employment, even if it means that private insurers often cover the healthiest in our population, a practice known as skimming. There are those who would prefer a totally public system of coverage, myself included, but private sector coverage picks up over 58 per cent of drug expenditures across Canada: private insurers, pharmaceutical manufacturers, and retail pharmacy corporations have somewhere between $3 billion and $11 billion to lose if Canada were to implement a universal, public pharmacare program (Gagnon 2014). Private insurers will not be in a hurry to give up their drug insurance business, but they are seeking to pay the lower public plan price, thereby having their cake and eating it too.

Essential medicines should not be viewed as just another commodity, akin to shopping for a pair of shoes, where you can go elsewhere if you don't like the price. If, however, we view essential medicines as integral to health care, and of no intrinsic value to the healthy person, then public health policy must enable the state to intervene and negotiate the best possible price for its public drug program. As Joel Lexchin suggested at a CTAC event I attended in fall 2015, the state should have the right to intervene when the main factor that influences price is, in his words, "patient desperation." While true innovation deserves to be rewarded, it is well understood that the relationship between the drug company list price and the actual cost of manufacture is completely opaque.

While there are many principled advocates who would agree that regulators should intervene to ensure the human right to essential medicines, there are others, equally principled, who take a more pragmatic approach, one recognizing that health system resources are finite. Rotenberg (2015) suggests patients need to work with their doctors to better distinguish between wants and needs, particularly with regard to frivolous use of diagnostic procedures, and the inappropriate use of antibiotics. In terms of coverage, we need a fairer process to determine what should or should not be covered.

From a community perspective, one barrier to access remains the application of co-pays and deductibles for those who can least afford them. Evidence suggests that providing effective medicines to such patients at little or no direct cost can improve adherence to treatments, improve health outcomes, and thereby lower medical and hospital costs. Even a $2 co-pay can prevent an individual with limited income from getting a prescription filled, and we should not be satisfied with any plan that perpetuates their use (Morgan, Daw, and Law 2014). In fact, the optimal policy response should not be to reduce benefits for seniors, but to increase benefits for non-seniors.

In my view, the dichotomy between income-based and age-based programs is a false one. The UPDP we envisage should be based on need, regardless of age. Fair and progressive taxation of all stakeholders should allay any concerns about equity in the system. That said, the imminent arrival to market of a host of novel and costly therapeutics ranging from cures for hepatitis C, to biologics, and immunotherapies for cancer will overwhelm what we currently have in place. Choices will still have to be made in what the health-care system is able to cover, but without a complete overhaul we can expect our options will continue to diminish.

Under current guidelines, patients can access the majority of Health Canada–approved treatments for HIV at time of diagnosis, regardless of degree of disease progression. This is not the case for people mono- or co-infected with hepatitis C who must wait until they are very sick before provincial or territorial systems will agree to cover the effective but costly new direct-acting antiviral medications.

## The Role for an Annual Guaranteed Income

There is an irony specific to HIV infection: HIV does not discriminate but manages nonetheless to search out the most vulnerable among us. It is a sad reality that the virus is often at the bottom of the list of social and economic challenges faced by many people living with HIV. While others are writing about the transitions imposed by episodic health concerns and the need for policies of accommodation in the workplace, there is one overarching social policy that deserves to be revisited, and that is the guaranteed annual income.

A GAI, also known as a negative income tax, would provide a basic liveable income for all citizens, without a means test or work require- ment. Various proposals have been circulating for years, based on the principle of establishing an income floor below which no person or family could fall, but with incentives for recipients to enter or remain in the workforce and to earn more than the guaranteed income would provide. The basic amount of annual income could be determined us- ing a formula such as the OECD Low Income Measure, which has been adopted by Ontario. It is not for this writer to suggest an amount, but it should be more than the $20,000 yearly income reported by approxi- mately one-third of Canadians. This would replace the maze of sepa- rate federal and provincial programs with a unified and unconditional benefit delivered through the tax system. As money is earned in excess of the basic level, it would gradually be taxed back until a break-even level is reached, and above which there is no further benefit.

Like the UPDP, a guaranteed income would be universal in the sense that it would not target certain groups or people of a certain age, such as seniors or children, but would be based on need across the lifespan. Best of all, it would do away with "welfare" and help reduce the stigma and disincentives associated with social assistance programs.

A GAI would complement a UPDP and replace federal transfers for disability supports, social assistance, and myriad programs sup- porting primarily seniors and children (the Old Age Supplement, the

Guaranteed Income Supplement for seniors, the Canadian Child Tax Benefit, and National Child Benefit Supplement). It would not make sense to replace the Canada Pension Plan or Employment Insurance, according to a majority of social policy experts and politicians.

How would you respond to the person who asks "What? You think the government should just hand out free money to everybody?"

There is the example of a GAI social experiment that took place in Dauphin, Manitoba, for four years in the 1970s. Forget's (2011) findings from the "MINCOME" Project show positive health outcomes during the time of the basic income regime, not just for recipients of the income, but also for the community as a whole. The results were also in line with similar North American experiments showing that fears that a guaranteed income would discourage a work effort were unfounded.

Support can be found for GAI across the political spectrum: environmentalists view it as a way to reduce emphasis on productivity, or to recognize collective ownership of natural resources. Anti-poverty groups recommend it for its redistributive impact on income. Feminists appreciate its recognition of the fact that unpaid caregiving in the home, disproportionately provided by women, is seldom recognized as "real work" or remunerated accordingly.

Today, Glen is back on his feet, thanks to excellent care, but struggling to return to work, and move to the Trillium program to get his medications. This is a scary and difficult transition that could have been made much easier with a GAI, together with a UPDP that would waive the deductible until he gets back on his feet.

Adisa is working again, but finds she must still make decisions between co-pays and deductibles for her medications or ensuring that she and her daughter can put food on the table.

As a society, there are many creative solutions we could adopt in addition to the ones discussed here – solutions that would have better supported Glen, Adisa, and many others living with HIV. These include but are not limited to free education and training for the poor, more affordable housing, microloans, better access to mental health supports, and harm-reduction programs.

As an advocate, more often than not, I feel like Sisyphus, the Greek character who was forced by the gods to roll a boulder over and over again to the top of the mountain, only to have it come crashing back down. Any sense of personal satisfaction is tempered by the knowledge that our achievements have been the result of a group effort. The Trillium Program in Ontario is a good example of people with HIV advocating for a catastrophic drug program, not just for one disease group, but rather for all citizens with excessively high drug costs in Ontario. Still, the larger policy changes that would truly result in a more just and equitable society seem to lie beyond our collective reach. If we are to be successful, then to move those really big boulders, we need more shoulders, in other sectors, to lean into the task. We must reach beyond HIV and work in much broader coalitions of mutual interest.

If you pick up this book in 2027, what, I wonder, will have changed? Will public health and social policies ten years from now support a race to the bottom or will they have raised the bar for everyone? I'd love to know how this book ends.

## REFERENCES

Canadian Institute for Health Information (CIHI). 2014. *National Health Expenditure Trends, 1975 to 2014.* Toronto: CIHI.

Council of the Federation. 2016. "The Pan-Canadian Pharmaceutical Alliance: Negotiations Being Considered by Each Province/Territory." http://www.pmprovincesterritoires.ca/phocadownload/pcpa/pcpa_considered_oct31_2015.pdf.

Forget, Evelyn L. 2011. "The Town with No Poverty: The Health Effects of a Canadian Guaranteed Annual Income Field Experiment." *Canadian Public Policy* 37 (3): 283–305. https://doi.org/10.3138/cpp.37.3.283.

Gagnon, Marc-André. 2014. *A Roadmap to a Rational Pharmacare Policy in Canada.* Ottawa: Canadian Federation of Nurses Unions.

Guaraldi, Giovanni, et al. 2014. "Morbidity in Older HIV-Infected Patients: Impact of Long-Term Antiretrovital use." *AIDS Reviews* 16 (2): 75–89.

Lohse, Nicolai, et al. 2009. "Survival of Persons with and without HIV Infection in Denmark, 1995–2005." *International Journal of Epidemiology* 38 (5): 1202–6.

Morgan, Steven G., et al. 2015. "Estimated Cost of Universal Public Coverage of Prescription Drugs in Canada." *Canadian Medical Association Journal* 187 (7): 491–7. https://doi.org/10.1503/cmaj.141564.

Morgan, Steven G., Jamie R. Daw, and Michael R. Law. 2014. *Are Income-Based Public Drug Benefit Programs Fit for an Aging Population?* Montreal: Institution for Research on Public Policy.

Rotenberg, Brian. 2015. "What Should Be Covered by Our Publicly Funded Health-Care System?" *Hill Times*, 11 December.

# 8 Charting the Course: Exploring HIV, Employment, and Income Security through an Episodic Disability Lens

WENDY PORCH AND TAMMY C. YATES

With the advent of antiretroviral combination treatment, for people living in Canada at least, HIV is no longer fatal. Most people living with HIV in Canada who adhere to treatment now have an average life expectancy of sixty-five (Patterson et al. 2015). This is an outcome few could have hoped for in the early days of the epidemic. To focus solely on life expectancy as an indicator of well-being, however, disregards the complicated and topsy-turvy reality of what it means to live, day by day, year by year, with HIV. Focusing on disease outcomes ignores the emotional, social, financial, and employment-related challenges associated with living with an unpredictable, stigmatized, and invisible episodic disability. This chapter examines some of the challenges people living with HIV have faced, and continue to confront, in employment and income security. This chapter also reflects on the often-limited role played by social policy and examines how new ways of thinking about HIV and disability might transform individual lives.

This chapter incorporates a case study in order to illuminate how the course of HIV and the associated opportunities for income security have changed over time. This case study is not based on a specific individual, but draws on a composite of individuals that Realize (formerly the Canadian Working Group on HIV and Rehabilitation) has encountered in our work since the organization was founded in 1998. The case study follows Henry from the early days of the epidemic to the current day. As you will note, Henry is a black Canadian. This is significant because we see Henry encounter barriers to HIV prevention and treatment that are directly related to intersecting forms of stigma, including homophobia, faced by members of Canada's African, Caribbean, and Black communities. Following each section of the case study is a discussion of relevant employment and income security issues, as well as the impact that social policy has on the opportunities and, at times, constrained choices available to people living with HIV.

## HIV as an Episodic Disability

HIV is often referred to as an "episodic disability." Episodic disabilities are marked by fluctuating periods and degrees of wellness and disability (Episodic Disabilities Employment Network 2016). These periods of wellness and disability are unpredictable. Advances in medical technologies have meant that many diseases and conditions are no longer imminently fatal, and disabling symptoms can often be reduced, managed, or delayed. This means that more and more Canadians are living longer with lifelong episodic disabilities. While the specific prevalence of episodic disability is not known, millions of Canadians live with diseases/conditions linked to episodic disability. The majority of people affected by episodic disabilities are in their prime working years and may move in and out of the labour force in an unpredictable manner. People with episodic disabilities face significant employment and income support issues. Most must rely on health and disability benefits and, as a result of the strict definitions and policies that govern these benefit programs, few people are able to participate in the workforce part-time or when their health allows (Realize 2016). Although this chapter examines issues related to an individual living with HIV, many of the policy barriers that Henry encountered are common to many people living with other episodic disabilities, such as multiple sclerosis, Crohn's and colitis, diabetes, etc., and are often caused by rigid definitions of disability that do not consider the needs of people living with fluctuating conditions. These will be further elaborated below.

In order to deepen our understanding of where hopes for employment and income security for people with episodic disabilities, such as HIV, may have strayed off-course, let's meet Henry.

## Diagnosis

Henry (a pseudonym) was born in Halifax in 1970. His mom and dad are both from Halifax, and Henry can trace his family roots back to the early days of the black refugees – early black settlers in Nova Scotia who escaped to freedom during the war of 1812. Henry is bisexual, but his relationships have mostly been with men. Henry's parents are very religious and he feels uncomfortable sharing his sexual orientation with his parents, and in particular with his dad. He keeps his relationships a secret from them and lives his life "on the down low." He gets the sense from his mom that she knows, but loves him anyway. When Henry was twenty-four, he tested positive for HIV. His mom was devastated and his dad stopped talking to him. Henry took the medication the doctors prescribed, in spite of how sick it made him feel. The reality was that this medication was his lifeline. Henry survived through those rough times, but saw many of his friends die of AIDS-related complications. In 1998, his doctors switched his treatment to highly active antiretroviral therapy, and his health stabilized.

When Henry first became sick, he had to stop university and dropped out without finishing his bachelor of science degree. Henry moved in with his parents and his mom looked after him until he could take care of himself again. Without a job or income, Henry went on Nova Scotia's income support/social assistance program. Although his health had largely stabilized, Henry found it very difficult to take part in all of the daily activities to which he had become accustomed. He was frequently nauseated and could not sleep properly at night. Some days were worse than others, and he found himself dealing with unpredictable periods of illness. He still lived with his parents and found it hard to have a social life, because his mom was always around and also because he did not know how to talk about his HIV status. He often felt depressed and lonely.

**Reflection**

For Henry, life as a young black man who has sex with men but does not identify as gay, is not an unusual occurrence. As the Black Coalition for AIDS Prevention's "Dealing with Being Different: Resource Guide for Gay, Lesbian, Bisexual, Transgender, Queer and Questioning Black Youth" states, "Black youth who believe that they may be gay, lesbian or bisexual may also be feeling that those labels don't quite relate to the experience they are going through. Some young people feel that you can't be both Black and gay or lesbian, and that it's either or" (Black-CAP 2008, 3).

Black youth represent an at-risk population for HIV and other STIs in part because of cultural ideas about gender and in part as the result of social determinants of health such as poverty, insecure housing, and access to education (Davis, Gahagan, and George 2013). Cultural beliefs in the Black, African, and Caribbean communities about the black male stereotype of black men only being heterosexual pressures young black men who have sex with men to keep their experiences to themselves and may limit their opportunities to seek sexual health–related advice, including information about HIV transmission and prevention. As noted in the *Lancet*, "The best biomedical and behavior change interventions cannot succeed without spaces in which men can safely seek care and services, communicate openly about their sexual lives, and be supported to adopt available preventive options" (Beyrer et al. 2012, 4).

In our case study, we see that Henry found himself at greater risk by virtue of his need for secrecy about his sexual activities.

For Henry, as for many diagnosed with AIDS in the mid-1990s, the diagnosis started a dramatic shift in his social and financial spheres. As Henry's health deteriorated, he withdrew from school and associated social supports. Withdrawal from life after a positive diagnosis was a common reaction. Many people diagnosed in the early days of the epidemic attributed their withdrawal from social supports post-diagnosis to "the perception that AIDS equalled death" (Conyers 2004, 8).

It is hard to surmise now how Henry's university would have reacted to him withdrawing from his program and whether he would have been eligible for a refund of his tuition fees. We do know that today there are still significant policy-related issues facing students living with HIV or other episodic disabilities. Students living with episodic, chronic health conditions are likely to face an additional financial burden when attending post-secondary education. These burdens are often the result of inflexible policies on how courses are structured and paid for (Harrison 2015). Students living with episodic disabilities, during periods of impairment, have had to reduce their course load. This can add substantially to tuition costs, especially at institutions at which fees are assessed for each semester basis, rather than by credit or by course. Students who are forced to quit their courses after withdrawal deadlines as the result of worsening health are sometimes ineligible for a refund of tuition fees. Some institutions do offer partial refunds for cases of medical withdrawal, and others make an appeals process available to students withdrawing from courses or from the institution for documented medical reasons.

Returning to Henry, while he may or may not have been refunded tuition fees, we do know that HIV affected his opportunity to complete his degree and earn a living. Without an income, Henry had to return home and apply for income supports.

Throughout Canada, access to provincial disability income supports varies significantly. Some provinces have separate disability-specific income support programs (e.g., Ontario), and some do not (Nova Scotia). Of those provinces that have separate disability income support programs, some consider a positive HIV test adequate to meet eligibility requirements. Other income support programs, such as the national Canada Pension Plan, use definitions of disability that stress that the disability must be "severe and prolonged" (Government of Canada, Service Canada 2016). The Disability Tax Credit, another significant part of federal programs intended to support people with disabilities, also uses a definition of disability that relies on "severe and prolonged" as the core criteria. People living with HIV, especially those on medication, have a hard time proving that HIV is a "severe and prolonged" disability. Policies surrounding the definition of disability in these cases do not allow for conditions that are episodic, no matter how severe they are during the episodes, to qualify as a disability. By not being able to access the Disability Tax Credit, people with HIV, who often have great difficulty acquiring stable employment anyway, are also locked out of the Registered Disability Savings Program (RDSP). The RDSP is intended to support people with disabilities in saving for the future. Many people with disabilities, such as Henry, receive social assistance. Normally, social assistance asset limits prevent people from acquiring any kind of savings, but the RSDP is exempt from this rule. RDSP amounts may also be matched by government funds, in some circumstances. Again, however, it is difficult for people with HIV to prove that they meet the eligibility requirements for these programs on the basis of static and rigid definitions of disability that are applied, which in turn contributes to many people with HIV living in poverty. Poverty, we know, exacerbates the effects of HIV and leads to a marked reduction in quality of life.

Adequacy of income remains a serious problem for people in Canada who rely on income support programs. Nova Scotia's current program, the Employment Support & Income Assistance Program, provides a single person, who is renting or owns a home, with $555 per month to pay for shelter and personal living expenses (Government of Nova Scotia 2013). Applicants may be eligible for additional income on the basis of special needs in transportation, employment, or health, but each must be justified separately. The Ontario Disability Support Program (ODSP) provides a single person with a maximum of $1098 per month, which includes a shelter allowance and a personal amount to cover everything else. Advocacy organizations in Canada have repeatedly called for a commitment to a minimum income standard for Canadians with disabilities, and have yet to see substantive changes in social policy. As noted by the Public Health Agency of Canada (2013, 2), "Income is a predictor of health-related quality of life for PHA for both mental health and health distress." Without a minimum income guarantee, and a clear and transparent system, people living with HIV continue to face significant challenges to maintaining their health and to achieving a decent standard of living.

In Henry's case, he was lucky to be able to rely on his parents to partially support his monthly expenses and his mother as a caregiver in his time of need. But not all Canadians living with HIV or other disabilities have a family to turn to, and many must live in a never-ending cycle of poverty that exacerbates their precarious health. Nevertheless, people living with HIV have managed to return to work once their health stabilized. We return to Henry several years down the road, to examine the challenges of returning to work while living with HIV.

### Returning to Work

In 2001, at the age of thirty-one, Henry decided to try re-entering the job market. He had spoken to people at the AIDS Committee of Nova Scotia about trying to get back to work, and felt he was ready to do something else with his life. There were many gaps in his résumé, however, that he could not easily explain. He never finished his university degree and had limited work experience. He was not even sure what to say if someone asked him about his health during a potential job interview. He didn't know how to get back into the job market or how to commit to being at work every day when some days he felt so nauseated and tired that he could hardly get out of bed in the morning. Henry also did not understand who would pay for his medications if he went back to work and stopped receiving social assistance, or what would happen if he got sick again.

Like many people diagnosed with HIV in the early days of the epidemic, Henry had to immediately withdraw from school and give up his social life in order to focus on trying to stabilize his health. In the mid-1990s, before the advent of antiretroviral combination treatment, an HIV diagnosis usually meant death. For those who eventually stabilized their health and found themselves alive years later, there was uncertainty about what to do next in their life.

As Conyers writes of her experiences with focus group participants who were diagnosed with HIV/AIDS, "These participants described varied periods of aimlessness as they awaited their fate, until they eventually realized that they might not die anytime soon and that it was becoming the norm to continue to work" (Conyers 2004, 8).

People living with HIV today still share many of Henry's concerns about work. Even where there is motivation and a willingness to seek out employment, there can be many barriers to returning to work, which can include, as in Henry's case, a lack of employment-related experience and concerns about explaining gaps in résumés.

Many people living with HIV who are on social assistance and contemplating a return to the workforce also face policy-based disincentives to return to work (RTW). Social assistance/income support programs in Canada often feature very confusing policies and rules on RTW. Recipients are often required to report any employment earnings monthly. Then, a percentage of earnings is deducted from their social assistance cheque for the following month. Some social assistance recipients have reported employment income incorrectly and then were notified that their assistance had been suspended. Administrative errors in calculating income to be clawed back as a result of reported employment income seem to be common and may be tied to the complexity of the policies that govern earned income and difficulties staff have in trying to apply these complex rules. The policies that govern the clawback of employment earnings are a serious disincentive to work, creating a climate of confusion and fear, in which people are more anxious about attempting to work and having their supports inadvertently cut off than they are about adjusting their lifestyles to living on an income below the poverty line.

Not all income support programs feature employment supports, and even in those that do, these supports are being eroded. Recently, in Ontario, recipients of the Ontario Disability Support Program (ODSP) found that their Work Related Benefit (WRB) was to be cut during restructuring. The new Employment Related Benefit that is to replace it, however, will apply only to people who are returning to work, but not to those who have already been attempting to supplement their income with work. As well, enormous technical issues that have accompanied the Ontario roll-out of a reporting system for ODSP offices has meant that, while the WRB was cut, the new benefit intended to replace it has not even been implemented yet.

Henry, as noted above, had fears about losing access to extended health benefits that he enjoyed while receiving provincial income supports. Many income support programs in Canada offer recipients access to universal health benefits that often include access to a drug card. Without access to these benefits, many people living with HIV and other episodic disabilities simply would not be able to afford their costly medications. People with HIV, like Henry and others with episodic disabilities, must think long and hard about whether or not returning to work and losing access to their extended health benefits would harm their health. Even for people who land a job with health benefits, there is often a probationary period that is not covered by the employer's group insurance coverage. Some income support programs allow recipients to maintain access to their health benefits even when they have started working, but not all do, so the uncertainty about having uninterrupted access to treatment definitely discourages some people living with HIV and other episodic disabilities from returning to work, even when they feel well enough to work.

## Thinking about Retirement

After looking for nine months, Henry was able to get a job with a community agency serving people living with HIV and other episodic disabilities. He was able to stay at work for fourteen years, but over time, he started to feel very fatigued. He had increasing numbness in his fingers and toes and was diagnosed with neuropathy. Aging with HIV has been very confusing for Henry. Although he is not yet fifty, he has been told by his doctors that he is at increased risk for cardiovascular disease related to his HIV medications. He has also been told that he has some neurocognitive problems related to HIV. At times he finds himself struggling to come up with the names of clients he has known for years. Nevertheless, Henry keeps working. He takes advantage of his right to accommodation at work to be able to have flexible work hours as well as extra breaks when he needs them. He feels better when he is working, as he feels part of something bigger than himself. He sometimes wonders though what will happen when he turns sixty-five. Will he be eligible for a retirement pension? How will he support himself when he is too old to work?

After living with HIV for more than twenty years, Henry is aging with HIV. Like many other long-term survivors, Henry never thought he would be in the position to ponder retirement, but now that he is doing so, he has more questions than answers. Many Canadians living with HIV share Henry's concerns about financial security. Without any other income upon which to rely, people living with HIV who depended on social assistance and/or have no savings will retire with an average income of less than $17,000 per year, far below the poverty line. Henry's medications, which have more recently been covered by his work benefits plan, will also need to be paid for after retirement. Nova Scotia does offer the Seniors' Pharmacare Program as long as Henry's income falls under $22,896 per year, and as a single senior he would not be required to pay a premium to join (Government of Nova Scotia 2016). However, he may still have to co-pay for his medication, and that would eat into his already very low income.

Worries for people aging with HIV are not restricted to income alone. Many people aging with HIV also have concerns about their health and future care needs. Henry is experiencing cognitive impairment related to HIV, but he does not know if his cognitive abilities will continue to decline or even if anything can be done to help him. Like Henry, many people aging with HIV wonder if there are care facilities to help manage their condition while still also protecting their privacy. However, knowledge of HIV within care homes is limited. For lesbian, gay, bisexual, transgender, and queer people aging with HIV, there are concerns about finding a care home that welcomes people who are not heterosexual.

### Conclusion

In the early days of the HIV epidemic, people like Henry who received a positive HIV diagnosis abandoned their hopes for the future, as they prepared themselves for what they thought was an inevitable death. Remarkable progress in antiretroviral therapy has allowed Henry – and most people in Canada today living with HIV who have access to treatment – to live long and productive lives and to manage the disease as a complex chronic condition. We have a growing population of people who are aging with HIV and who, over the past twenty years and more, have been trying to live the most normal life possible with the sometimes disabling effects of their condition. As people living with HIV with access to effective medication continue to live longer, their dreams have had to shift, be remoulded and transformed. However, social policy in Canada has not kept up with the changing nature of HIV and the increased numbers of people living longer with episodic disabilities.

Canadian social policy has to respond to this changing reality by becoming more flexible and recognizing the myriad spaces between well and sick, and the resulting degrees of disability, that people living with HIV may embody over their life course.

REFERENCES

Black Coalition for AIDS Prevention (Black-CAP). 2008. "Dealing with Being Different: A Resource Guide for Gay, Lesbian, Bisexual, Transgender, Queer and Questioning Black Youth." http://www.black-cap.com/downloads/Dealing_With_Being_Different.pdf.

Beyrer, Chris, et al. 2012. "A Call to Action for Comprehensive HIV Services for Men Who Have Sex with Men." *Lancet* 380 (9839): 424–38. https://doi.org/10.1016/S0140-6736(12)61022-8.

Conyers, L.M. 2004. "Expanding Understanding of HIV/AIDS and Employment: Perspectives of Focus Groups." *Rehabilitation Counseling Bulletin* 48 (1): 5–18. https://doi.org/10.1177/00343552040480010201.

Davis, Antoinette N., Jacqueline C. Gahagan, and Clemon George. 2013. "'Everyone Just Keeps Their Eyes Closed and Their Fingers Crossed': Sexual Health Communication among Black Parents and Children in Nova Scotia, Canada." *International Journal for Equity in Health* 12 (1). https://doi.org/10.1186/1475-9276-12-55.

Episodic Disabilities Employment Network (EDEN). 2016. "About Episodic Disabilities." http://www.edencanada.ca/en/episodicdisabilities.

Government of Canada, Service Canada. 2016. "Canada Pension Plan Disability Benefit: Overview." https://www.canada.ca/en/services/benefits/publicpensions/cpp/cpp-disability-benefit.html.

Government of Nova Scotia. 2013. "Basic Income Assistance Rates." http://novascotia.ca/coms/employment/income_assistance/BasicAssistance.html

– 2016. " Seniors' Pharmacare Program." https://novascotia.ca/dhw/pharmacare/seniors-pharmacare.asp.

Harrison, Elizabeth. 2015. *Episodic Disabilities and Post-secondary Education in Canada: A Review of the Literature.* Canadian Working Group on HIV and Rehabilitation. http://realizecanada.org/wp-content/uploads/FINAL_Lit_Review.pdf.

Patterson, S., et al. 2015. "Life Expectancy of HIV-Positive Individuals on Combination Antiretroviral Therapy in Canada." *BMC Infectious Diseases*

15 (24). http://bmcinfectdis.biomedcentral.com/articles/10.1186/s12879-015-0969-x.

Public Health Agency of Canada (PHAC). 2013."Chapter 4: Current Evidence on Social Determinants of Health Affecting People Living with HIV/AIDS." In *Population-Specific HIV/AIDS Status Report: People Living with HIV/AIDS.* http://www.phac-aspc.gc.ca/aids-sida/publication/ps-pd/people-personnes/chapter-chapitre-4-eng.php.

Realize. 2016. "Episodic Disabilities." http://www.realizecanada.org/en/our-work/episodic-disabilities/.

# PART THREE

Populations

# 9 Governing Participation: A Critical Analysis of International and Canadian Texts Promoting the Greater Involvement of People Living with HIV and AIDS

ALEX McCLELLAND, ADRIAN GUTA,
AND NICOLE R. GREENSPAN

Into its third decade, the HIV epidemic remains a leading health crisis in Canada and around the world. The response to HIV is now orchestrated through a complex assemblage of provincial and federal governments, non-governmental organizations, corporations, philanthropic organizations, as well as large global multilateral institutions and aid agencies. This type of response is in stark contrast to the early days of the Canadian epidemic when HIV was assumed to affect only those on the margins (e.g., gay men, Haitian migrants, hemophiliacs and injection drug users) (Triechler 1999). The current institutionalization and corporatizations of the HIV response have been critiqued as undermining the original goals of the AIDS movement (Comaroff 2007; Guta, Murray, and McClelland 2011). Taking our lead from these critiques, we revisit and interrogate key policy developments that led to this shift and consider the consequences for the Canadian AIDS movement and key actors.

Specifically, we will examine policy documents that conceptualize and articulate the principle of "greater involvement of people living with HIV and AIDS" (GIPA). This internationally recognized principle is meant to underpin programmatic responses to the HIV epidemic in Canada and around the world (UNAIDS 1999, 2004b; Stephens 2004). GIPA is foremost a participatory principle that promotes the inclusion of people living with HIV[1] and recognizes them as important stakeholders who bring knowledge rooted in lived experience (Cabassi 2004, 24). However, our interest in critically examining GIPA began out of a collective concern that the *freedom* to participate is obscuring the troubling reality of the ongoing marginalization and exclusion of the very people it was meant to place at the centre of the AIDS response. With our analysis we ask, What role, if any, is there for a range of diversely marginalized people in today's institutionalized vision of a singular AIDS response?

Proponents of GIPA have argued that including people living with HIV in decision-making improves the quality of prevention, health promotion, care, programming, and policy development. Increasingly GIPA is becoming measured and enumerated as an indicator of success for the funding of programmatic initiatives. While first elaborated in international guidance documents, GIPA is now listed as an indicator in monitoring and evaluation frameworks for both the federally administered Public Health Agency of Canada AIDS Community Action Program, and in regional contexts, such as in Ontario's Community HIV and AIDS Reporting Tool. Intervention-based research has demonstrated that GIPA reduces stigma and isolation for people living with HIV and AIDS (Wingood and DiClemente 2000), and promotes increased feelings of personal development and self-worth (Barker 2005; Roy and Cain 2001). Canadian researchers in concert with AIDS service organizations have led in documenting the integration of GIPA into their programing (see, for example, Collins et al. 2007; Ontario AIDS Network 2011). While Canadian scholars have led in developing research on GIPA, there has been surprisingly little scholarship about GIPA, compared to the volume of research produced on the social, behavioural, and biomedical aspects of HIV (for a few notable exceptions see Roy and Cain 2001; Kinsman 1996; Altman 1994; Travers et al. 2008).

In Canada, when GIPA has been examined, the focus is on the normative evaluation of the negative consequences of not implementing GIPA "meaningfully" or "effectively" in AIDS service organizations, support services, or research interventions (Roy and Cain 2001; Travers et al. 2008; Roy 1995). For example, the influential study *Living and Serving* (Collins et al. 2007) outlines the ways in which Ontario's community-based HIV organizations involve people living with HIV in the HIV response, and identifies barriers to their engagement. The study does not interrogate the assumptions underpinning the GIPA principle, but rather outlines a range of recommendations on how community-based organizations can work to better integrate people living with HIV in their work. Similarly, Travers et al. (2008) identified barriers to the involvement of people living with HIV, particularly in Canadian community-based participatory research projects on HIV. This normative evaluation of the implementation of GIPA in participatory research projects outlines a range of barriers to achieving the "meaningful" involvement of people living with HIV, including stigma and discrimination, the disclosure of HIV-positive status, health challenges, credentialism, practical skills, capacity building, trust, and other priorities such as income and food security (ibid.).

These Canadian studies have provided important insight into the changing nature of AIDS work within a neoliberal context and the increasing trajectory towards formalization, professionalization, funding austerity, and needs for efficiency. This reflects the broader growth of neoliberal policy in the health and education sectors since the 1970s and their encroachment into people's everyday lives (Luxton and Braedley 2010). Now, health interventions are treated as business ventures that seek a maximum possible return on the investments made by state institutions and taxpayers. However, in the aforementioned studies GIPA is seldom interrogated and assumed to be unchanged, politically neutral, and both necessary and beneficial, without much discussion or debate. The underlying assumption here is that if international declarations and community-based organizational policies on GIPA were realized, social problems that are reproduced in community-based organizations, interventions, and research projects would be resolved.

The objective of this chapter is to offer a critical contribution by problematizing the rationalities that have guided the development and deployment of GIPA. We examine key GIPA policy and programmatic documents with attention to what forms of participation for people with HIV these texts enable or constrain. The goal of this analysis is to surface alternative readings of GIPA documents and offer a critical interpretation of what they represent for the engagement of people living with HIV in the Canadian and global response. We further aim to contribute to a growing critical re-engagement in HIV studies in opposition to the ongoing privileging of biomedical perspectives (Mykhalovskiy and Rosengarten 2009; Adam 2011; Mykhalovskiy 2010; Patton 2011).

**Guiding Theory**

Our analysis of GIPA policy documents is informed by Michel Foucault's (1980) writings about the complex relationship between power and knowledge in shaping discourse, knowledge, and systems of social control. Foucault's (2002) orientation to discourse provides a useful

approach for investigating GIPA and the growing inducement to involve people living with HIV. For Foucault, discourse provides a way of
reconciling what one says ("language") and what one does ("practice") within larger systems of representation and meaning (Hall 2001,
72). Specifically, Foucault (2003, 138) was interested in how individual
and collective conduct is orchestrated through what he terms "governmentality" (or the "conduct of conducts") through which ideolo-
gies and discourses are used to promote and secure particular conceptions of social order. Dean (2010, 18) explains that governmentality
employs "a variety of techniques and forms of knowledge, that seek
to shape conduct by working through the desires, aspirations, interests and beliefs of various actors." A number of scholars have observed
such techniques manifested in citizenship projects aimed at creating
"communities" who mobilize to promote safety, health, and economic
prosperity (Miller and Rose 2008; Cruikshank 1999; Cooke and Kothari
2001; Rose 1999).

We take our lead from earlier critical HIV studies that identified strategies for governing people living with, and affected by, HIV through
subtle and overt public health surveillance, health promotion, medical
treatment, and claims of shared culture and purpose (Liesch and Patton
2010; Geary 2007; Keogh 2008; Elbe 2005; Ingram 2010). Much of this
literature has noted the key role played by neoliberal discourses about
health and citizenship wherein individuals become entrepreneurs of
themselves through a combination of health seeking and individual
capacity building (Rose 2007; Miller and Rose 2008; Hamann 2009).
On a programmatic level this can be seen in microfinance schemes
that turn women in "developing" contexts into entrepreneurs (Rankin
2002), and in health promotion (Gastaldo 1997) and community-based
participatory research (Guta, Flicker, and Roche 2013; Guta et al. 2014)
where communities are mobilized to improve their own health conditions through self-initiated research. The HIV sector continues to lead
in developing and implementing such techniques for active citizenship
internationally.

## A Discursive Analysis of GIPA Texts

We analysed key international policy and programmatic guidance
documents and a series of Canadian texts to examine current concep-
tualizations and definitions of GIPA. The international documents are

prominent in conceptualizing how GIPA has been taken up in the Canadian context. The texts examined represent a subset from a sample of forty-five GIPA documents selected as part of a global review of GIPA to inform the development of a "best practice" guide from program workers in the AIDS response (McClelland and De Pauw 2010). The original review identified examples of GIPA in organizational policy-making, programing and research, education, peer-support, campaigns and public speaking, advocacy, and the experiences of workers with HIV, and synthesized them for a programming audience. The results of this broad review were developed into a guide to inform the daily practices of front-line HIV intervention staff in organizations around the world. The documents we focus on in our secondary review for this chapter were selected for their prominence and role as coordinating texts in GIPA initiatives. The international texts we selected have been widely cited in the Canadian literature on GIPA – where GIPA is often described in relation to international policies and declarations – and have guided how GIPA is taken up and conceptualized at the local level, where key actors shape how the response to AIDS is organized. In the current analysis, we pay attention to what forms of engagement the texts conceptually enable or constrain.

This discourse method is used to elucidate how GIPA is discursively conceptualized, and problematize key aspects of its deployment. However, such an analysis cannot offer a "true" or "authentic" account of subjective experiences of people living with HIV. Nor can it account for how texts come to be activated in the social realm. Our approach instead offers insights into how conduct may be shaped by the neoliberal logic of corporatism, managerialism, and rationality that circulate in the AIDS industry. We argue that these documents produce possibility for the participation of people living with HIV in the current response to the Canadian epidemic. In the nearly twenty-five years since Cindy Patton (1990) first described the emergence of the AIDS industry, we continue to see the impact of shifting from community AIDS responses to formalized governmental approaches. Our textual analysis does not call into question whether people living with HIV should be involved in the AIDS movement, but instead challenges the kind of engagement prescribed by a programmatic, managerial, and self-help discourse of GIPA. We complement our discursive reading with insights from our own lived, practised, and professional experience in the tradition of Cooke and Kothari (2001), who call for greater *reflexivity* among those engaged in participatory work to ensure complex and nuanced power relations are revealed. We draw on our collective experience to inform our reading of GIPA documents.

## The Denver Principles

> The idea that personal experiences should shape the AIDS response was first voiced by people living with HIV in Denver in 1983. The GIPA Principle was formalized at the 1994 Paris AIDS Summit when 42 countries agreed to "support a greater involvement of people living with HIV at all ... levels ... and to ... stimulate the creation of supportive political, legal and social environments." (UNAIDS 2007)

In our review of documents we trace the trajectory and development of notions of participation in the HIV response. Through this development we see participation first being understood as a *right*, as described in the Denver Principles, then becoming a *responsibility* for people living with HIV. At the same time, the outcomes of GIPA as it is now discursively elaborated include improved relevance, efficiency, and acceptability of HIV interventions. The documents we examine promote the idea that people living with HIV should remain closely connected to AIDS service organizations and should be constantly reminded about their responsibility to reduce further transmissions. Here people living with HIV come to be understood as an instrumental resource in the response to the epidemic (Geary 2007; Holt 2013). In this review, we also identify the emergence of a managerial discourse of efficiency, self-help, and capacity building that has become the central goal of many HIV-related participatory interventions. From Denver to Paris to UN policy and program guidance documents, the developments we trace have come to shape and frame how GIPA is discursively conceptualized in the Canadian response.

The discursive conditions of possibility that produced the form of GIPA we see in policy and programmatic documents today can be traced to the Denver Principles declaration (1983). The statement was written by American AIDS activists living with HIV who attended the 1983 Second National AIDS Forum hosted by the National Lesbian and Gay Health Conference in response to their exclusion from official decision-making. This one-page declaration of the rights and responsibilities of people living with HIV is written in a collective voice of anger and protest. This early text predated the codified form of GIPA we see today, but situated HIV in the social context of crisis, mass death, and lack of state response. The Denver Principles demand entry into the corridors of power to ensure expedited responses to the growing epidemic. The text of the Denver Principles rhetorically claims space and identity for HIV-positive people. The language throughout is emotive and impassioned; it reflects the context in which it was developed where people were dying en masse and being discriminated against. The text further calls on decision-makers (the American medical establishment for whom the statement was intended) to radically change their approach to caring for people who had contracted the virus: "We condemn attempts to label us as 'victims,' a term which implies defeat, and we are only occasionally 'patients,' a term which implies passivity, helplessness, and dependence upon the care of others. We are 'People with AIDS'" (Advisory Committee of the People with AIDS 1983).

The Denver Principles reject an identity based on the labels of "patients" or "victims" and instead uses "people with AIDS," an identity entitled to the dignity and rights accorded to all people. The text claims space by calling for participation as equals in the production of knowledge in the responses to HIV. This text was the first time that this identity was asserted and defined, and this language is widely used today in the HIV response (including the Canadian programmatic documents discussed below). Explicitly, it calls for people living with HIV to "be involved at every level of decision-making and specifically serve on the boards of directors of provider organizations." This tactic was widely used among treatment activists at a time when the overarching demonstration mantra was "drugs into bodies" (Smith and Siplon 2006). Treatment activists worked tirelessly to get a "seat at the table" with government funders, regulatory bodies, and pharmaceutical companies to ensure the development and rollout of life-saving medications. While the Denver Principles are written in impassioned activist language, the authors were attuned to the language of the medical and state institutional structures they wanted to win over. This activism saved countless lives and laid the groundwork for organizational engagement that we see today in more recent GIPA policies.

Although the Denver Principles were produced out of a social context very different from the institutional policy and programmatic documents that follow, we believe it is important to frame our analysis in relation to this text to address how GIPA policies have been taken up and practised more than twenty years later in the current AIDS industry.

## GIPA as International Policy Framework

In the decade following the Denver Principles, the HIV sector witnessed increased political mobilizing by people living with and affected by HIV. The increased mobilization culminated in the 1994 Paris AIDS Summit, where forty-two countries (including Canada) agreed to recognize the principle of the greater involvement of people living with HIV and AIDS (GIPA) in the Paris Declaration (UNAIDS 1999; 2004b; Stephens 2004). The document is just two pages long and comprises four sections. The first section notes that HIV "constitutes a threat to humanity" and "is hindering social and economic development" and "that new local, national and international forms of solidarity are emerging, involving in particular people living with HIV/AIDS and community-based organizations" (1994). Here we see the emergence of economic rationality alongside community-based solidarity.

In the next section of the Paris Declaration, signing countries "solemnly declare" to make "our obligation as political leaders to make the fight against HIV/AIDS a priority." Thus, while community and civil society are introduced earlier, leadership now comes from political leaders of nation states. These leaders further determine to "mobilize all of society – the public and private sectors, community-based organizations and people living with HIV/AIDS – in a spirit of true partnership." These partnerships will involve "activities and work carried out by multilateral, intergovernmental, non-governmental and community-based organizations," which will be coordinated and sustained "by the joint and cosponsored United Nations programme on HIV/AIDS" (Paris AIDS Summit 1994). What starts as a political enterprise at the state level moves out to become a global coordinating and regulatory system based on the structure of nation states.

Overall, what becomes apparent in this text is the increasing bureaucratization of the author's voice. The language moves away from the passionate activist language of life and death in the Denver Principles to discussions of developing the "capacity" and "coordination" of organizations of people living with HIV. In this policy document, the language of "we" shifts from people living with HIV to "We, the Heads of Government or Representatives of the 42 States assembled in Paris on 1 December 1994." These leaders and representatives "solemnly declared" it *their* obligation to make fighting HIV and AIDS a priority and to "mobilize all of society – the public and private sectors, community based organizations and people living with HIV/AIDS – in a spirit of true partnership" (Paris AIDS Summit 1994). The text sets the role of people living with HIV within the organizing hub of community-based organizations, and emphasizes that individual goals should be aligned with organizational goals. Whereas in the Denver Principles people living with HIV did not want to be separated from their communities, the Paris Declaration text created a form of professional space within the programmatic response to HIV for people living with HIV.

Following the Paris Summit, UNAIDS (1999) developed a policy guidance document entitled *From Principle to Practice: Greater Involvement of People Living with or Affected by HIV/AIDS (GIPA)*. The document is helpful in defining GIPA (which includes introducing the acronym into popular use) as "recognizing the important contribution people infected or affected by HIV/AIDS can make in the response to the epidemic"; and "creating space within society for their involvement and active participation in all aspects of that response" (2). Moreover, "this contribution can be made at all levels, from the individual to the organizational, and in all sectors from the social and cultural to the economic and political" (2). The document includes a pyramid of involvement, with the highest form including the participation of people living with HIV "in decision-making or policy-making bodies, and their inputs are valued equally with all the other members of these bodies," but it notes that too often their role is limited "to observer or educational functions" (2–3). In this model of engagement, the greater the specialized "expertise" of a person with HIV, the greater that person's capacity to contribute and be recognized as contributing towards AIDS responses. The document further identifies early "challenges to implementing GIPA at higher levels," including acknowledging HIV status publicly, lack of organizational preparedness, lack of personal skills and preparation, lack of proper conditions within organizations, and questions of sustainability for working roles (5–6). In this section of the document, we find the first discussion of "capacity" and the proposal that the need for "communication and personal empowerment counselling should be part of a generic training package for people participating in GIPA initiatives. As well, such training must be reinforced by ongoing support for PWHAs [people living with HIV/AIDS] if their effectiveness is to remain high and their motivation strong" (5). Later, the importance of the private sector is introduced, and the point that while people living with HIV may not have the necessary technical skills, they should be considered for jobs (8). However, ongoing training and support for individuals is needed, as well as "GIPA training packages for PWHAs," which should include personal empowerment, communication, and presentation skills (8–9).

In 2001, the United Nations held a General Assembly Special Session on HIV/AIDS (UNGASS), and a Declaration of Commitment (DoC) was adopted by all member states at the conclusion of the meeting where 189 countries endorsed the GIPA principle. The fifty-two-page DoC is "the first comprehensive set of principles and targets ever adopted internationally for confronting HIV/AIDS" and presents itself as a formal report (UNAIDS 2001). Starting with "We, heads of State and Government and representatives of States and Governments," the report identifies 103 specific sections, among which member states commit to "acknowledging the particular role and significant contribution of people living with HIV/AIDS ... in addressing the problem of HIV/AIDS in all its aspects, and recognizing that their full involvement and participation in the design, planning, implementation and evaluation of programmes is crucial to the development of effective responses to the HIV/AIDS epidemic" (UNAIDS 2001).

Participation in this sense becomes highly strategic and instrumental. With this declaration, GIPA is recognized as making responses to HIV "effective," and this builds upon what was introduced in the Paris Declaration about improving the response. As this declaration became the international monitoring mechanism for country progress in the response to HIV, GIPA then became a "progress indicator" applied and integrated into national AIDS plans – in which progress is documented and monitored by the UN annually.

In the UNAIDS' *Position Paper: Greater Involvement of People Living with or Affected by HIV/AIDS (GIPA)* (2004b) and the four-page *Policy Brief: The Greater Involvement of People Living with HIV/AIDS (GIPA)* (2007), GIPA is elaborated and discussed in detail beyond the Paris Declaration and the DoC. A notable addition is the need for "sustained support for people doing GIPA work" (UNAIDS 2004a, 2). These documents explain that to undertake "GIPA work," people living with HIV need training and skills, because "the motivation of individual persons or groups is not enough to sustain GIPA" (ibid.). Another important aspect of this brief is that "persons living with HIV" are described as "probably the greatest resource in the global response to the epidemic" (1). Their human capital becomes something to harness and mobilize – a kind of commodity. Here again, GIPA is credited with improving the "relevance, acceptability and effectiveness" of HIV responses (UNAIDS 2007, 1). The position paper also states that GIPA "aims to realize the rights and responsibilities of people living with HIV, including their right to self-determination" (ibid.). Notably, GIPA becomes more strongly linked to universal access to treatment: "The engagement of people living with HIV is all the more urgent as countries scale up their national AIDS responses to achieve the goal of universal access to prevention, treatment, care and support services" (ibid.), and that involvement includes "people living with HIV ... actively involved in their own health and welfare. They take an active role in decisions about treatment, self-education about therapies, opportunistic infections and adherence, and positive prevention" (2).

## GIPA as National Policy Framework: The Canadian Example

We now examine modules of *One Foot Forward: A GIPA Training Toolkit* by the Canadian AIDS Society (CAS) (2009a). These documents are the primary GIPA program guidance documents developed for a national context in Canada, and they provide a comprehensive example of localized participatory policy and program guidance, which continually references the international policy documents that were encompassed in our review to frame conceptions of the GIPA. The toolkit uses the UNAIDS (2007) definition of GIPA. CAS describes this training toolkit as a series of documents that are "designed by and for PHAs (people living with HIV and AIDS) to assist them in building capacity and in acquiring leadership skills that promote their greater and more meaningful involvement in communities across the country" (2009a). While we understand that CAS has gone through turmoil in recent times, we read these texts as standing apart from the organization itself. The toolkit is distributed online and via the CATIE ordering centre, Canada's leading organization for knowledge on HIV. The modules have been developed continually since 2009 through a range of committees consisting of people living with HIV. Recent editions have addressed participation for youth and for aging populations living with HIV. The modules provide exercises to help people living with HIV "gain a better sense of where [they] are in the process of choosing where to concentrate [their] greater and meaningful involvement" and a self-assessment questionnaire at the end of each module to help them "reflect on how well [they] have taken in the information" (Canadian AIDS Society 2009b, 2).

Module 1 provides people living with HIV with an introduction and overview of community-based organizations, common programs and activities, and organizational structures available to them (Canadian

AIDS Society 2009c). The nature of "conflict" is introduced in this section, and readers are warned to avoid "gossip; rumour; innuendo;
name-calling; and getting dragged into politics" (13). Module 2 encourages people living with HIV to assess their agency's capacity to involve
them, and encourages "getting to know your agency" (Canadian AIDS
Society 2009d, 9). However, participating in agency life has acknowledged "pitfalls," which people living with HIV need to be aware of:
"When you become involved in the work of an agency, whatever the
program or area of involvement, you run the risk of being emotionally
involved because you yourself are living with HIV every day. Being
that close to a particular issue may cloud your judgment, cause you to
become involved in the internal politics of the agency, bring on stress
that you don't want and otherwise turn the experience sour for you.
Always be aware of how getting caught up in office politics will affect
you personally and try your best to avoid it" (10).

The groundwork in modules 1 and 2 prepare people living with HIV
to become "leaders" in module 3 (Canadian AIDS Society 2009e). Leadership is described as "not so much about making things happen as it is
about helping things to happen" and "some of the best leaders are those
who are quiet and listen" (2–3). This is in stark contrast to the tactics of
early AIDS activists who recognized their struggle as inherently and
unavoidably political and used strategies like die-ins that shut down
government, medical, economic, and media institutions to draw attention to their cause. The importance of listening is further emphasized
by the abrupt introduction of an exercise that asks the reader to

> Put down this module, or pause the CD.
> Sit comfortably, wherever you are.
> Now, listen. Listen for one minute.
> What did you hear?
> What sounds were near you? A clock? Your breath?
> What sounds were beyond those sounds? Traffic? Creaking in your house?
> Learn to really listen. Try this exercise once each day. It only takes a
>    minute and you can do it wherever you happen to be. Pay close atten-
>    tion to what you hear. That's what listening and hearing is about. (3)

In the difficult task of "influencing the influencers" (leaders) the reader is reminded to "be happy, regardless of the outcome. The only person
you can really, truly change is you" (Canadian AIDS Society 2009e, 5).
This is further elaborated through discussion of "basic communication

skills" and advice on posture and commonly misread body cues like "fidgeting" (13–14). This continues in module 6, where people living with HIV are encouraged to assess their transferable skills (Canadian AIDS Society 2009f). In module 7 the reader is reminded, "When working on your résumé, you need to think about your skills and not your sero-status. Unless you experience recurrent illness, you are as fit to work as the next person" (Canadian AIDS Society 2009g, 6).

## Discussion

Through this review of international and Canadian GIPA policy and program documents, we have identified the ways in which this participatory principle has come to represent a managerial framework prescribing how people living with HIV should respond to the epidemic. We argue that the texts we have analysed discursively constrain the response of people living with HIV, and endorse a particular orientation to the self and others. These documents serve a very real function in structuring operations and organization of AIDS responses.

The documents reviewed create an international script that is taken up locally, as we see with the development of the Canadian AIDS Society toolkit, which relies on its explication of GIPA through UNAIDS GIPA policy documents. In our own engagement within HIV responses, we have seen this script taken up within a range of HIV interventions, which tells HIV-positive people to form or join advisory committees, evaluate services, compete for program and research dollars, and build "capacity" to become more productive in the fight against AIDS – all while staying clear of issues that are deemed "political." In this script, governments and politicians can be trusted to worry about structural inequities and the resulting racism, classism, homophobia, transphobia, drug user stigma, and gender-based violence that fuel the global epidemic. All the while, this script consigns people living with HIV to keep doing and promoting "GIPA work." What we see here is the sublimation of attempts at earlier radical forms of democracy that characterized the beginnings of the movement, into more governable forms of citizenship that can be mobilized to achieve the goals of state and extra-state institutions (Brown 1997). As we have argued elsewhere (Guta, Murray, and McClelland 2011), this shift leads to restricted opportunities for resistance to a singular version of the global AIDS response.

An important trend we have identified in these documents is the introduction and deployment of corporatist managerial language, logic, and rationalities – *efficiency, benchmarks, progress indicators, capacity-building, skills development, etc.* This market logic can be seen in the description of people living with HIV as a "resource" to be tapped to make the global AIDS response more effective. However, this efficiency has little to do with large-scale aid investments, reducing trade patents, or national interventions that might seek to equalize income. Rather, they take the form of increasing the individual human capital of people living with HIV through capacity building that enables them to be more efficient GIPA workers. These documents fail to question for whom and for what purpose this "capacity" is being built, as in much of the literature that merges health promotion and economic interests (Labonte and Laverack 2001). More than just enabling people living with HIV to undertake GIPA work, it instils a particular ethical relation between them, their human capital, and others within their communities, within systems of governance (Hamann 2009). These texts invite the individual subject living with HIV to seek out self-determination by participating in processes and mechanisms designed by states and multilateral institutions. The discourse of empowerment belies the subtle aims to manage and discipline a "disorganized" seropositive subject and make it more productive – to enable it to *do* that GIPA work. Kinsman (1996, 400) tells us, "The strategy to produce self-managing, self-regulating individuals with HIV/AIDS, who will be much easier for social and medical agencies to handle, is in part a shifting of demands for empowerment. There was activist pressure for this – an impetus 'from below.' As in other areas, 'empowerment' has been transformed from a critique of professional powers into a new mode of 'professional' activity."

In particular, the Canadian AIDS Society *One Foot Forward* modules perpetuate the belief that people living with HIV are unruly and need to be trained to fit into the system that supposedly serves them. On its website, the Canadian AIDS Society calls itself "the national voice of people living with HIV/AIDS in Canada. Representing community-based AIDS organizations across the country." The organization regularly organizes national and regional events where the *One Foot Forward* series are mobilized to train people living with HIV. But as we have outlined, this toolkit is an explicit example of how individuals with HIV are made to recognize the ways in which their bodies, habits, skills, feelings, etc. are disorganized, and how they could turn these into something more productive. These documents focus on describing the skills individuals might need to fit into professional environments (as a worker or a volunteer), and how to succeed within those environments that are underpinned by a logic of accountability and professionaliza-tion. In Foucault's terms (1994, 225), these forms of capacity-building are "technologies of power" that require people living with HIV to submit to forms of domination. Yet we acknowledge the supposed transformative effect GIPA on some people's lives, giving them a sense of purpose and meaning. From a Foucaultian perspective (ibid.), they reflect "technologies of the self, which permit individuals to effect by their own means or with the help of others a certain number of opera-tions on their own bodies and souls, thoughts, conduct, and way of be-ing, so as to transform themselves." However, regardless of how we choose to frame this approach to GIPA, as technologies of domination or technologies of the self, they are both techniques of governing self and others and cannot be separated from the operations of power.

In the *One Foot Forward* series we are especially troubled by the no-tion that "good leaders" do not speak, do not involve themselves in politics, and do not get emotional. Emotional political engagement and disruption were once central aspects of the AIDS response and changed the relationship between health-care recipients and care-providers, and between citizens and the state. This shift has enabled engagement and participation from individuals who had been marginalized, and some have been able to find a "voice," including people who use drugs, peo ple who are co-infected with hepatitis C and/or TB, and people who live in extreme poverty. However, many other people on the margins cannot, will not, or refuse to become "good listeners" and sit quietly, and, despite investments in their "capacity" and human capital, will never be good candidates for "GIPA work."

## Conclusion

We posit that the concept of GIPA has not evolved through debate and discussion because there was concern that critiques would take us back to the beginnings of the epidemic when people living with HIV were silenced and without a "seat at the table." This, we fear, has led to sus-picions that anyone who raises concerns is a threat. Elisabeth Pisani (2008, 195) has argued that one risks being labelled a "monster" when challenging long-held beliefs within the HIV response. In our experi-ence of presenting this work, we were struck by claims that we were "against GIPA." We are not against GIPA, but we find ourselves in a position similar to that of Foucault (1994, 256), who famously said, "My point is not that everything is bad, but that everything is dangerous."

To reiterate, our argument has not been that GIPA is "bad." Rather, we call for the examination of the assumptions that underpin emancipatory discourse, especially those which may result in stifling dialogue and constraining our ability to challenge the inequities fuelling the ongoing AIDS epidemic. Cruikshank (1999, 68–9) tells us, "The will to empower may be well intentioned, but it is a strategy for constituting and regulating the political subjectivities of the 'empowered.'" As has been observed elsewhere, simply giving community a "seat at the table" will not result in change if those with greater authority dictate the limits of participation (Stern and Green 2008).

NOTE

1 We do not use the acronym *PHA* or other such acronym in our work (PLHIV, PLHA, PWA, etc.) as we believe this is a reductive practice that can dehumanize people with HIV. These terms are used in this chapter only when quoting others' texts. As the HIV response is heavily regulated by medicine and science, we have adopted the use of epidemiological terms and acronyms for many things in our work. The use of the acronym *PHA*, which is widely used in the Canadian context, assumes that people living with HIV are a homogeneous group with the same needs and experiences. Using terms like this helps make the jobs of bureaucrats and researchers easier, but this check-box logic for representation creates false assumptions about who we are looking at and the people we are working with. People living with HIV are widely diverse, with divergent needs and lives.

REFERENCES

Adam, Barry D. 2011. "Epistemic Fault Lines in Biomedical and Social Approaches to HIV Prevention." In "Bridging the Social and the Biomedical: Engaging the Social and Political Sciences in HIV Research," supplement, *Journal of the International AIDS Society* 14 (S2). https://doi.org/10.1186/1758-2652-14-S2-S2.
Advisory Committee of the People with AIDS. 1983. "Denver Principles." http://www.thebody.com/content/art30903.html.
Altman, Dennis. 1994. *Power and Community: Organizational and Cultural Responses to AIDS, Social Aspects of AIDS*. London: Taylor & Francis.
Barker, A. 2005. *Volunteers in Action: Engaging Volunteers in the HIV/AIDS Sector. Findings from the 2005 British Columbia Assessment*. Vancouver: AIDS Vancouver.

Brown, Michael P. 1997. *Replacing Citizenship: AIDS Activism and Radical Democracy*. New York: Guilford.

Cabassi, J. 2004. *Renewing Our Voice: Code of Practice for NGOs Responding to HIV/AIDS*. Geneva: International Federation of Red Cross and Red Crescent Societies. https://doi.org/10.3362/9780855988388.

Canadian AIDS Society. 2009a. *One Foot Forward: A GIPA Training Toolkit*. Ottawa: Canadian AIDS Society.

– 2009b. *One Foot Forward: A GIPA Training Toolkit. Module i: Introduction*. http://www.cdnaids.ca/wp-content/uploads/Module-i-2.pdf.

– 2009c. *One Foot Forward: A GIPA Training Toolkit. Module 1: Community-Based Groups*. http://www.cdnaids.ca/wp-content/uploads/Module-1.pdf.

– 2009d. *One Foot Forward: A GIPA Training Toolkit. Module 2: Assessing Your Agency*. http://www.cdnaids.ca/wp-content/uploads/Module-2-2.pdf.

– 2009e. *One Foot Forward: A GIPA Training Toolkit. Module 3: Leadership*. http://www.cdnaids.ca/wp-content/uploads/Module-3-2.pdf.

– 2009f. *One Foot Forward: A GIPA Training Toolkit. Module 6: What about ME?* http://www.cdnaids.ca/wp-content/uploads/Module-6-2.pdf.

– 2009g. *One Foot Forward: A GIPA Training Toolkit. Module 7: Is That All There Is?* http://www.cdnaids.ca/wp-content/uploads/Module-7-2.pdf.

Collins, E., et al. 2007. *Living and Serving II: 10 Years Later: The Involvement of People Living with HIV/AIDS in the Community AIDS Movement in Ontario*. Toronto: Ontario HIV Treatment Network.

Comaroff, Jean. 2007. "Beyond Bare Life: AIDS, (Bio)Politics, and the Neoliberal Order." *Public Culture* 19 (1): 197–219. https://doi.org/10.1215/08992363-2006-030.

Cooke, Bill, and Uma Kothari, eds. 2001. *Participation: The New Tyranny?* London: Zed Books.

Cruikshank, Barbara. 1999. *The Will to Empower: Democratic Citizens and Other Subjects*. Ithaca, NY: Cornell University Press.

Dean, Mitchell. 2010. *Governmentality: Power and Rule in Modern Society*. 2nd ed. Los Angeles: Sage.

Elbe, Stefan. 2005. "AIDS, Security, Biopolitics." *International Relations* 19 (4): 403–19. https://doi.org/10.1177/0047117805058532.

Foucault, Michel. 1980. *Power/Knowledge: Selected Interviews and Other Writings*. Toronto: Random House of Canada.

– 1994. *Ethics: Subjectivity and Truth*, edited by Paul Rabinow. New York: New Press.

– 2002. *Archaeology of Knowledge*. Routledge Classics. London: Routledge.

– 2003. *The Essential Foucault: Selections from Essential Works of Foucault, 1954–1984*, edited by Paul Rabinow and Nikolas Rose. New York: New Press.

Gastaldo, Denise. 1997. "Is Health Education Good for You? Re-thinking Health Education through the Concept of Biopower." In *Foucault: Health and Medicine*, edited by A. Peterson and R. Bunton, 113–33. New York: Routledge.

Geary, A.M. 2007. "Culture as an Object of Ethical Governance in AIDS Prevention." *Cultural Studies* 21 (4–5): 672–94.

Guta, Adrian, Sarah Flicker, and Brenda Roche. 2013. "Governing through Community Allegiance: A Qualitative Examination of Peer Research in Community-Based Participatory Research." *Critical Public Health* 23 (4): 432–51. https://doi.org/10.1080/09581596.2012.761675.

Guta, Adrian, Stuart J. Murray, and Alexander McClelland. 2011. "Global AIDS Governance, Biofascism, and the Difficult Freedom of Expression." *Aporia* 3 (4): 15–29.

Guta, Adrian, et al. 2014. "Governing through Community-Based Research: Lessons from the Canadian HIV Research Sector." *Social Science & Medicine* 123:250–61. https://doi.org/10.1016/j.socscimed.2014.07.028.

Hall, Stuart. 2001. "Foucault: Power, Knowledge, and Discourse." In *Discourse Theory and Practice*, edited by Margaret Wetherell, Stephanie Taylor, and Simeon Yates, 72–81. London: Sage.

Hamann, Trent, H. 2009. "Neoliberalism, Governmentality, and Ethics." *Foucault Studies* 6:37–59. https://doi.org/10.22439/fs.v0i0.2471.

Holt, Martin. 2013. "Enacting and Imagining Gay Men: The Looping Effects of Behavioural HIV Surveillance in Australia." *Critical Public Health* 23 (4): 404–17. https://doi.org/10.1080/09581596.2013.796038.

Ingram, Alan. 2010. "Governmentality and Security in the US President's Emergency Plan for AIDS Relief (PEPFAR)." *Geoforum* 41 (4): 607–16. https://doi.org/10.1016/j.geoforum.2010.02.002.

Keogh, Peter. 2008. "How to Be a Healthy Homosexual: HIV Health Promotion and the Social Regulation of Gay Men in the United Kingdom." *Journal of Homosexuality* 55 (4): 581–605. https://doi.org/10.1080/00918360802421692.

Kinsman, Gary. 1996. "'Responsibility' as a Strategy of Governance: Regulating People Living with AIDS and Lesbians and Gay Men in Ontario." *Economy and Society* 25 (3): 393–409. https://doi.org/10.1080/03085149600000021.

Labonte, Ronald, and Glenn Laverack. 2001. "Capacity Building in Health Promotion, Part 1: For Whom? And for What Purpose?" *Critical Public Health* 11 (2): 111–27. https://doi.org/10.1080/09581590110039838.

Liesch, John, and Cindy Patton. 2010. "Clinic or Spa? Facial Surgery in the Context of AIDS Related Facial Wasting." In *Rebirth of the Clinic: Places* and Agents in Contemporary Health Care, edited by Cindy Patton, 1–16. Minneapolis: University of Minnesota Press.

Luxton, Meg, and Susan Braedley. 2010. Neoliberalism and Everyday Life. Montreal and Kingston: McGill-Queen's University Press.

McClelland, Alexander, and Lia De Pauw. 2010. Greater Involvement of People Living with HIV (GIPA): Good Practice Guide. Amsterdam: International HIV/ AIDS Alliance and the Global Network of People Living with HIV (GNP+).

Miller, Peter, and Nikolas S. Rose. 2008. Governing the Present: Administering Economic, Social and Personal Life. Cambridge: Polity.

Mykhalovskiy, Eric. 2010. "Integrating HIV Treatment and Prevention: Shifts in Community-Based Organising and Biopolitics in the Canadian Context." In HIV Treatment and Prevention Technologies in International Perspective, edited by Mark Davis and Corinne Squire, 61–86. Basingstoke, UK: Palgrave Macmillan. https://doi.org/10.1057/9780230297050_4.

Mykhalovskiy, Eric, and Marsha Rosengarten. 2009. "HIV/AIDS in Its Third Decade: Renewed Critique in Social and Cultural Analysis – An Introduction." Social Theory & Health 7 (3): 187–95. https://doi.org/10.1057/ sth.2009.13.

Ontario AIDS Network. 2011. Living and Serving 3: GIPA Engagement Guide and Framework for Ontario ASOs. Toronto: Ontario AIDS Network.

Paris AIDS Summit. 1994. "Paris Declaration, 1 December."

Patton, Cindy. 1990. Inventing AIDS. New York: Routledge.

– 2011. "Rights Language and HIV Treatment: Universal Care or Population Control?" Rhetoric Society Quarterly 41 (3): 250–66. https://doi.org/10.1080/ 02773945.2011.575328.

Pisani, Elizabeth. 2008. The Wisdom of Whores: Bureaucrats, Brothels and the Business of AIDS. Toronto: Penguin Group Canada.

Rankin, Katherine N. 2002. "Social Capital, Microfinance, and the Politics of Development." Feminist Economics 8 (1): 1–24. https://doi.org/10.1080/ 13545700210125167.

Rose, Nikolas S. 1999. Governing the Soul: The Shaping of the Private Self. 2nd ed. London: Free Association Books.

– 2007. The Politics of Life Itself: Biomedicine, Power, and Subjectivity in the Twenty-First Century. Information series. Princeton, NJ: Princeton University Press. https://doi.org/10.1515/9781400827503.

Roy, Charles. 1995. Living and Serving: Persons with HIV in the Canadian AIDS Movement. New York: University of New York.

Roy, Charles, and Roy Cain. 2001. "The Involvement of People Living with HIV/AIDS in Community-Based Organizations: Contributions and

Constraints." *AIDS Care* 13 (4): 421–32. https://doi.org/10.1080/09540120120057950.

Smith, Raymond A., and Patricia D. Siplon. 2006. *Drugs into bodies: Global AIDS Treatment Activism*. Westport, CT: Greenwood Publishing Group.

Stephens, David. 2004. *Out of the Shadows: Greater Involvement of People Living with HIV/AIDS (GIPA) in Policy*. Washington, DC: Policy Project.

Stern, Ruth, and Judith Green. 2008. "A Seat at the Table? A Study of Community Participation in Two Healthy Cities Projects." *Critical Public Health* 18 (3): 391–403. https://doi.org/10.1080/09581590801959337.

Travers, Robb, et al. 2008. "The Greater Involvement of People Living with AIDS Principle: Theory versus Practice in Ontario's HIV/AIDS Community-Based Research Sector." *AIDS Care* 20 (6): 615–24. https://doi.org/10.1080/09540120701661690.

Triechler, Paula A. 1999. *How to Have Theory in an Epidemic: Cultural Chronicles of AIDS*. Durham, NC: Duke University Press.

UNAIDS. 1999. *From Principle to Practice: Greater Involvement of People Living with or Affected by HIV/AIDS*. Geneva: UNAIDS.

– 2001. "Declaration of Commitment on HIV/AIDS: Global Crisis – Global Action." http://www.un.org/ga/aids/coverage/FinalDeclaration HIVAIDS.html.

– 2004a. *Position Paper: Greater Involvement of Person Living with or Affected by HIV/AIDS*. Geneva: UNAIDS.

– 2004b. *Report on the Global AIDS Epidemic*. http://data.unaids.org/global-reports/bangkok-2004/unaidsbangkokpress/gar2004html/gar2004_00_en.htm.

– 2007. *Policy Brief: The Greater Involvement of People Living with HIV/AIDS*. Geneva: UNAIDS.

Wingood, G., and R. DiClemente. 2000. "The WiLLOW Program: Mobilizing Social Networks of Women Living with HIV to Enhance Coping and Reduce Sexual Risk Behaviour." In *Working with Families in the Era of HIV/AIDS*, edited by W. Pequegnat and J. Szapocznik, 281–98. London: Sage Publications.

# 10 What a Mess! Viewing Trans Women Living with HIV as Managers of Policy Mess

NATALIE DUCHESNE

The topic of HIV/AIDS and trans people has not received nearly as much attention as it deserves in Canada, or at least not from academics, policymakers, and mainstream HIV organizations. It is a step in the right direction that this edited volume addresses the issue of trans people and HIV. While this chapter can only begin to scratch the surface, I hope to demonstrate how trans women living with HIV navigate various policy spheres.[1] If readers take away anything from this chapter, let it be the need for more careful consideration of trans women's experiences and needs as they relate to HIV policy.

This chapter is based primarily on interviews with four trans women living with HIV in Toronto and Montréal. I will discuss how these women make their way through a rapidly changing and unpredictable policy landscape in order to not only survive but also thrive. I address health and welfare primarily, but also touch on some intertwining issues such as aging and migration. I take for granted that HIV, health, and welfare policy will remain complex, fuzzy, and at times contradictory. As such, no matter the improvements we make to policy, trans people will continue to need to manage the policy messes they encounter. For this reason, I argue one of our priorities should be to better understand the conditions under which trans people are able to do so successfully. What can we do to minimize the volatility they face? How can we increase the policy options available to them?

## Context: Trans Women and HIV

Transsexual women have been facing the HIV epidemic since the 1980s. In Canada, trans people responded in the 1990s by forming community organizations such as the High Risk Society in Vancouver, or Action santé travesti(e)s et transsexue(le)s du Québec (ASTT[e]Q) in Montréal (see Laframboise 2014; Namaste 1998). Trans women, and especially sex workers, have also played a key role in ensuring that trans people have been included in organizations such as the Prisoners' HIV/AIDS Support Action Network (Toronto), Maggie's: The Toronto Sex Workers Action Project, and Stella (a sex-worker organization in Montréal).[2]

Meanwhile, epidemiology, public health, and policy have been woefully late arriving on the scene. Trans people have tended to fall through the cracks of epidemiological data. One reason is that official statistics generally follow a population model that is organized by categories (e.g., "men who have sex with men") that fail to account for trans people (see Namaste 2015). There are no national Canadian data specific to trans people (see PHAC 2014b). According to a meta-analysis in the United States, 27.7 per cent of trans women are living with HIV (Herbst et al. 2008). In the absence of Canadian data, the Public Health Agency of Canada (2014b) has estimated the same percentage for Canada (27.7 per cent) in their *Population-Specific HIV/AIDS Status Report: Women*.[3] They specify that rates may be higher in some cities like Montréal and Vancouver. International studies have found that prevalence tends to be higher among trans women who are international migrants, racialized, or sex workers (Giami and Bail 2011).[4]

Trans women did not need epidemiological data to know that AIDS ravaged an entire generation. As one participant in Namaste's research on transsexual and transvestite[5] performers in Montréal put it, "If I look at my generation [the second generation of transsexuals in Québec], well, most of my friends from my generation are all dead. So they are pretty much all dead from AIDS, or they were killed, or they committed suicide. So from my own generation, and that there, it's really, there are not many left. From, I dunno, a number like, just like that, let's say we were twenty, well today there are only five left. It's as bad as that" (interview participant in Namaste 2005, 71, translated from French by the author)

Despite its slow start, PHAC's inclusion of trans women in its population-specific report on women goes a long way to adding trans women to the Canadian HIV policy agenda. AIDS service organizations (ASOs) are also starting to note trans people, but they often struggle to adapt their services. Luckily, a few trans-led initiatives, mostly in Canadian urban centres, can assist ASOs. A few examples from ASTT(e)Q will illustrate. ASTT(e)Q is a community organization in Montréal that aims to improve trans people's access to social and health services. As part of this work, ASTT(e)Q has published a guide for health care and social service providers (Ezra 2012). The guide not only explains trans issues in general terms, but also includes specific HIV/AIDS content. In addition, the organization offers training sessions for front-line workers. ASTT(e)Q has also developed the CHARGE Peer Support and Leadership program. Trans peers are trained and then inserted into local ASOs looking to better tailor their services to trans people (including youth and sex workers). The program has had promising results thus far. Through their guidebook, training sessions, and peer program, ASTT(e)Q is helping ASOs and other service providers become better allies for trans people. One can hope that such trans-led initiatives will encourage mainstream ASOs, which for the most part do not work on trans issues, to widen their mandates.

A few notes are in order about the specificity of trans women and HIV, especially since few readers may be familiar with these realities (see also Duchesne 2011; Ezra 2012, 47–57). Trans people often have trouble accessing health-care services; trans women who are living with HIV face the added barrier of finding health-care professionals who are knowledgeable about both trans and HIV issues (Schilder et al. 1998). For example, trans women may need a doctor who can monitor the interactions between hormones and antiretrovirals. Trans women also experience certain side effects differently from others. Lypodystrophy, the redistribution of body fat, can masculinize one's facial features. This visible sign of HIV treatment can be difficult for anyone, but it is especially hard for trans women who have made great sacrifices to feminize their bodies (Namaste 2015). Finally, stigma within trans communities still makes talking about HIV taboo.

## Methods

The data presented in this chapter are drawn from a larger study about trans people's interactions with public policies in Montréal and Toronto. The empirical work comprised thirty one-on-one interviews with trans people in the spring of 2012. These semi-structured interviews centred on participants' day-to-day lives, including work, social life, and other regular activities. Special attention was given to government interactions, including those with health and social services. I worked from interviewees' day-to-day experiences to identify the policies with which they interacted (typically twenty to forty per interview) and to analyse the skills and capacities trans people employ in their policy encounters.

At times I will reference interviews from the larger project to provide context and examples, but will for the most part focus on four interviews with trans women who discussed HIV/AIDS. Since I did not ask systematically about participants' sero-status, other participants might also have been living with HIV but did not mention it during our interview, either because it was not a part of their day-to-day living or the result of stigma.

I also chose not to ask participants about socio-demographic traits such as gender, age, and race/ethnicity. Instead, I probed for such details when they were relevant to what the participants were saying. This is a methodological choice that needs some explanation. During two years of preliminary work getting to know trans people and communities in Montréal and Toronto, it became evident that one of the biggest assumptions made about trans people was that their gender is always central to their lives. This assumption creates a confirmation bias that discourages us from asking about the relative importance of gender in diverse trans people's lives or policy contexts. In fact very little research looks at other dimensions of their lives. A parallel can be made to epidemiological data and trans people. At first trans people were invisible to researchers and public health officials, because their reality did not fit into accepted population models.

Bourdieu (1990, 2004) has argued that scholars tend to forget that our models are not the same thing as the phenomenon we study. In a research context where we frame our questions, methods, and analysis through social categories of difference, such as gender, we forget that in the real world, things are not so clear-cut. My work follows a Bourdieusian approach to reflexivity, where methods and analysis are constructed to make visible the world beyond our current intellectual models. Trans people are used to being asked about their gender, but I wanted to know what would come up if I let their day-to-day lives frame interviews. I thus decided to not systematically ask participants about their socio-demographic traits.

While I acknowledge that this choice has meant that I may have missed valuable data from other participants potentially living with HIV/AIDS, the benefits arguably outweigh the cost. I got a closer look at participants' lives in their own terms (be it gender or not), instead of by exploring who they are in my models or what they already represent to scholarship. Some interesting points came out of this approach.

Fabienne,[6] one of four interviewees discussed in this chapter, mentioned HIV only once, in passing near the end of the interview. She had been discussing community groups with which she had come into contact. When asked if there were any others, at first she answered no. Then, almost as an afterthought, she added that she had volunteered at an AIDS hospice. It was only when I asked why that she explained that she had previously been a resident. Fabienne had been healthy for some time and her present was filled with other priorities. How might our research and policies account for this shifting importance? I will discuss this later in the chapter, but first I present the analytical framework that is used to explore how trans women manage the policy messes they encounter.

**Policy Messes**

Most policy analysis centres on policy actors (policymakers, managers, front-line workers). It is easy to forget that policymakers and policy users do not necessarily differ from one another. In order to successfully navigate policy, trans people must act in the midst of confusion, contradicting information, and rapidly changing program offerings and services. In other words, they must deal with the messiness of policy. This is the same messiness that policymakers, managers, and analysts must face. While policy scholars have long attempted to make sense of this complexity, Roe (2013) offers the most direct examination of policy messes.[7] He has developed a conceptual toolkit that allows us to analyse messes in productive ways. While Roe's work is centred on traditional policy actors, it can nonetheless help us bridge the gap between our understanding of policymakers and policy users.

Specifically, Roe's work examines reliability and mess professionals, or mess managers for short. Within the policymaking domain, mess managers find themselves somewhere between macro policy design and front-line implementation. They manage complex policy systems: electricity grids, health care, finance, and so on. Their job? To keep the lights on. Unlike a traditional approach to priority setting, which defines and solves problems, reliability and mess professionals work with messes. Unlike problems, messes can't be solved, they must be managed.

As Roe describes it, "Issues are a mess not only when they are complex, but also when they are uncertain, incomplete, and disputed. They are uncertain when causal processes are unclear or not easily comprehended. They are complex when more numerous, varied, and interdependent than before. Issues are incomplete when efforts to address them are left interrupted, unfinished, or partially fulfilled. Issues are disputed when individuals take different positions on them because of their uncertainty, complexity, and incompleteness. A policy mess is an amalgam of these contingencies that has become so accident-prone along its multiple dimensions that it has to be managed" (8).

Already, this definition gives us a lot to work with. Let us consider the Canadian welfare mess: its uncertain, complex, incomplete, and disputed elements. First, the welfare system is filled with uncertainty. While we might have good reasons to support the creation of a national housing strategy or to argue in favour of incorporating the notion of a liveable wage into welfare policy, we do not know exactly what the outcomes of these initiatives might be. There are hundreds if not thousands of variables to consider. Furthermore, policies on the minimum wage, taxes, zoning, and federal social transfers, to name a few, affect welfare policy and needs. For example, zoning by-laws affect the affordability of housing, and federal social transfers in part determine what services provinces can offer. These policy systems are interconnected across every sphere of government. It should go without saying that decades of welfare programs and initiatives have failed to alleviate poverty. Welfare is highly disputed, if only because of varying values about *who* and *what* matters most. The reliability and mess managers who deal with the welfare mess can be found in various spheres of government, ensuring that social housing units are maintained and that benefits are paid out.

Importantly, policymakers are not alone in dealing with this mess. Millions of Canadians battle poverty and deal with uncertain access to food and shelter (Segaert 2012; Tarasuk, Mitchell, and Dachner 2014; Wellesley Institute 2010). They face the complexity of agencies and service bureaus, bureaucrats and rules, forms and decisions. Moreover, they have to string together incomplete policy "solutions" to make ends meet: diet supplements, medical equipment reimbursements, tax credits, allowed supplementary income, disability recognition, etc. As they navigate these turbulent policy waters, policy users must convince front-line workers, community organizers, landlords, neighbours, and the public at large that they deserve to live with dignity and that they are eligible for social and health services. In dealing with the uncertainty and complexity of policy, policy users, such as trans women living with HIV, share an uncanny resemblance to Roe's professional mess managers.

There are, however, some important differences between professional mess managers and policy users. Reliability and mess professionals form networks that can span policy messes, but ultimately they are responsible for one policy mess (e.g., welfare). Not so with policy users. The complexity and uncertainty faced by policy users expands as they face multiple policy messes simultaneously. The trans women I will discuss below dealt with the welfare mess, the health-care mess, the HIV-response mess, and a plethora of other policy issues, depending on their individual circumstances. In addition, the skills trans women employ to manage messes are not the same as professional mess managers, a topic addressed in the last section of this chapter.

Despite their differences, both professional mess managers and policy users have a lot to gain from good mess management. Roe's professionals can be assessed by their ability to provide a reliable service (electricity, health care, etc.). Reliability entails keeping critical policy systems running and avoiding crisis; keeping the lights on. As Roe notes, even the best mess managers cannot guarantee that systems will continue to function. Sometimes these professionals do not have the resources to overcome the challenges before them. But while good mess management cannot guarantee reliability, it goes a long way to ensure that systems keep moving.

Likewise, trans women living with HIV/AIDS have varying ability to manage policy messes. And like their professional counterparts, their best work often goes unnoticed. Ultimately the system that they must keep running is their lives. For policy users, reliability is related to survival and a meaningful life – things like stable access to food, shelter, health care, and social services, as well as the opportunity to contribute, be valued, and grow as individuals, are indicators of success. Like mess managers, at times even the most talented trans women are unable to avoid crises: violence, discrimination, or unavailable services can make for impossible conditions. Still, we might examine what makes some trans women successful when with dealing with fickle policy arenas such as welfare, HIV policies, or trans-specific policies.

To be clear, I am not suggesting that we stop trying to improve the policy landscapes of HIV and welfare. Indeed, we have much work to do. But the complexity and uncertainty of these policy spheres will not disappear. Sometimes the best thing policymakers and users alike can hope for is to manage the messes before them. Creating conditions that are conducive to good mess management should be on our radar.

Again the work of Roe (2013) is useful. He has developed the notions of volatility and options variety to describe mess management contexts. As he defines it, "Volatility is the extent to which system managers and operators confront uncontrollable or unpredictable conditions that threaten their ability to provide the critical service. Some periods are of low volatility: There are no surprising or unscheduled interruptions in the electricity supply, water provisions, or financial services. Other periods are one of high volatility: Temperatures go up, causing increased difficulties to the providers of electricity, water, or health services" (18).

Highly volatile situations are those where conditions change quickly and unpredictably, affecting a manager's ability to provide a reliable service. To continue with Roe's example, if temperatures suddenly rise, it puts a strain on our electrical system (e.g., a higher than expected energy demand). It increases the chances that a mess manager will have to act (e.g., divert power, call for energy conservation) and threatens reliability. Simply put, more things can go wrong.

The effects of volatility on policy systems are not so different from its effects on policy users. Obviously, some groups and life trajectories are more likely to face instability. But they need not be stuck in a continuous cycle of insecurity. A trans woman will face heightened volatility when she transitions, but a few years down the line, her life may have settled.

Importantly, not all turbulent periods in people's lives are policy relevant, but many are. In what follows, I focus on policy-induced volatility, or when changing life circumstances affect policy needs. A couple of examples will help to illustrate. They are relatively straightforward but will add some complexity and nuance in the following section that examines trans women's mess management in more detail.

The first example is from Jenny. She was worried about changing attitudes towards the criminalization of HIV non-disclosure. She explained,

> It also goes into the disclosure law ... it opens up a whole other ballpark, for anybody that is HIV-positive. If you are having sex with somebody, you need to disclose. If you don't, you are arrested. There have been several cases recently in the news where people have not disclosed and stuff ... And even for somebody, a trans person like myself, that is a bit scary. Because if I get involved in a relationship with somebody and I have

disclosed, and then a year later we have a big fight and break up, he can go to the police and say, "She never disclosed," I get arrested. I have no backup on that at all, which is really scary.

At the time of the interviews (spring 2012), the *R v Mabior* case was before the Supreme Court of Canada and this had raised the public profile of recent cases (see Gagnon and Vézina in this volume). Jenny explained that a loving relationship gone sour could lead to future accusations. The unpredictability of charges (even if she discloses) along with the feeling of not being able to control the situation scared her. The current policy context of the criminalization of HIV non-disclosure made her life more volatile.

The second example is from an interview with Roxanne, who had begun a physical and social transition. While I have spoken with trans people who had relative ease in their transition, I have yet to come across a trans person who did not face volatility. A first dimension of volatility is other people's reactions (friends, family, work colleagues, as well as health-care professionals and bureaucrats). Second, there is a period of adjustment while the individual learns about what services are available and decides what she wants. Third, a trans person must make her way through the policies that stand between her and where she wants to be. Depending on what the person wants, this might include civil status change(s), access to hormones, mental health services, as well as state-funded surgeries. Roxanne was facing all three types of volatility at the time of the interview. She had recently moved to Toronto to surround herself with supportive people (friends, community, and health professionals). She was learning about what was available and accessing the services she wanted. For instance, she wanted to take hormones and was frustrated by the time it took to access them. A transition entails a big life change, which increases volatility and affects policy needs.

The criminalization of HIV non-disclosure and transitioning are easily recognizable as issues faced by trans women living with HIV. There were, however, many other events in the lives of participants that increased volatility: the sudden death of a relative, a difficult breakup, a changing job market, or an accident leading to injury. Sometimes, life just happens.

A few characteristics of the volatility faced by participants are useful to keep in mind. First, volatility is not an all-or-nothing value; it's best to think of it as moving along a spectrum and as being composed of multiple factors. For instance, Roxanne had just started her transition, but she also had medium-term housing as well as a regular income (I will give more details below). The overall level of volatility in Roxanne's life was made up of all of these details and more. Second, volatility is in constant flux. Approaches that focus on social categories (e.g., trans), linking them to discrimination and injustice, have a tendency to hide this fact. Individuals who make up marginalized populations aren't necessarily vulnerable all the time. Many trans people have successfully transitioned and lead perfectly stable and meaningful lives; some even lead privileged lives. Third, volatility is not always a bad thing nor can it be avoided altogether. It is a part of life. A transition increases the volatility in an individual's life, but also opens the door to a more meaningful life. Fourth, an increase in volatility means more things *could* go wrong, but it does not predetermine that they will.

The second dimension of a policy mess context, as developed by Roe (2013), is option variety. He describes options as the "different resources in terms of money, personnel, and strategies" (18–19) that professional mess managers have at their disposal. In the case of policy users, we might say that option variety is related to money, social networks, and strategies. To explain, we can come back to the examples above (criminalization and transitioning).

Jenny was worried about potentially facing HIV non-disclosure charges. Despite being generally well connected to ASOs that could give her up-to-date information about how to best shield herself from criminal prosecution, there is no strategy that could fully protect her against the threat. Her option variety is low (at least relative to criminalization). As for Roxanne and her transition, she was well connected to service providers and community workers, and in particular had a social worker and a doctor who helped her plan the best course of action to get what she wanted (strategy). She had a high option variety.

Volatility and option variety come together to form an individual's reliability and mess management context. Someone who experiences low volatility but has access to a lot of resources can prepare for the future. Roe calls this the *just-in-case* mode. When in this mode, a policy user can save up money, network to find people who could help if things become more difficult, or think about what to do if a doctor was no longer available. Someone who experiences high volatility in combination with high choice variety is in a *just-on-time* mode. This individual has a lot to manage but also has the resources to navigate the policy messes along the way. The most dangerous mode is called *just-for-now*. It occurs when someone is facing high volatility but low choice variety. This mode can easily slide into a full-blown crisis.

The four women being studied here were not in a just-for-now mode at the time of the interview. But many of the thirty participants in the larger project did face high volatility and few options. For example, one woman was unable to find stable housing. There were no available shelter beds. Her only option was to sleep on her nephew's couch, but she could only stay there a few days (just-for-now). She had been stuck in this mode for several years.

Roe explains that when professionals are in the just-for-now mode for prolonged periods of time, their capacity to manage messes is affected. As they constantly face emergencies, they eventually lose the ability to switch to just-on-time or just-in-case modes, even when the situation would warrant it. Unfortunately, I observed something similar with trans people. A few participants in the study had survived over a decade of high volatility and low options. This state of being had harsh effects on their mental health; they were isolated, under-housed, and in difficult economic situations. Their skills and capacities had suffered: their interpersonal skills, their ability to manage stress, to formulate strategies, and to find information. Just like Roe's professionals who find themselves unable manage policy messes, these participants (mostly trans women) were no longer able to manage the policy messes they encountered. A few of them mentioned that they were losing hope. Trans people stuck in a just-for-now mode for extended periods of time see their quality of life deteriorate dramatically. This is one of the reasons that it is so important for us to think about what conditions are conducive to good mess management. Looking at the experiences of trans women who are talented mess managers is a good starting point.

**Four Mess Managers**

*Roxanne*

At the time of the interview, Roxanne was in her early sixties. She had been living with HIV for over a decade, but had just started her transition. She had recently moved from the Québec countryside to Toronto, because she needed a change of air and was looking to improve her English. The biggest factor was, however, her desire to transition. Like many other trans people from her generation, she had gone through most of her life not knowing that she could indeed live as a woman.

She had first started to find information about transsexuality via the Internet a couple years before the interview. During this process, she made a friend in Toronto, who told her about the community and services available there. Roxanne now lived in medium-term HIV/AIDS housing and had nine months to find a more permanent apartment. Her income was composed of the Québec disability pension plan and Ontario Disability Support Program benefits (ODSP).[8] At the time of the interview, her life was filled with appointments with doctors, an aesthetician (hair removal), and community workers. She also attended Meal Trans, a weekly dinner and social held at the 519 Church Street Community Centre (The 519) in Toronto.

Overall, Roxanne's level of volatility was high because of her temporary housing situation as well as her transition. Her housing situation was greatly improved by having a nine-month lease, which gave her time to find something more permanent. It increased her options and shielded her from even greater uncertainty. Nonetheless, finding an apartment within her means would be a challenge. Wait times for social housing are generally longer than nine months and Toronto rental rates are high. However, Roxanne was well connected with community workers. A couple of participants from the larger study were able to secure social housing much faster than the average wait time, because they had the right people in their corner. Roxanne might have the same luck.

The second source of volatility in Roxanne's life was her transition. She was still getting to know what was available. Trans-specific policies have been shifting quickly over the past decade. This makes finding accurate and current information harder. Roxanne had heard that the Ontario government no longer paid for sex reassignment surgery. However, these surgeries had been re-listed by the government in 2008. Luckily, a physician at the Sherbourne Health Centre had corrected the mistake.[9] The next steps were still a little vague: "So I guess that my doctors will send me to see the doctors over there, or some psychiatrists, some specialists, I don't know what, and then they will put me in a program for what I want to get, to get money from them, from the government, I don't know, from [the Centre for Addiction and Mental Health], it's a little vague for the moment" (translation from French).

Roxanne still had a way to go in order to qualify for state-funded surgery, but she was on the right track. Being connected to The 519 would help. Several participants I spoke with had received help from

The 519 staff while navigating their transition. Roxanne had a lot of resources at her disposal.

While Roxanne faced a high level of volatility, she also had a high variety of options. She had a social worker and a doctor who were helping her develop a plan of attack to get housing and access trans-specific health care. It was not by chance that she had found herself so well connected. Several years ago, at a time when her HIV status caused more volatility, she had learned the importance of being connected. She explained, "In Montréal, I would access those services as well, the organizations that were there, and it's because with HIV, we feel so isolated in society, sometimes face stigmatization, so when we go in these organizations like that, we feel like we are with family, we feel, well, there is a sentiment of belonging and friendship that feels good" (translation from French).

Knowing that community organizations and the services they offer were beneficial, Roxanne had sought out what groups were present in Toronto as soon as she arrived. This initiative was part of what made Roxanne a good mess manager. It also indicates the advantage of a just-in-case mode.

From a policy perspective we can point to the existence of the medium-term housing project as well as the presence of the Sherbourne Health Centre (which specializes in trans-related health care) as setting up conditions for Roxanne's success. The housing reduced her current volatility by giving her reprieve while finding an apartment. The housing social worker would help her avoid future volatility (by assisting her in her search for a place to live). Being a client at the Sherbourne Health Centre gave Roxanne access to the most qualified doctors to guide her through her transition. This would likely save her time and diminish the window of volatility in her life.

*Jenny*

Jenny is a transgender woman who was in her early sixties at the time of the interview. She was born and raised in Toronto and joked that anything beyond the downtown core was the country. She had transitioned in the 1990s, had been living with HIV for many years, and had been living in the same subsidized apartment for over a decade. Her income was made up of her Canadian disability pension as well as ODSP benefits. She supplemented this income by cleaning houses.

Jenny volunteered three to four days a week for community organizations or by giving talks about her experiences as a transgender woman and as a person living with HIV. Indeed, she was very much involved and this gave her a sense of fulfilment. Altogether, Jenny had a solid base from which to address policy messes.

Jenny mostly faced the welfare mess and the health care mess. In the past year, her ODSP payments had suddenly stopped five times. She explained,

> Oh they are terrible, I was cut off five times last year, it's frustrating ... What they do is, when I do my [guest talks for community groups] I get an honorarium and stuff. [Ontario works] will enter it in and they won't push send or something. And then I get letter saying, "You did not declare income for the month of August" or something. And that happened five times last year. I had a really good worker there, who has moved on to another spot right now. I hope she is coming back. All I would have to say is "Hi, it's Jenny" and she would say, "Oh shit, again?" I'd say, "Yup," and she would fix it right there and then.

Jenny also recounted a few incidents with health-care professionals. For example,

> It's devastating sometimes. I can be sitting waiting in a lab for blood work, and they will look at the health card, and instead of looking at the name, will look at the gender, and come out and say "Mr Smith," or something, and I know it's me they are talking about, and I usually throw a hissy fit. I have done that a few times. A few months ago, I had to go for a prostate exam, and I am settled-in the little cubicle with one of the gowns, you know, when you go for a medical, and there are like ten cubicles. And a man walks up and says, "Jenny." And I walk out, and he looks at the paperwork and looks up and "Oh! you're a man!" 'Cause he looked at the health card thing, eh, the hospital card. And I looked at him and I said, "Well, I know that, and you know that, now everybody else in here knows that." So he was pretty good. He did the exam and stuff and I was leaving and I got the elevator and I came back in and I looked at the receptionist and I said, "I need to see a supervisor." And a supervisor came out and I told her what happened. And she said, "I'm really sorry. That should not have happened." I said, "No, this is 2010, it should not be happening," and she really apologized.

Despite a couple of spikes in volatility over the past year (when her benefit payments stopped or she faced certain health professionals), Jenny was enjoying a period of low volatility. She also had a lot of options. Of the four women being presented here, she was the best placed. She had a solid network of support, but she was also very skilled in diffusing difficult situations and working with bureaucrats, doctors, etc. Jenny also knew how to keep her options high. For example, working under the table not only increased her available income but also helped her when ODSP payments suddenly stopped. It was just-in-case planning. The vast majority of participants I spoke with who had received welfare or disability benefits had food security issues. To her credit, Jenny did not.

## Fabienne

Fabienne arrived in Canada as a refugee from Mexico six years before the interview. At the time, she had an AIDS-related illness and was hospitalized and then sent to a Montréal AIDS hospice for three months. Her original refugee claim had been rejected, and it was only on appeal that she gained the right to stay in Canada. While her arrival to Canada was followed by a period of volatility (illness and the refugee process), her life had since stabilized. Fabienne was now a permanent resident and in the process of applying for full citizenship. She worked in the hotel industry and had good working conditions, although she wished she could find full-time employment. At the time of the interview, she was in convalescence, as she had recently had sex reassignment surgery. She had been receiving employment insurance disability benefits, but these had run out. She was in the process of applying for welfare benefits to cover the reminder of her convalescence.

Fabienne recently separated from her husband and was heartbroken. She had sponsored his immigration to Canada, but shortly after he gained his permanent resident status, he accused her of assault. He called police and they arrested her. The timing of this caused problems, as she had just had sex reassignment surgery (including vaginoplasty). Post-surgery care, such as dilation four times a day, is crucial for a successful outcome, as is rest. Although her life situation had previously been stable, the resulting assault charge and the separation from her husband were wreaking havoc in her life. She had exhausted her savings on legal fees, all the while not working because of her convalescence. She worried that she would not qualify for social assistance. It was a complicated case, as she was married and would have to prove that her husband did not have the means to support her. She also had to face the potential of being financially responsible for her husband because she had sponsored his immigration. Finally, despite having convinced a judge of her innocence in relation to the alleged assault, her citizenship application was on hold until matters were settled. Fabienne's future was thus uncertain, but mostly she was heartbroken.

After a period of stability, the level of volatility in Fabienne's life had increased. She had no income and was unsure if she would qualify for welfare benefits. Her ability to obtain citizenship was threatened. From a policy perspective, we might hypothesize about what would have happened had it not taken six years for her to be able to apply for citizenship, or to access sex-reassignment surgery. We might also wonder how the police officers who arrested Fabienne came to think that a woman who had just had sex-reassignment surgery could physically assault her husband. But beyond these reflections, one must admit that there is no policy that can fix a broken heart or bad timing. Fabienne had been a skilled mess manager in the past (dealing with the refugee process, for instance). Once she was ready to face divorce, it is likely that she would be able to face the other messes in her life as well. Otherwise, she might eventually confront the same fate as trans people who are a stuck in a just-for-now mode for too long.

*Vanessa*

Vanessa had come to Canada as a refugee from Venezuela many years ago and had been living with HIV for twenty years. A few years before the interview, she had been hospitalized with life-threatening meningitis. She had since recovered, but was unable work. She lived on ODSP benefits and in a subsidized apartment. She also volunteered in a few Toronto-based community organizations as well as with a Latin HIV/AIDS network. It was important to Vanessa that I know about the ways she supported members of her communities. My interview with her underlined the importance of creating opportunities for people who are unable to work. Although to be fair, Vanessa made her own opportunities happen.

Vanessa is another example of a highly skilled mess manager. Her specialties were planning for the future and diffusing volatility. She explained to me that she kept a back-up doctor.

VANESSA: I have a family doctor, a general doctor. I have HIV doctor.
I have backup, just in case.
NATALIE: A backup HIV doctor?
VANESSA: Yes, just in case.

Vanessa was very satisfied with her primary HIV doctor. Despite being very busy, this doctor made time for her. However, Vanessa also had a backup in case she needed care when her primary doctor was unavailable. She was not going to leave her health to chance.

But even Vanessa sometimes faced volatility. Recently, she had been in a social housing unit far away from her community (the Toronto gay village). She had been beaten up in the street and no longer felt at ease in her neighbourhood. This had contributed to a depression and a loss of motivation in her volunteer work. Vanessa is a great communicator. She was able to convince her housing worker that she needed a transfer to another housing unit as soon as possible. In consequence, she was able to move closer to the village (near her friends and the services she used). Her quality of life quickly improved.

**Conclusion**

Vanessa, Roxanne, Jenny, and Fabienne had all faced important challenges. They had experienced violence, discrimination, poverty, and maladapted services. They had to manage the welfare mess, the HIV mess, and trans-specific policy messes. And yet they had all not only survived but thrived. They are success stories in a world of imperfect policies. In sharing their stories, I want to further our understanding of what makes for good managers as well as make a case for prioritizing policies that can create favourable conditions for policy users who are dealing with messes.

Policy and life situations are in constant flux. Trans-specific policies such as funding for sex-reassignment surgeries or civil status changes have evolved substantially in the past decade. As this and other chapters in this volume show, HIV policy and welfare policy are also changing rapidly. These policy areas are exceptionally complex, not only for policymakers and analysts, but also for policy users. Trans women living with HIV/AIDS must navigate a world of policy messes that are unpredictable and uncontrollable. Meanwhile, they must also live their lives and weather the ups and downs.

More than ever, trans women are on the policy radar. Governments, ASOs, and researchers are looking for ways to adapt their policies, services, and analysis to meet the needs of this population. Just as ASOs have much to learn from the trans women who fought back against the AIDS epidemic, so too can policymakers and researchers learn from trans women's abilities to manage messes. In short, the first step to crafting future actions is to draw on the expertise of trans women.

Good mess management occurs in fluctuating volatility and option variety. Two general aims are to reduce unnecessary volatility and to increase option variety. For example, we can shorten the length of a volatile period by ensuring that trans women can access trans-related health care and especially transition-related health care in a timely fashion. We can increase trans women's option variety by funding the community workers (including social workers) and front-line bureaucrats who guide policy users. We can also prioritize creating opportunities for trans women living with HIV to give back to their communities and to develop the skills needed to manage the messiness of policy.

## NOTES

1  I am limiting myself to trans women in this chapter, but trans men remain understudied (Scheim et al. 2014).

2  The Prisoners' HIV/AIDS Support Action Network, which supports prisoners and ex-prisoners, has included trans people since their creation in 1991. Both Maggie's and Stella, which offer services for sex workers and advocate for their rights, include trans sex workers.

3  In comparison, data on men who have sex with men indicate a prevalence of 15.1 per cent in Canada (PHAC 2014a).

4  The studies that are summarized in the above metadata analysis have limitations. They tend to be centred on trans populations that are most visible, such as street sex workers, or those who use ASOs' services (such as testing) (see Giami and Bail 2011; Melendez, Bonem, and Sember 2006).

5  Today in anglophone contexts, the term *crossdresser* is generally preferred rather than *transvestite*. However, out of respect for the self-identification of participants in the referred study (*travestis*), I used *transvestite*.

6  All names were changed to protect confidentiality.

7  Two examples would be "muddling through" (Lindblom 1959) and the "garbage can model" (Cohen, March, and Olsen 1972).

8 While she now lived in Ontario, the participant had previously contributed to the Québec pension plan. As a result, she received pension payments from Québec and an adjusted sum from the Ontario Disability Support Program.
9 Most trans people I spoke with in Toronto were or had been clients at the Sherbourne Health Centre. This clinic specializes in trans-related care.

REFERENCES

Bourdieu, Pierre. 1990. "The Scholastic Point of View." *Cultural Anthropology* 5 (4): 380–91. https://doi.org/10.1525/can.1990.5.4.02a00030.
– 2004. *Esquisse pour une auto-analyse*. Paris: Éditions raisons d'agir.
Cohen, Michael D., James G. March, and Johan P. Olsen. 1972. "A Garbage Can Model of Organizational Choice." *Administrative Science Quarterly* 17 (1): 1–25. https://doi.org/10.2307/2392088.
Duchesne, Natalie. 2011. *HIV and Transgendered/Transsexual Communities*. Interagency Coalition on AIDS and Development. https://egale.ca/wp-content/uploads/2011/08/HIV_and_Trans_Communities_EN.pdf.
Ezra, Jackson. 2012. *Taking Charge: A Handbook for Health Care and Social Service Providers Working with Trans People*. Montréal: Action santé travesti(e)s transsexuel(le)s du Québec.
Giami, Alain, and J. Le Bail. 2011. "HIV Infection and STI in the Trans Population: A Critical Review." *Revue d'Épidémiologie et de Sante Publique* 59 (4): 259–68. https://doi.org/10.1016/j.respe.2011.02.102.
Herbst, Jeffrey H., et al. 2008. "Estimating HIV Prevalence and Risk Behaviors of Transgender Persons in the United States: A Systematic Review." *AIDS and Behavior* 12 (1): 1–17. https://doi.org/10.1007/s10461-007-9299-3.
Laframboise, Sandy Leo. 2014. "Finding My Place: The High Risk Project Society." In *Trans Activism in Canada: A Reader*, edited by Dan Irving and Rupert Raj, 51–6. Toronto: Canadian Scholars' Press.
Lindblom, Charles E. 1959. "The Science of 'Muddling Through.'" *Public Administration Review* 19 (2): 79–88. https://doi.org/10.2307/973677.
Melendez, Rita M., Lathem A. Bonem, and Robert Sember. 2006. "On Bodies and Research: Transgender Issues in Health and HIV Research Articles." *Sexuality Research & Social Policy* 3 (4): 21–38. https://doi.org/10.1525/srsp.2006.3.4.21.
Namaste, Viviane. 1998. *Évaluation des besoins: Les travesti(e)s et les transsexuel(le)s au Québec à l'égard du VIH/Sida*. Montréal: Cactus.
– 2005. *C'était du spectacle! L'histoire des artistes transsexuelles à Montréal, 1955–1985*. Montréal and Kingston: McGill-Queen's University Press.

– 2015. *Oversight: Critical Thoughts on Feminist Research and Politics*. Toronto: Women's Press.

Public Health Agency of Canada (PHAC). 2014a. *Population-Specific HIV/AIDS Status Report: Gay, Bisexual, Two-Spirit and Other Men Who Have Sex with Men*. http://www.phac-aspc.gc.ca/aids-sida/publication/ps-pd/men-hommes/index-eng.php.

– 2014b. *Population-Specific HIV/AIDS Status Report: Women*. http://www.phac-aspc.gc.ca/aids-sida/publication/ps-pd/women-femmes/es-sommaire-eng.php.

Roe, Emery. 2013. *Making the Most of Mess: Reliability and Policy in Today's Management Challenges*. Durham, NC: Duke University Press. https://doi.org/10.1215/9780822395690.

Scheim, Ayden, et al. 2014. "Sexual Health on Our Own Terms: The Gay, Bi, Queer Trans Mens' Working Group." In *Trans Activism in Canada: A Reader*, edited by Dan Irving and Rupert Raj, 247–58. Toronto: Canadian Scholars' Press.

Schilder, Arn J., et al. 1998. "'They Don't See Our Feelings': The Health Care Experiences of HIV-Positive Transgendered Persons." *Journal of the Gay and Lesbian Medical Association* 2 (3): 103–11. https://doi.org/10.1023/B:JOLA.0000004052.12136.1b.

Segaert, Aaron. 2012. *The National Shelter Study 2005–2009*. Homelessness Partnering Strategy, Human Resources and Skills Development Canada. http://www.homelesshub.ca/resource/national-shelter-study-2005-2009.

Tarasuk, Valerie, Andy Mitchell, and Naomi Dachner. 2014. *Household Food Insecurity in Canada, 2012*. http://proof.utoronto.ca/resources/proof-annual-reports/annual-report-2012/.

Wellesley Institute. 2010. *Precarious Housing in Canada*. http://www.wellesleyinstitute.com/publications/new-report-precarious-housing-in-canada-2010/.

# 11 "Good Medicine": Decolonizing HIV Policy for Indigenous Women in Canada

TRACEY PRENTICE, DORIS PELTIER,
ELIZABETH BENSON, KERRIGAN JOHNSON,
KECIA LARKIN, KRISTA SHORE,
AND RENÉE MASCHING[1]

We live by stories [and] we also live in them. One way or another we are living the stories planted in us early or along the way, or we are also living the stories we planted – knowingly or unknowingly – in ourselves. We live stories that either give our lives meaning or negate it with meaninglessness. If we change the stories we live by, quite possibly we change our lives.

Ben Okri as cited in King 2003, 154

## Introduction

In this chapter, we suggest that responding to HIV among Indigenous[2] women in Canada is most effective when beginning with a strengths-based perspective: one that centres the voices and experiences of HIV-positive Indigenous women, is grounded in Indigenous knowledge and ways of knowing, and places social and structural strategies for addressing HIV on equal footing with biomedical interventions. In doing so, we challenge current models of HIV policy development and implementation that are deficit-based, emphasize behavioural determinants, and are almost always framed by a biomedical perspective that pathologizes women, sacrifices cultural diversity, and hinders Indigenous self-determination.

Our work adds to the growing critique of the vast majority of health policy, and the research from which it flows, that is grounded in a pathogenic model that highlights the "problems" of Indigenous people and communities, their illness-related gaps and needs, and the "risks" and "vulnerabilities" for Indigenous ill-health (Richmond, Ross, and Egeland 2007). This pathologizing practice is typical of a Western scientific, positivistic, and biomedical approach to understanding the world (Ahenakew 2011) that is deeply embedded in Eurocentric values, structures, and methods. Further, this practice reinforces unequal power relations by constructing Indigenous peoples as sick, "deviant from an assumed normal state" (Shields, Bishop, and Mazawi 2005, x), passive, dependent, and powerless, while settlers are constructed as self-sufficient and powerful. Such "portraits of Aboriginal sickness and misery" (O'Neil, Reading, and Leader 1998, 230) can then be used to justify neocolonial interventions that "govern, regulate, manage, marginalize, or minoritize" (Shields, Bishop, and Mazawi 2005, x) Indigenous individuals and communities.

Pathologizing practices and research also locate the roots of a perceived "sickness" or "trauma" in individual behaviours, thereby erasing centuries of colonial context and the ongoing settler colonialism that benefits from such representations (Greensmith 2015). This research has undoubtedly contributed to our understanding of the inequitable burden of HIV and AIDS on Indigenous women and informed public policies to address the negative health outcomes associated with these "risks" and "vulnerabilities." The solutions that flow from such practices, however, have focused largely on downstream interventions that focus on mitigating risk at the individual level. While women's shelters, addiction treatment programs, and harm reduction programs, for example, are essential elements in a comprehensive response to HIV, they emerge from a fundamentally pathogenic orientation that responds to disease over health, illness over wellness, and HIV risk factors over HIV protective factors. On their own, however, they do little to recognize or mitigate the harms associated with centuries of colonialism – a context that continues to create the conditions that contribute to the need for such programs in the first place.

Pathologizing practices, then, have had the harmful consequence of constructing a dehumanizing, stigmatizing, and ultimately negative narrative of HIV-positive Indigenous women as dying, diseased, dysfunctional, and disconnected, from themselves, their families, communities, and cultures. In turn, the production and reproduction of such a narrative has helped support and justify settler colonialism, including policies that are largely imposed upon them, that continue to construct positive Indigenous women as powerless and in need of help from mostly white, mostly HIV-negative experts. Millon (as cited in Greensmith 2015), for example, argues, "The contemporary service provisional sector has been set up to support and help Indigenous peoples based on their 'injury' and indeed has become an industry created out of their trauma" (1).

The HIV sector in Canada has not been immune to reinforcing the narrative of Indigenous peoples as "at risk" and "vulnerable." In a complex interplay between accessing funding that targets those in greatest need and responding to the needs of community, Indigenous organizations themselves have been implicated in contributing to the narrative of the sorrows of Indigenous peoples. Too often the compelling justification for this work is grounded in the burden of disease within the community. Organizations such as the Canadian Aboriginal AIDS Network (CAAN) have advocated for dedicated Aboriginal funding, for instance, and undertaken problem-focused research to produce evidence of direct relevance to Aboriginal community-based AIDS organizations. To counter this narrative, Aboriginal strategies have been developed at the provincial, territorial, national, and international level that highlight community capacity and resilience in the response to HIV and AIDS. Environments of Nurturing Safety (EONS) (Peltier 2010) specifically responds to the needs of Indigenous women. Over the course of recent years, CAAN's research and programming focus has also shifted towards increasingly strengths-based approaches.

In the following pages we contextualize HIV among Indigenous women and provide an overview of Visioning Health, a culturally grounded, strengths-based, arts-informed, and community-based participatory research project that some co-researchers[3] referred to as "good medicine." We believe Visioning Health represents an alternative approach. We also share findings from our research and point to policy and practice implications using an Indigenous intersectionality-based policy analysis framework. Recommendations include centring the voices and lived experience of positive Indigenous women in policy development; supporting and developing leadership by positive Indigenous women; supporting strengths-based policy development that is grounded in Indigenous notions of holistic health; Indigenizing the process, content, and methodology of policy development; developing policies and practices that support connectedness for positive Indigenous women at multiple levels; creating safe spaces; and developing policies that incorporate a colonial analysis.

## HIV among Indigenous Women in Canada

Indigenous women comprise approximately 4 per cent of the Canadian female population. In 2013, however, Indigenous women accounted for 32 per cent of HIV reports among women (PHAC 2014). Since 2001, the proportion of Indigenous AIDS diagnoses attributed to women has averaged 26.5 per cent, reaching a peak of 50 per cent in 2008, versus 9.1 per cent for women of other ethnicities (PHAC 2006, 2012). Indigenous women also tend to be diagnosed at a younger age (15–29 years) than their non-Indigenous counterparts, perhaps reflecting that they have a median age of 27.7 years compared to 40.6 years for non-Aboriginal women (O'Donnell and Wallace 2011), and have a larger percentage of HIV transmissions from injection drug use (PHAC 2014).

Indigenous and allied scholars agree, however – despite the overwhelming focus on behavioural determinants, as noted above – that the inequitable impact of HIV and AIDS on Indigenous women in Canada is fundamentally linked to the cumulative and ongoing impacts of colonization as a social determinant of health for Indigenous peoples, including the residential school system and the policy environment that created it (Pearce et al. 2008). The effects of the imposition of these institutions and their values on Indigenous peoples have been widely felt in the form of intergenerational or historical trauma, cultural disconnection, the interruption of traditional gender roles, and the devaluing of Indigenous women, both within Indigenous communities and without (Bourassa, McKay-McNabb, and Hampton 2004). This, in turn, has had serious and well-documented consequences for Indigenous women's health, including higher rates of trauma-induced mental illness, substance use, sexual abuse and intimate partner violence, incarceration, and HIV and AIDS.

## Towards a Strengths-Based Understanding of HIV-Positive Indigenous Women's Health: The Visioning Health Response

Responding to the community-identified need for research that focused on health instead of illness, on strengths and assets instead of deficits (Prentice 2004; Peltier 2010), a team of positive Indigenous women, Indigenous community partners, and academics developed a culturally grounded, decolonizing, strengths-based, arts-informed, women-centred, and community-based participatory research project. Our goal was to create an opportunity for the positive Indigenous women in our project to change the policy narrative; to tell a kind of story about themselves that was different from what has typically been told by others – their/our[4] own stories; using photos and other kinds of art; stories of what it means to be "healthy" as a positive Indigenous woman, and the role that culture and gender can play in supporting or maintaining health.

With the ongoing guidance of Traditional Knowledge Keeper Wanda Whitebird, and *oshkaabewis*[5] Sharp Dopler, we worked with thirteen positive Indigenous women in three locations (Toronto [$n$ = 5], Montreal [$n$ = 4], and one "virtual" group [$n$ = 4]) in intensive arts-informed and culturally grounded group research. We used a modified photovoice process that included cultural teachings and protocols, such as prayer, smudging, sharing circles, sweat lodges, drum-making, and drumming/singing in our research design. Two groups used digital photography to answer the research questions, and one group made and decorated traditional First Nations hand drums. Instead of focus groups, all groups participated in three sharing circles (Bartlett et al. 2007), a culturally resonant form of focus groups that embody and reflect the storytelling traditions of Indigenous peoples and Indigenous values such as egalitarianism, sharing, support, non-judgment, non-interference, and spirituality.

All sharing circles were digitally recorded with permission. Co-researchers were asked to share stories of (1) what it means to be healthy as a positive Indigenous woman, and what strategies help to create or maintain health; (2) what the role of culture and gender is in supporting health for positive Indigenous women; and (3) what the photos or artworks they created say about health for positive Indigenous women. Groups met for forty to sixty hours each, ranging from four full days to six months of biweekly meetings, depending on their preferences. At the end of the project, all co-researchers met for an all-groups meeting in which they/we participated in ceremony, shared their/our artworks (photos or drums) and experiences of participating in the project, participated in collaborative data analysis, and celebrated the end of our project. VH co-researchers produced more than fifty photo-stories (photos or traditional hand drums and accompanying narratives) on what it means to be healthy as a positive Indigenous woman, the role that culture and gender can play in supporting their/our health, and additional health-enabling strategies. Transcripts from nine sharing circles (three per group) supplemented our dataset.

An additional goal of Visioning Health was to develop policy recommendations from our work using an Indigenous intersectionality-based policy analysis framework. Intersectionality "refers to the idea that gender is experienced by women simultaneously with their experiences of class, race, sexual orientation, and other forms of social difference" (Varcoe, Hankivsky, and Morrow 2007, 19). While recognizing gender as an important determinant of health for positive Indigenous women, intersectionality resists the homogenization of gendered experiences of HIV, and rejects the primacy of gender as *the* most important social characteristic. Instead, intersectionality is about the interpenetrating, mutually constitutive, historically and socially situated ways in which multiple social indicators interact. Particularly in regards to Indigenous women, intersectionality reminds us that a gender-based analysis alone is often insensitive to "the multiple needs of Aboriginal women, who suffer not only from gendered discrimination, but racism and other forms of oppression" (NWAC 2007, 6). Thus, an intersectional analysis can help us understand the various ways that culture and gender intersect with each other, with other determinants, and with "broader historical and current systems of discrimination such as colonialism" (CRIAW 2006, 5) to shape and inform the lives of positive Indigenous women.

As Clark reminds us, though, "Intersectionality remains rooted in western notions of democracy and sovereignty that do not recognize the importance of tribal knowledge, spirituality and interconnectedness of past, present and future generations" (2012, 141). Neither does it recognize the pervasive and pernicious impact of colonization on Indigenous lives; the importance of families, communities, and "all my relations"; the inherent right of Indigenous peoples to self-determination; or the essential roles of agency and activism in achieving self-determination.

An Indigenous intersectionality-based policy analysis, then, urges us to also consider (1) the ways in which policies and policy intersections are embedded in Western world views; (2) the ways in which gender and culture or gender and colonization are deeply implicated; (3) the broader context of families and communities and the ways in which they are impacted or affect the individual; (4) the ways in which individual or community agency is enabled or constricted; and (5) the degree to which resistance is acknowledged or erased (Clark 2012, 141). Attending to these elements will help to decolonize existing policies and practices and point to policy solutions that are holistic and relational, acknowledge and support Indigenous self-determination, emerge from the strengths of individuals and communities, and build on the activism and resistance that has always existed in Indigenous communities.

## Health and Health-Enabling Strategies
## for Positive Indigenous Women

Positive Indigenous women co-researchers were a diverse group, representing a range of First Nations and Inuit identities, geographic locations, ages, gender identities, time since diagnosis, and life experiences. Each woman brought a unique perspective to our project; however, they/we shared three common experiences: self-identification as Indigenous and therefore a common experience of colonization, self-identification as women, and HIV-positive. While we cannot claim to have identified a homogeneous definition of positive Indigenous women's health – to do so would mask the diversity of our group – we have identified common characteristics of health for the positive Indigenous women in our project. Following Adelson (1998), we suggest that these be understood as "a depiction of an ideal state ... an idealized image, a prototype against which to gauge [positive Indigenous women's] state of being" (14). In other words, health as we define it below is aspirational rather than concrete, an ideal to strive towards rather than an accurate representation of current realities.

For the positive Indigenous women of Visioning Health, health was understood as holistic, relational, collectivist, and integrally tied to an individual and collective identity as Indigenous women. Individual health for positive Indigenous women includes components of physical, mental, emotional, and spiritual health, but it also includes family, community, social, and environmental dimensions. Health entails the interrelatedness of all these dimensions; finding a dynamic balance between them and in relation to life circumstances. This means that health is a process rather than a state of being, and the responsibility for driving that process lies with positive Indigenous women. The notion of self-determination, of taking responsibility for, and taking control of, health is a cross-cutting theme.

Health for positive Indigenous women co-researchers, however, is constituted through relationships at multiple intersecting levels. According to Wilson, "The relational way of being was at the heart of what it means to be Indigenous," and this extends beyond human relationships to encompass relationships to the land, the environment, the cosmos, and ideas (2008, 80). Being healthy for positive Indigenous women then means being connected or in relationship with oneself – physically, mentally, emotionally, and spiritually – and with others, including peers, friends, family, and community. It means being connected or in relationship to the land, environment, and the natural world, regardless of where one lives, and with culture through Elders, ceremonies, and traditional teachings. Being healthy for positive Indigenous women also means being in relationship with Spirit or Creator, in whatever way that makes sense for them. Each of these levels is interrelated, of course, and positive Indigenous women's relationships at each level are bidirectional and mutually constitutive. This is the meaning of "all my relations." In other words, the individual health of the positive Indigenous women in our study is integrally connected to, influences, and is influenced by the health of all other levels. As Adelson asks in her seminal work on health beliefs and Cree well-being, "Can we 'be alive well' [healthy] if the land is not?" (1998, 13).

These findings are interesting in a number of ways. While what constitutes health for positive Indigenous women is not radically different from what constitutes health for Indigenous peoples generally, it is nonetheless the first strengths-based articulation of positive Indigenous women's understanding of health in the literature. As such, our findings can be considered an initial step towards documenting positive Indigenous women's perceptions of health. This can, in turn, be used to design strengths-based policy and practice that better meets the needs of positive Indigenous women. More broadly, it can also be used to design strengths-based HIV prevention policy for Indigenous women and girls who are not positive.

To this end, our findings highlight a clear disconnect between the vast majority of research, policy, and practice for positive Indigenous women that has sought to understand and address their/our experiences using a far more limited and limiting concept of health than the one articulated by the Visioning Health co-researchers. Too many studies, policies, and programs focus on problems, deficit, and disease reduction, prioritize physical health and to a lesser extent mental health, while all but ignoring emotional and spiritual dimensions, and almost exclusively promote biomedical "fixes" for positive Indigenous women's health issues that are devoid of socio-cultural context and content. Further, it is clear from our findings that these approaches are experienced as inadequate, unbalanced, disempowering, and in some cases counterproductive. Instead, the stories that the Visioning Health co-researchers shared guide us to ground our research, policy, and practice in positive Indigenous women's notions of health that are culturally grounded, holistic, collectivist, and rooted in relationship at multiple levels.

We also identified several health-enabling strategies in Visioning Health that co-researchers use to support their self-identified health and to help them move towards their self-defined vision of thriving health. Each of these strategies is interconnected and often overlapping. While they were originally identified in the photos and narratives of individual women, these strategies were collectively identified by co-researchers as key elements of support during our participatory analysis.

"Understanding colonization," or understanding how positive Indigenous women are "shaped by [their] environment" is a key element of supporting positive Indigenous women's health and a necessary condition for moving towards greater health, as defined by the women in our project. In Visioning Health, this was typically talked about in the context of intergenerational trauma that has ongoing and sometimes devastating impacts on Indigenous families and communities, and structural violence including deliberate disruption and demonization of cultural norms, values, beliefs, and knowledges; repression and loss of Indigenous languages and gender roles; banning of traditional practices and ceremonies; forced adoption of Indigenous children into non-Indigenous families now known as "the sixties scoop"; and ongoing stigma and discrimination that point to deeply embedded racist and sexist policies, practices, and social structures. Coming to understand that these experiences are also gendered and are linked to "contemporary health and health behaviors including those associated with HIV risk, such as interpersonal violence and substance abuse" (Walters at al. 2011, S262) is crucial for positive Indigenous women. As Krista Shore suggested in our all-groups meeting, "There is more to us than all of a sudden being a statistic and being HIV positive. You know, there are circumstances, there's a pathway, there is a history." For positive Indigenous women to move towards thriving health, this negative impact of colonization and the many ways that it has shaped and continues to shape their/our lives must be understood.

"Resistance and resilience" and "awakening voice and identity" are related to and interconnected with "understanding colonization" and in combination can be seen as cyclical and iterative. In contrast to the dominant narratives of positive Indigenous women as vulnerable, diseased, and dysfunctional, the positive Indigenous women in our project spoke passionately about confronting the negative impacts of colonization, of overcoming hardships, of adapting to new and difficult situations, and of carrying on despite these challenges. In the face of conscious and unconscious attempts to demean, belittle, pathologize, medicalize, delegitimize, erase, or render their experiences invisible, positive Indigenous women regularly stand their ground and assert, "We're still here!" From individual to collective acts of resistance, positive Indigenous women are pushing back and changing the "language, metaphors and images through which they come to be (re)known" (Culhane 2003, 593).

Building on these acts of resistance, positive Indigenous women are also reclaiming their voice and reclaiming their identity. Connecting with culture, honouring themselves as women, and reconstituting HIV-positive status as a strength instead of weakness, as a teacher instead of a punishment, have all emerged as significant health-enabling strategies for positive Indigenous women. This means standing in their strengths as positive Indigenous women, being proud of who they/we are, and defining themselves/ourselves on their/our own terms, not in response to an externally imposed identity. As Kecia Larkin asserts and others affirmed, "You can't tell me who I am!" Reclaiming voice and identity for positive Indigenous women was "empowering," life-affirming, and "an important strategy for individuals in terms of developing a positive sense of one's self and promoting changes in one's community" (McCall, Browne, and Reimer-Kirkham 2009, 29).

"In a climate where stigma is arguably harder to cope with than the actual disease" (Burtch 2015), safe spaces at individual, organizational, and community levels, including social support, is another important strategy for supporting positive Indigenous women's health. In one of the first journal articles in Canada on HIV among Indigenous women, Ship and Norton reported that stigma was a considerable barrier for women, as they fought "for a place in society, in our communities, to feel normal, just to feel accepted and loved, and respected" (2001, 78). Sadly, things have not changed much in the fifteen years since that article was published. Some of the women in Visioning Health were still struggling to "feel normal," "to live as normal a life as possible without any kind of having to have people fear us when we are with them" (LB). Other women kept their HIV-status to themselves. Safe spaces for positive Indigenous women, then, including support from children, family, peers, service providers, and community, are an essential element of creating and maintaining health. These can range from personally safe spaces, to organizational safe spaces, to institutional and community safe spaces that help to remove structural and systemic barriers to positive Indigenous women's health (Peltier 2010). Providing childcare or child-friendly spaces for positive Indigenous women in research or programs is one small example. Designing culturally relevant and women-specific services is another (see CAAN's PAW-licy

Statement (2012) on creating safe spaces for positive Indigenous women for more examples).

Spirituality was identified as a cross-cutting theme in Visioning Health and a core element of positive Indigenous women's health, but most co-researchers had gone through a period in their lives in which they were disconnected from their spiritual selves. Reconnecting with Spirit marked a turning point in their lives. For many of the Visioning Health women, spirituality was grounded in Indigenous cultures, including connecting with and honouring the Creator, Elders, ancestors and spirit helpers, prayer, participating in ceremonies, and receiving traditional teachings. Connecting to nature, including trees, water, animals, the Sacred Sun, Grandmother Moon, Mother Earth, and Grandfather Rocks was also considered connecting to Spirit. Policy directions that support spirituality – for instance through ceremony, access to Elders and ceremonial events, as a foundation of health for positive Indigenous women, and therefore, the inclusion of spirituality in programs and research – are encouraged.

## Culture and Gender as Determinants of Health for Positive Indigenous Women

We began Visioning Health by asking what the role is of culture and gender and their intersections in supporting the health of positive Indigenous women. As evidenced above, culture and gender intersect at every moment of women's lives to influence the health-related choices that are available to them and the possibility that they will create a healthy future. They are mutually constituted and experienced simultaneously, not just by Indigenous women, but by everyone. As Mohawk scholar Patricia Monture-Angus writes, "To artificially separate my gender (or any other part of my being) from my race and culture forces me to deny the way I experience the world" (1995,178). However, as Halseth (2013) has suggested, culture, in its many guises, holds the greatest potential to both understand and intervene in Indigenous women's lives.

As a distal determinant, culture affects every aspect of positive Indigenous women's lives, from the moment they/we are born to the time they/we pass into the spirit world (Loppie Reading and Wein 2009). Culture – or more to the point, the suppression of one culture by another culture, otherwise known as colonization – and its intersection with gender plays a significant role in creating the conditions of social, economic, and political marginalization that increases some Indigenous women's vulnerability to HIV infection in the first place. Visioning Health co-researchers point to the legacy of residential schools, the loss of traditional gender roles, and particularly the decentring of women from their rightful place as the "hearts of our nations" as an indirect but primary cause of what Simoni, Sehgal, and Walters call the "triangle of risk" (2004) for Indigenous women; of sexual trauma, injection drug use, and HIV sexual risk behaviours.

Culture and gender, however, are also implicated in all health-enabling strategies identified in this research. From understanding colonization to reclaiming culture, traditions, ceremonies and identity, culture and gender play a central role in supporting positive Indigenous women's health. The many ways that they/we interrupted and resisted the negative stories and stereotypes that other people tell, and the ways in which they/we reclaim voice and identity were focused on culture. Culture also underpinned spiritual resources that positive Indigenous women drew on to support their health, including connecting to/through the land and the natural environment in particularly gendered ways.

### Decolonizing Policy and Practice for Positive Indigenous Women

Visioning Health profoundly affected the positive Indigenous women in our project and was a poignant example of how research can "bring life" to Indigenous communities. After a century of Indigenous peoples being "researched to death," Visioning Health is at the vanguard of a larger movement in Indigenous HIV research that is using Indigenous knowledge and cultures, including strengths and arts-based approaches, to understand and to resist colonial practices, to reclaim, rekindle, and reinvigorate Indigenous culture and traditions, to revitalize communities, and to change the stories they/we live by. The implications for policy and practice are substantial, given that, at least in part, policy and practice reflect the research and methodologies that inform it (NCCHPP 2014). The following policy directions are drawn from our final sharing circle on "key messages" that co-researchers hoped audiences would take away from Visioning Health, and ongoing discussions with research team members. Consistent with an Indigenous intersectionality-based policy analysis framework, however, these policy directions should be understood as interconnected, intersectional, and mutually constituted.

*"Reclaiming Voice": Policy and Practice for Positive Indigenous
Women Should Incorporate an Anti-Colonial Analysis*

Colonization is a historical and ongoing oppressive practice that continues to shape and constrain the lives and choices of Indigenous women. Understanding the multiple ways that colonization shapes HIV policy and practice, including the perpetuation of pathologizing practices that demean and dehumanize Indigenous women and focus on individual behaviours instead of structural inequities, is a crucial step towards "reclaiming voice and identity" for positive Indigenous women, resisting negative stereotypes, rebuilding positive identities, and revitalizing communities.

Policies and practice that make space for discussions of colonization as oppressive practice, and support positive Indigenous women in understanding and overcoming the impact that colonization has on their/our lives, will be important for the health of positive Indigenous women. A good start would be implementing recommendation 18, the first "health" recommendation, from the Truth and Reconciliation Final Report (2015, 2), which states in part, "We call upon the federal, provincial, territorial, and Aboriginal governments to acknowledge that the current state of Aboriginal health in Canada is a direct result of previous Canadian government policies, including residential schools." Ensuring that all levels of government and public servants involved with Indigenous peoples receive training on the impact of colonization will also move this policy direction forward. Finally, recognizing the impact of colonial history on program development and design and sharing control over programs with Indigenous leaders and organizations directly supports self-determination in contrast to the imposition of services and support from outside the Indigenous community.

*"Creator Gives Us What We Need": Policy and Practice
for Positive Indigenous Women Should Be Grounded
in Local Indigenous Knowledge and Culture*

With few exceptions (see CAAN 2012), policy and practice for positive Indigenous women has typically grown out of research that was grounded in non-Indigenous methodologies and modes of inquiry that often produced results that were consistent with the norms and values of a Western research paradigm but inconsistent with the norms and values of Indigenous communities. As Kovach reminds us, "The proposition is that methodology itself necessarily influences outcomes. Indigenous research frameworks have the potential to improve relevance in policy and practice within Indigenous contexts" (2009, 13). Hence, a major corrective to the policy and program failure for positive Indigenous women is to ground it in local approaches to and expressions of Indigenous knowledge, culture, and ways of being. This includes the use of storytelling.

In Indigenous communities, stories, and traditional teachings from Elders, spiritual beliefs and ceremonies, the land, and lived experiences are important sources of knowledge. History, customs, values, and life lessons are taught and shared through stories, as are one's relationship to place, to Creation, and to family (Archibald 2008). Stories are vessels that carry important information about how to be human, and how to deal with life's challenges. In a modern context, however, stories are also "decolonization theory in its most natural form" (Sium and Ritskes 2013, iii). Consistent with the principles of Indigenous intersectionality-based policy analysis, using stories in our work centres the experiences of positive Indigenous women and demands that their/our voices be heard. Stories give space and light to issues of importance to them/ us, and in these ways, stories are acts of resistance and resilience, of insurgence and resurgence (McIsaac 2002). They are also revolutionary and disrupt dominant notions of scholarship, objectivity, intellectual rigour. Stories and storytelling challenge our notions of "evidence," of what counts as knowledge. As Sium and Ritskes (2013) note, "Stories as Indigenous knowledge work to not only regenerate Indigenous traditions and knowledge production, but also work against the colonial epistemic frame to subvert and recreate possibilities and spaces for resistance" (iii). Therefore, evidence-informed policy and practice for positive Indigenous women must include stories and narrative as legitimate forms of evidence.

*"Shaped Like a Woman": Policy and Practice for*
*Positive Indigenous Women Should Be Women-Centred*

Visioning Health has shown that gendered experiences of HIV require gendered responses. Building on the experience of Visioning Health and CAAN's five-year strategy on HIV and AIDS for Indigenous women (Peltier 2010), an essential component of the Canadian and the Indigenous response to HIV should be a focus on creating culturally, physically, emotionally, spiritually, and mentally "safe spaces" for positive Indigenous women in which they can take stock of their lives, "bear witness" (Kecia Larkin) to each other's experiences, learn about their culture, rally their resources, feed their spirits, nurture their souls, and collectively vision a healthy future. These should be non-judgmental, non-shaming spaces in which positive Indigenous women can "come together to help each other, like we're doing now ... teach each other" (Stacy), and in which confidentiality is ensured. In many cities, towns, and communities, it is not yet safe for positive Indigenous women to be openly HIV-positive, to disclose to friends and family, and in many cases to health-care and social service providers. This makes creating women-centred services particularly important but extremely challenging. Policy and practice should make services more accessible for positive Indigenous women by ensuring confidentiality so that "what was said here, doesn't go out there" (LA).

Visioning Health has also shown, however, that the experience of gender is intricately tied to culture and colonization. As previously noted, women traditionally occupy a central place in Indigenous communities as "the heart of our nations" and this means they have a central role and responsibility in creating change, not just for themselves but also for their families and communities. Elder Art Solomon's teaching that "when women pick up their medicine bundles, nations will begin to heal" (Peltier et al. 2013, 85) implies that "Aboriginal women must bring policy into focus through their [traditional roles] as women. The women are the moral guardians of the society and the ones to lead initiatives for positive social change" (Kenny 2004, 1). This interpretation of women's roles as guardians of society and as agents of change is further reflected in CAAN's five-year strategy on HIV and AIDS for Aboriginal women, which advocates for a women-specific but inclusive strategy that begins with women and then "ripples[s] out [to] touch the lives of all within our communities" (Peltier 2010, 20). As the Visioning Health co-researchers shared, it's about "the inclusion of our children" (Doris Peltier), "our families" (Kecia Larkin), "our whole community" (Krista Shore). "It's not about a women's approach, it's about a community approach, led by women" (Doris Peltier). Policy and practice should nurture and support the inclusion of women in leadership across the board.

*"Having that information in one place when you need it is huge": Policy and Practice for Positive Indigenous Women Should Be Holistic, Relational, and Intersectional*

The health and lives of positive Indigenous women are simultaneously affected by intersecting issues that are experienced as interconnected, and therefore policies and practice for positive Indigenous women that focus on singular aspects of their lives are ineffective. Instead, policies and practices to address positive Indigenous women's health must reflect their notions of health as holistic, encompassing mental, physical, emotional, and spiritual elements. This means challenging the notion that HIV is primarily a biomedical issue that requires a biomedical response. Policy initiatives must recognize and correct this imbalance, bringing equal attention to mental, emotional, and spiritual aspects of positive Indigenous women's lives, as well as social and structural aspects.

As Kecia Larkin observed, "Having access to information and resources is huge," but frequently this information is fragmented and resources are scattered, or services for one aspect of positive Indigenous women's lives do not include other aspects. For example, positive Indigenous women in our project experienced HIV stigma and discrimination while attending substance-use treatment programs, and they frequently report that housing is difficult to find because of racist and HIV-discriminatory attitudes of landlords. Policies that recognize and address these experiences are sorely needed, including policy interventions that counter racism and HIV-related stigma and discrimination for those who deliver services to positive Indigenous women. Given that health for positive Indigenous women is rooted in relationships with self, family, community, nature, and Creator, policy interventions and services should also nurture and support women's relationships at each of these levels.

*"What are the good things?": Policy and Practice*
*for Positive Indigenous Women Should Be Strengths-Based*

Visioning Health guides us to take a strengths-based approach to research and to the policy and practice that flows from it. This means "no more fear tactics" (Kecia Larkin). No more policies that position positive Indigenous women as reckless or irresponsible. No more criminalization. Krista Shore adds, "Instead of looking at the negative and examining all the wrong things and what's wrong with us, what are the right things? What are the good things about us?" Policies that build on "the good things" constitute an important shift towards an approach that understands, explains, and nurtures health, instead of illness (Richmond, Ross, and Egeland 2007), "empowers" positive Indigenous women (Kecia Larkin), and positions them as active agents within their own lives and the lives of their communities. Policies that support meeting the needs of women and recognize and support this agency – such as policies that support positive Indigenous women to keep their children instead of being taken into the care of the state – are crucial to positive Indigenous women's pursuit of self-determination.

To be clear, though, this does not mean that we abandon problem-focused policy or research completely. As noted earlier, these have resulted in many life-saving interventions, including needle exchange programs and substance-use treatment programs. The suggestion, rather, is to balance and contextualize this approach with strengths-based approaches that honour women's journeys, recognize their unique gifts, and support them to find their way.

*"Get out of my chair!": Policy and Practice for Positive Indigenous Women Should Be Driven by and Have Leadership from Positive Indigenous Women*

Positive Indigenous women have been and continue to be silenced, marginalized, tokenized, or ignored. The call has typically been for community-based or community-driven policy and practice for positive Indigenous women, in which communities are engaged in design, development, and implementation. The experience of Visioning Health, however, compels us to shift this call from community-driven initiatives to those in which positive Indigenous women are directly and meaningfully engaged in all aspects. Leadership in policy and practice will support positive Indigenous women's self-determination and ensure that initiatives are timely and relevant to their needs. Recognizing that positive Indigenous women are diverse in age, times since diagnosis, experience of HIV, gender identities, nations, geographic region, and personal life experiences, this means engaging established and emerging positive Indigenous women leaders in developing policy and practice, and investing in future leaders through peer support and peer-mentoring programs and capacity-building initiatives. It means not just asking positive Indigenous women what they want, but also ensuring that they have the resources to make it happen. It means taking a back seat to their leadership, actually listening to what they tell us, and using our resources to support their vision. As Doris Peltier suggests and Kecia Larkin confirms, "We're here and we're not going away," so "Get out of my chair!"

## Conclusion

We need a radical rethink of the way that HIV policy for Indigenous women is developed and implemented. As long as policies and programs are grounded in a biomedical model that is underpinned by Euro-centric values and structures, it will continue to fail Indigenous women. In contrast to the way Visioning Health co-researchers conceptualized "health" as holistic, relational, and grounded in cultural identity, current HIV policy isolates and elevates physical health over all other aspects. The new UNAIDS target of 90 per cent of people living with HIV will know their status, 90 per cent of those with an HIV diagnosis will receive antiretroviral therapy, and 90 per cent of those on therapy will achieve viral suppression is but one example of biomedical supremacy in the response to HIV. Treatment as Prevention, a model that originated in Vancouver, is another. While these policy interventions have the potential to make a dent in the HIV epidemic, they do nothing to address the pre-existing and ongoing historical, social, political, and cultural factors that create HIV vulnerability for Indigenous women in the first place. Likewise for the pathogenic practices that currently characterize HIV policy. Future research and policy directions must be grounded in strengths-based perspectives. This is not to say that research and policy must not tackle the grievous physical, mental, emotional, spiritual, and social harms that are a part of many positive Indigenous women's lives. Rather, addressing these concerns must be framed by a historical perspective that recognizes the on-going impacts of colonization and a strengths-based perspective that acknowledges and builds on the multiple strengths and assets that Indigenous women possess.

In an era that marks the end of AIDS exceptionalism, and the beginning of integration with hepatitis C, sexually transmitted and blood-borne infections, TB, mental health, aging, and related comorbidities, stories and storytelling that keep the voices and experiences of positive Indigenous women at the forefront will become increasingly important. For example, as CAAN expands its organization mandate, all work will continue to place the needs and issues of positive Indigenous peoples at the centre of all initiatives.

We conclude by acknowledging the ancestors who have come before us on a well-traversed pathway, carrying many gifts and tools. These include ceremonies, stories, Indigenous languages, teachings, culture, dreams, and visions, and most importantly the gift of connections, relationships, and interconnectedness to all of Creation and to the land. All of these gifts intrinsically shaped Indigenous world views and should be the foundation of a new response to HIV among Indigenous women.

NOTES

1 Indigenous protocols and our critical Indigenous and decolonizing approach to this chapter guide us to position ourselves as authors. This chapter is intensely personal, purposeful, and grounded in our intersecting identities, relationships, and experiences. We are a team of Indigenous and non-Indigenous researchers, both academic and community-based, who worked together on Visioning Health, the project that is the empirical grounding for this chapter. Visioning Health was the subject of Tracy Prentice's PhD thesis work, co-developed with Doris Peltier, the women's leadership coordinator at the Canadian Aboriginal AIDS Network (CAAN) and an openly HIV-positive Anishinabe woman. Kecia Larkin (Blackfoot and Kwa' Kwa' Ka' Wakw), Krista Shore (Cree), and Elizabeth Benson (Gitskan) are HIV-positive Indigenous women with long histories of advocacy and activism in the Indigenous HIV community. They were also co-researchers in the Visioning project. Kerrigan Johnson was the Visioning Health peer research associate and a two-spirited Anishinabe woman. Renée Masching, an Indigenous woman of Iroquois and Irish bloodlines, is the director of the Research and Policy Unit at CAAN and a Visioning Health community partner.
2 In this chapter we use the terms *Indigenous* and *Aboriginal* interchangeably to indicate the original peoples of Canada, including First Nations, Métis, and Inuit. We recognize that this remains a contentious issue, even within our own writing team, and respect the right of individuals to self-identify in whichever way they choose.
3 Throughout this project, we refer to the positive Indigenous women who participated in Visioning Health as co-researchers. This is a reference to the participatory nature of our project and to the central decision-making role that was shared with all positive Indigenous women in our project. It is an explicit recognition of their roles as researchers, as co-creators of new knowledge, rather than passive participants.
4 Following the convention used by Tuck and Yang (2012), an Indigenous/ non-Indigenous writing team, we use a forward slash for pronouns to acknowledge that some of us are Indigenous and others are not; some of us are HIV-positive and others are not.

5 *Oshkaabewis* is a ceremonial attendant or a "helper." This honoured and
traditional role is grounded in the principle of generosity, one of the Seven
Sacred Teachings (Elder Lillian Pitawanakwat 2006).

## REFERENCES

Adelson, N. 1998. "Health Beliefs and the Politics of Cree Well-being." *Health* 2
(1): 5–22. https://doi.org/10.1177/136345939800200101.
Ahenakew, C. 2011. "The Birth of the 'Windigo': The Construction of
Aboriginal Health in Biomedical and Traditional Indigenous Models of
Medicine." *Critical Literacy: Theories and Practices* 5 (1): 14–26.
Archibald, J. 2008. "An Indigenous Storywork Methodology." In *Handbook of
the Arts in Qualitative Research*, edited by G. Knowles and A. Cole, 371–84.
Los Angeles: Sage.
Bartlett, J., et al. 2007. "Framework for Aboriginal-Guided Decolonizing
Research Involving Métis and First Nations Persons with Diabetes." *Social
Science & Medicine* 65 (11): 2371–82. https://doi.org/10.1016/j.socscimed
.2007.06.011.
Bourassa, C., K. McKay-McNabb, and M. Hampton. 2004. "Racism, Sexism and
Colonialism: The Impact on the Health of Aboriginal Women in Canada."
*Canadian Woman Studies* 24 (1): 23–39.
Burtch, M. 2015. "Ottawa Health Ad Stigmatizes HIV Status." *Daily Extra*,
13 March. https://www.dailyxtra.com/ottawa-health-ad-stigmatizes-
hiv-status-66714.
Canadian Aboriginal AIDS Network (CAAN). 2012. *PAW Den PAW-licy
Statement*. Vancouver, BC: CAAN.
Canadian Research Institute for the Advancement of Women (CRIAW). 2006.
*Intersectional Feminist Frameworks: An Emerging Vision*. Ottawa: CRIAW.
Clark, N. 2012. "Perseverance, Determination and Resistance: An Indigenous
Intersectional-Based Policy Analysis of Violence in the Lives of Indigenous
Girls." In *An Intersectionality-Based Policy Analysis Framework*, edited by O.
Hankivsky, 133–59. Vancouver, BC: Institute for Intersectionality Research
and Policy, Simon Fraser University.
Culhane, D. 2003. "Their Spirits Live within Us: Aboriginal Women in
Downtown Eastside Vancouver Emerging into Visibility." *American Indian
Quarterly* 27 (3 and 4): 593–606. https://doi.org/10.1353/aiq.2004.0073.
Greensmith, C. 2015. "The Management of Indigenous Difference in Toronto's
Queer Service Sector." *Settler Colonial Studies*. https://doi.org/10.1080/
2201473X.2015.1079182.

Halseth, R. 2013. *Aboriginal Women in Canada: Gender, Socio-economic Determinants of Health, and Initiatives to Close the Gap*. Prince George, BC: National Collaborating Centre for Aboriginal Health.

Kenny, C. 2004. *A Holistic Framework for Aboriginal Policy Research*. Ottawa: Status of Women Canada.

King, T. 2003. *The Truth about Stories: A Native Narrative*. Toronto: House of Anansi.

Kovach, M. 2009. *Indigenous Methodologies: Characteristics, Conversations, and Contexts*. Toronto: University of Toronto Press.

Loppie Reading, C., and F. Wein. 2009. *Health Inequalities and Social Determinants of Aboriginal Peoples' Health*. Halifax: National Collaborating Centre for Aboriginal Health.

McCall, J., A. Browne, and S. Reimer-Kirkham. 2009. "Struggling to Survive: The Difficult Reality of Aboriginal Women Living with HIV/AIDS." *Qualitative Health Research* 19 (12): 1769–82. https://doi.org/10.1177/1049732309353907.

McIsaac, E. 2002. "Oral Narratives as a Site of Resistance: Indigenous Knowledge, Colonialism, and Western Discourse." In *Indigenous Knowledges in Global Contexts: Multiple Readings of Our World*, edited by G. Sefa Dei, B. Hall, and D. Goldin Rosenberg, 89–101. Toronto: University of Toronto Press.

Monture-Angus, P. 1995. *Thunder in My Soul: A Mohawk Woman Speaks*. Halifax, NS: Fernwood Publishing.

National Collaborating Centre for Health Public Policy (NCCHPP). 2014. "Briefing Note: Understanding Policy Developments and Choices through the '3-i' Framework: Interests, Ideas and Institutions." Montreal: NCCHPP.

National Women's Association of Canada (NWAC). 2007. "Aboriginal Women and Traditional Healing: An Issues Paper." Ottawa: NWAC.

O'Donnell, V., and S. Wallace. 2011. *Women in Canada: A Gender-Based Statistical Analysis. First Nations, Métis and Inuit Women*. Ottawa: Social and Aboriginal Statistics Division, Statistics Canada.

O'Neil, J., J. Reading, and A. Leader. 1998. "Changing the Relations of Surveillance: The Development of a Discourse on Resistance in Aboriginal Epidemiology." *Human Organization* 57 (2): 230–7. https://doi.org/10.17730/humo.57.2.b7628vwvg7q127m8.

Pearce, M., et al. 2008. "The Cedar Project: Historical Trauma, Sexual Abuse and HIV Risk among Young Aboriginal People Who Use Injection and Non-Injection Drugs in Two Canadian Cities." *Social Science & Medicine* 66 (11): 2185–94. https://doi.org/10.1016/j.socscimed.2008.03.034.

Peltier, D. 2010. *Environments of Nurturing Safety (EONS): A Five Year Strategy on HIV and AIDS for Positive Aboriginal Women*. Vancouver: Canadian Aboriginal AIDS Network.

Peltier, D., et al. 2013. "'When Women Pick Up Their Bundles': HIV Prevention and Related Services for Aboriginal Women." In *Women and HIV Prevention in Canada*, edited by J. Gahagan, 85–103. Toronto: Canadian Scholars' Press.

Prentice, T. 2004. *HIV/AIDS and Aboriginal Women, Children and Families: A Position Statement*. Ottawa: Canadian Aboriginal AIDS Network.

Public Health Agency of Canada (PHAC). 2006. *HIV/AIDS Epi Update*. Ottawa: PHAC.

– 2012. *Population-Specific HIV/AIDS Status Report: Women*. Ottawa: PHAC.

– 2014. *HIV and AIDS in Canada: Surveillance Report to December 31, 2013*. Ottawa: PHAC.

Richmond, C., Nancy A. Ross, and Grace M. Egeland. 2007. "Social Support and Thriving Health: A New Approach to Understanding the Health of Indigenous Canadians." *American Journal of Public Health* 97 (10): 1827–33. https://doi.org/10.2105/AJPH.2006.096917.

Shields, C., R. Bishop, and A. Mazawi. 2005. *Pathologising Practices: The Impact of Deficit Thinking on Education*. New York: Zed Books.

Ship, J., and L. Norton. 2001. "HIV/AIDS and Aboriginal Women in Canada." *Canadian Woman Studies* 21 (2): 25–31.

Simoni, J., S. Sehgal, and K. Walters. 2004. "Triangle of Risk: Urban American Indian Women's Sexual Trauma, Injection Drug Use, and HIV Sexual Risk Behaviours." *AIDS and Behavior* 8 (1): 33–45. https://doi.org/10.1023/B:AIBE.0000017524.40093.6b.

Sium, A., and E. Ritskes. 2013. "Speaking Truth to Power: Indigenous Storytelling as an Act of Living Resistance." *Decolonization* 2 (1): i–x.

Tuck, E., and W. Yang. 2012. "Decolonization Is Not a Metaphor." *Decolonization: Indigeneity, Education & Society* 1 (1): 1–40.

Truth and Reconciliation Canada. 2015. *Honouring the Truth, Reconciling for the Future: Summary of the Final Report of the Truth and Reconciliation Commission of Canada*. Winnipeg: Truth and Reconciliation Commission of Canada.

Varcoe, C., O. Hankivsky, and M. Morrow. 2007. "Introduction: Beyond Gender Matters." In *Women's Health in Canada: Critical Perspectives on Theory and Policy*, edited by Morrow, Hankivsky and Varcoe, 3–30. Toronto: University of Toronto Press.

Walters, K., et al. 2011. "Keeping Our Hearts from Touching the Ground: HIV/AIDS in American Indian and Alaska Native Women." *Women's Health Issues* 21 (S6): S261–5. https://doi.org/10.1016/j.whi.2011.08.005.

Wilson, S. 2008. *Research Is Ceremony: Indigenous Research Methods*. Halifax: Fernwood Publishing.

# 12 Do It in a Good Way: Recommendations for Research and Policy in Indigenous Communities Aging with HIV/AIDS

CHELSEA GABEL, RANDY JACKSON, AND CHANEESA RYAN

Canada is one of the healthiest countries in the world; however, it has one of the most dramatic examples of social inequalities in health (Adelson 2005). In 2012, Canadian Indigenous peoples accounted for 4.3 per cent of Canada's population, or approximately 1.2 million people; they are the fastest growing segment of the population (PHAC 2014). Indicators of economic, social, and health status among Indigenous Canadians compare unfavourably with the Canadian population overall (Adelson 2005; Cooke et al. 2007). Indigenous peoples experience lower life expectancy, higher rates of substance abuse, suicide, and addiction, higher incidence of chronic diseases, and higher rates of infectious diseases than the non-Indigenous population in Canada (Adelson 2005). The gap in health status between Indigenous and non-Indigenous populations is an enduring legacy of colonization and encroachment of industrial forces on traditional lifestyles, sustained by the continuing political, social, and economic marginalization of Indigenous peoples.

Specifically, the rate of HIV infections among Indigenous peoples has risen dramatically, approaching epidemic proportions (PHAC 2014). According to the Public Health Agency of Canada, Indigenous peoples made up 8.9 per cent of the HIV-positive population in Canada at the end of 2011, and 12.2 per cent of all new diagnoses that year. There are a number of HIV/AIDS characteristics unique to the Indigenous population in Canada: (1) between 1998 and 2012, Indigenous women made up 47.3 per cent of HIV cases within the Indigenous population, whereas women of other ethnicities only made up 20.1 per cent of the total cases; (2) injection drug use remains the main mode of transmission for Indigenous peoples at 58.9 per cent , compared with 17.7 per cent of people from other ethnicities; and (3) between 1998 and 2012, almost one-third

(31.6 per cent) of HIV cases in the Indigenous population were within fifteen to twenty-nine years old, and over two-thirds (67.4 per cent) were less than forty years old. In comparison to HIV cases of other ethnicities, the proportion of HIV cases in younger age groups are lower. The data suggest that Indigenous peoples are infected with HIV at a much younger age than their non-Indigenous counterparts (PHAC 2014). While the HIV-positive Indigenous population is younger than their non-Indigenous counterparts, 69.3 per cent of Indigenous peoples with HIV are thirty to forty-nine years old. This suggests that over the next two decades, the number of older Indigenous peoples living with HIV/AIDS is going to rapidly increase.

We begin with a brief overview of the jurisdictional complexities involved in health-care services for Indigenous peoples, to contextualize the analysis that follows. We then present an overview of policy responses to and literature about Indigenous people, HIV, and aging, drawing attention to the lack of focus on resiliency and successful aging. The rest of the chapter presents findings from sharing circles conducted with older Indigenous people living with HIV, showing that resiliency is often described as holistic. Findings suggest implications for policy and research. Our hope is that this knowledge can be used to influence community and primary health services to structure themselves in ways that will promote successful aging with HIV/AIDS in ways that are congruent with Indigenous culturally defined notions of health and well-being.

## Challenges of Indigenous Health Policy

The relationship between the government of Canada and Indigenous peoples is unique, characterized by a complicated legislative and constitutional regime. Consequently, "the outcome has been that of jurisdictional confusion and policy vacuums regarding many aspects of Aboriginal peoples' lives" (Macintosh 2006, 193). In Canada, primary health-care services for on-reserve First Nations are under federal jurisdiction, while primary health care for other Canadians is under provincial jurisdiction. Furthermore, the Indian Act, the principal regulator of Indigenous life in Canada, sets out in rather limiting ways the legal category of Indian, which determines the right to live on-reserve and to qualify for certain individual-based benefits (Coates and Morrison 1986). In most cases where the question of jurisdiction arises, both federal and provincial/territorial levels of government claim to hold power and the authority to assert a governance regime. It is not surprising to see that most provinces view Indigenous health as an "Indian" issue, and as such within federal jurisdiction, and an issue to be addressed through federal funding and programming (Macintosh 2006, 197). Thus, Ottawa's position on the jurisdictional question is highly complex.

The participation of federal, provincial, and territorial levels of government creates a highly complicated and uncoordinated system characterized by gaps in service and overlapping coverage. It also results in funding duplication and inconsistencies. Being an Indigenous person without legal status also denies access to certain health-care services, such as access to HIV treatment under the Non-Insured Health Benefit Program. In addition, funding for health-care services to Indigenous communities and organizations often comes in the form of program-specific envelopes. In the context of multiple health challenges, HIV is not given priority equal to other chronic diseases such as diabetes. This means that there are different lines of accountability, and each program has its own purpose-designed format for processing information. Minore and Katt write, "This generates a great deal of time-consuming paperwork at the local level, which is a source of constant complaint" (2007, 9). It is often difficult to attract and retain staff, not knowing whether funding will continue past the fiscal year-end. In addition, in order to receive funding, communities are often required to write proposals and make a case for new and renewed monies. This can often lead to administrative complexities and situational uncertainties.

It is also within this health policy context that Indigenous individuals living with HIV/AIDS and health providers must navigate. The Canadian response to HIV and AIDS is guided by the Federal Initiative to Address HIV/AIDS in Canada (FI) (PHAC 2004). Introduced in 2004 following extensive stakeholder consultations, the FI addresses four goals: (1) to prevent the spread of HIV, (2) address the quality of life for those already living with HIV, (3) contribute to the global HIV response, and (4) reduce associated social and economic impacts of HIV. Bolstering these broad national efforts, and recognizing that Indigenous peoples require a culturally relevant response, with support under the FI the Canadian Aboriginal AIDS Network (CAAN) developed a companion Aboriginal Strategy on HIV and AIDS in Canada II (ASHAC II) (CAAN 2009). This Indigenous-focused strategy espouses several strategic areas: (1) identifying the needs of Indigenous peoples, both on and off-reserve, (2) developing policies and program approaches to meet these needs, (3) grounding such approaches in the world views of Indigenous peoples, and (4) working to secure resources to develop and fully implement culturally based health approaches. Further, in supporting the Toronto Charter: Indigenous Peoples Action Plan on HIV/AIDS, ASHAC II also emphasizes the importance of Indigenous stakeholder involvement, particularly those living with HIV, advocates for implementation of the Toronto Charter, and monitors government inaction on HIV affecting Indigenous peoples. The Toronto Charter (International Indigenous Working Group on HIV/AIDS 2006), developed by Indigenous activists attending the International AIDS Conference in Toronto in 2006, promotes the meaningful inclusion of Indigenous peoples in identifying and responding to HIV. An evaluation of the FI highlights the need for continued collaboration and priority setting, the need to bolster knowledge translation, continued work to reduce barriers across the continuum of HIV-related health services, and the need to better identify, collect, and use internal information to enhance the national response to HIV/AIDS. In light of shifts in the nature and complexity of HIV and AIDS in Canada, both the FI and ASHAC II strategies urgently require updating.

While the FI and ASHAC II represent steps in the right direction in recognition of the epidemic within the Indigenous population and the recommendation of policies and programs specific to this population, both fail to address the "greying of the epidemic." In July 2010, the Public Health Agency of Canada published an *HIV/AIDS Epidemic Update*, which included a chapter on older Canadians (chapter 6). The report clearly illustrated the increasing proportion of positive HIV tests among older adults: "The number of annual positive HIV test reports has increased among those 50 years old and over by 76.5% since 1999" (PHAC 2010, 3). Trends in HIV/AIDS prevention, diagnosis, and treatment/outcomes among the older population have been identified in the research. Chapter 6 highlighted important trends, such as (1) research has shown that older Canadians are less informed about HIV/AIDS transmission than their younger counterparts, (2) physicians are less likely to discuss sexual health with older patients, (3) the over-fifty age group has the highest percentage reporting unprotected sex, putting them at higher risk of HIV infection, and (4) in addition to the limited knowledge of HIV transmission, older Canadians are less likely to be tested for HIV (PHAC 2010). Despite these findings, a focus on HIV/AIDS among the aging population is absent from the Federal Initiative on HIV/AIDS.

## Resiliency and Successful Aging

While there is a growing body of literature on HIV and aging, research tends to focus on the biomedical aspects of aging with HIV/AIDS. Therefore, there is a dearth of information on the social aspects of aging with HIV/AIDS (Roger, Mignone, and Kirkland 2013; Sankar et al. 2011; Vance, Struzick, and Masten 2008). The information that does exist fails to address the needs of the growing Indigenous population aging with HIV/AIDS. Given what we know about the health of the Indigenous population, and more specifically, the proportion of the population with HIV, the knowledge gap in this area should be of great concern (Duncan et al. 2011). Further research is needed to gain a better understanding of the lived experiences of this diverse population so that we can work towards effective, culturally resonating strategies that can help facilitate successful aging among older Indigenous peoples already living with HIV and/or AIDS.

While much of the literature examines the challenges of aging with HIV/AIDS, only a handful of articles highlight the resiliency of older people living with HIV/AIDS (PHA) and their abilities to cope. A study conducted by Siegel, Raveis, and Karus (1998) appears to be the earliest research to look at the strengths of older PHAs. Participants in their study spoke about advantages they perceived in being an older adult with HIV/AIDS. Siegel and colleagues found the "most notable were the emphasis on the value of wisdom and enhanced problem solving abilities that were believed to accompany aging" (705). Emlet et al. (2013) found that as individuals live longer with HIV, it may become a decreasing focus in their life and thus less internalized. Therefore, it is possible that individuals living over the long term with HIV develop vital stigma-management strategies, enhancing their quality of life and obtaining a level of successful aging (Emlet et al. 2013; Psaros et al. 2015). Psaros et al. (2015) found that concepts such as resilience, optimism, and problem-focused coping are essential to successful aging. Throughout the literature, protective factors for aging with HIV were identified, including social support (Owen and Catalan 2012; Poindexter 2004), acceptance of the disease and oneself (Emlet, Tozay, and Raveis 2010; Foster and Gaskins 2009), generativity (Emlet, Tozay, and Raveis 2010; Owen and Catalan 2012; Poindexter 2004; Sankar et al. 2011), self-esteem (Beuthin, Bruce, and Sheilds 2015), spirituality (Brennan 2008; Siegel and Schrimshaw 2002; Hampton et al. 2013), and drawing on cultural resources (Sankar et al. 2011).

Kahana and Kahana (2001) developed a model of successful aging that was applicable to adults aging with chronic, debilitating, and life-threatening conditions such as HIV/AIDS. This model suggests using psychological and social outcomes as measures of high quality of life, rather than the traditional measures of absence of disease and maintaining high levels of mental and physical functioning. Emlet et al. (2010) support Kahana and Kahana's (2001) preventative-corrective proactivity (PCP) model of successful aging. Vance and Robinson (2004) identify cognitive efficiency, hardiness, and a "can do" attitude as psychological components of successful aging. In addition, they identify social support and financial well-being as social components necessary for successful aging. Lastly, they discuss the importance of mobility, autonomy, and minimal disease as physical components that contribute to successful aging. Vance, Struzick, and Masten (2008) discuss the importance of hardiness in aging with HIV, concluding that it can mitigate aging and HIV-related decline. Further research is needed to build on the current findings on the resiliency that already exists within the older HIV-positive population, in order to translate these findings into strategies to help others with HIV to age successfully.

From reviewing the literature, we know that the successful aging discourse was based on Western values, and therefore its application to other cultures is questionable (Liang and Luo 2012). Thus, it is also important to consider what successful aging looks like in the context of aging with HIV through an Indigenous lens.

## Indigenous Peoples, Resiliency, and Successful Aging

One Canadian study that explored resilience among two-spirit men living over the long term with HIV in Ontario found that responses were culturally grounded (Jackson et al. 2015). Despite challenges, two-spirit men were adopting approaches that draw on the strengths of their culture. Resilient responses were grounded in Indigenous world views and include taking care of oneself (e.g., attending to physical, emotional, mental, and spiritual aspects of self), accepting life's challenges (e.g., gay identity, negative effects of colonization, HIV status), recognizing one's sense of agency to respond to challenges (e.g., developing community-involved strategies to minimize challenges), connecting to one's community (e.g., volunteerism, accessing Indigenous HIV/AIDS services and supports programs), and drawing on principles *mino-bimaadiziwin* (i.e., living the way of a good life). Results of this study highlight the need for further research to build on the findings on resiliency that already exists within the older PHA population, in order to translate these findings into strategies to help others with HIV to age successfully. With this in mind, and given the dearth of literature specific to Indigenous peoples aging with HIV/AIDS, our team explored this issue in more detail specific to aging with HIV and AIDS.

## Methods

In exploring Indigenous lived experience of aging from the perspective of those living over the long term with HIV, we drew on principles of community-based research (CBR) embedding both decolonizing and Indigenous methodologies. The use of these two additional approaches can be "summarized as research by and for Indigenous peoples, using techniques and methods drawn from the traditions of those peoples" (Evans et al. 2009, 894). As such, we decided early in our process to pivot the focus group method and we re-envisioned our approach to gathering participant data through the cultural protocols embedded in sharing circles (Poff 2006; Rothe, Ozegovic, and Carroll 2009). With our community partner (the Canadian Aboriginal AIDS Network) providing recruitment assistance, during each of the sharing circles we asked participants a broad series of questions on experiences of aging with HIV. In using sharing circles rather than focus groups, we intended to emphasize the importance of oral tradition and storytelling among Indigenous peoples (Poff 2006; Rothe, Ozegovic, and Carroll 2009). Sharing circles, common among Indigenous peoples in Canada, resonate with participants as egalitarian, supportive of cultural identity, and nonconfrontational, and they are structured to solicit collective identification of challenges and potential solutions (Rothe Ozegovic and Carroll 2009). In our sharing circles, moderated by a graduate student and a faculty member, an Indigenous Elder assisted in an effort to foster a sense of safety and establish trust. Our goal in adopting this approach was to create a "mutually respectful, win-win relationship with the research population – a relationship in which people are pleased to participate in research and the community at large regards the research as constructive" (Poff 2006, 28). Research plans and process, as well as sharing circle questions, were vetted through our community representatives prior to submission to the McMaster University Research Ethics Board.

All sharing circles and interviews were audio-recorded and transcribed verbatim. Consistent with recommendations offered by Onwuegbuzie and colleagues (2009) for analysing focus group data, we used constant comparison to braid the sharing circles stories of aging and HIV together and draw out themes. Transcripts of all focus groups/interviews were shared with community/academic representatives on our team, and they contributed to the analysis. Analysis of data involved three stages. The first step – open coding – is "the part of analysis that pertains specifically to the naming or categorizing of phenomena through close examination of the data" (Strauss and Corbin 1990, 62). Here, working alongside our community partners, we shared and read transcripts in ways that were meant to inform the development of codes to be used in grouping the data. Key codes developed through this method include participants' discussions, for example, that highlight healthy eating, exercise, and avoiding alcohol/drugs. In other words, working across all transcripts, we grouped smaller units of narratives from our transcripts in codes that expressed properties similar to one another. In the second stage of our analysis – axial coding – we grouped codes "back together in new way by making connections between a category and its subcategories" (97). Here, for example, we used group codes that expressed a relationship to one another into new categories. In other words, healthy eating, exercise, and avoiding alcohol/drugs were grouped as health-maintenance strategies promoting successful aging. The final stage of analysis – selective coding – refers to themes that emerge from the previous two steps. It is the process of "selecting the code category, relating it to other categories, validating those relationships, and filling in categories that need further refinement and development" (116). Key themes developed through this process include participants' discussions about aging as it relates to the physical, emotional, mental, spiritual, and social engagement. The findings are summarized below.

**Findings**

*What Is Successful Aging?*

Several interconnected themes emerged in our analysis as important in successful aging for Indigenous people living with HIV: physical, emotional, spiritual, mental, and social engagement. While all of the dimensions that an individual must embrace in order to achieve successful aging are intricately connected, the emphasis that one places on each individual dimension is subjectively determined. Therefore, successful aging does not rely upon an equitable balance between dimensions and can be represented by an overemphasis on some and an under-emphasis on others. The way in which individuals find their own balance of the five dimensions manifests in a nonlinear way. Recognition of the inter-connectedness of the five dimensions means that individuals can move freely from one dimension to the next, and back again, until the individual finds the right balance necessary to actualize successful aging. This means that there is no standard order in which the dimensions of successful aging need to be achieved, and the degree to which an individual will accept or embrace each dimension will vary considerably.

*Physical*

When participants were asked what successful aging means to them, most individuals recognized the importance of their physical health. Many people spoke about their physical health in relation to living with HIV and the impact the disease has had on their body. Participants spoke about the importance of treating their physical body well with greater regularity than an individual who is not living with a life-threatening disease. This dimension was often discussed in relation to a proper diet, physical exercise, maintenance of comorbidities, adherence to medications, and abstinence from drugs and alcohol.

> "I learned to eat well, to eat healthy food ... to try and eat so that I don't get diabetes, which is really prevalent in our communities. And I think part of why diabetes is so prevalent in our communities is because of the poverty diet that people are forced to eat" (Carol).

> "Exercise is my thing that really releases everything for me. I could be having the worst day possible and then I go to the gym and work out and it releases everything. It is really important" (John).

> "To me healthy aging is very plain and simple, not drinking as much as I have been. It's been really hard on my body. Since I have tested positive I am just starting to really understand that and do it in a good way. So that to me, my main goal is to stop my drinking so I can really live healthy" (James).

*Emotional*

Many of the sharing circle participants and interviewees could relate to one another on the basis of the adversities they experienced throughout their lives. They also shared similar beliefs and strategies about the importance of overcoming such challenges. They understood the impact of cumulative disadvantages on their health, therefore they understood the connection between overcoming these challenges in order to nurture their emotional well-being and subsequently their happiness. A majority of the participants spoke about the importance of self-love and acceptance as key to one's emotional health and thus as a determinant of successful aging.

> "I'm going to feed myself emotionally by being real with where I am at and owning it, and letting it go and voicing it and letting it go and letting the healing come in with every time that I share my story, because that's medicine you know" (Cindy).

> "It's being healthy, being happy, loving yourself, and loving everyone around you" (Mike).

> "My main goal is to embrace life itself, to appreciate life, and to appreciate yourself first, because if you don't love yourself first, you can't love nobody else and you can't embrace anybody else's thoughts and feelings" (Matt).

### Mental

Often participants spoke to the importance of working towards good mental health in relation to their ability to maintain a clear mind that is without the influence of drugs or alcohol. Individuals discussed the need to re-evaluate their lives since first becoming diagnosed, which was most often equated with death, then coming to the realization that they can now live a full life. Accepting this new reality and formulating a way to deal with it was fundamental to participants' ability to age successfully. Participants spoke about the challenge of having multiple stigmatizing identities such as being HIV-positive, older, and Indigenous, and how these factors can harm their self-esteem. More importantly, participants spoke about the need to overcome these stigmas in order to accept themselves. They recognized that gaining confidence and self-esteem was important for their mental health.

> "Successful aging for me is that I will be confident, and my self-esteem remains intact, and ... self-acceptance, which is very hard to do, especially when your hair is greying and you have to dye it all the time, and your

wrinkles are starting to come from everywhere, and when you are not used to it and the process is like, OK is it from the HIV medications – you know, the lipodystrophy thing – or is it from aging?" (Laura).

"Now that I am clearly thinking because I am not using alcohol or anything else to cloud my judgement, it has given me a more healthy approach to longevity" (Tom).

"HIV has affected me in many ways, to the point where, until the problems are resolved, I can't drive, I can't get behind the wheel of a car. I am dealing with a number of diagnoses, as surrounding the mental illness, two of them. But I don't let that define really what I am doing on this earth. It's a challenge yes, but it's solely finding that, although HIV has affected me in that way, it doesn't mean that I have to continue to being that unstable or an unstable, stigmatized person living with HIV. So I use that as an opportunity to learn about it, but to again keep myself on track" (Frank).

### Spiritual

Many participants spoke about the role of spirituality in their ability to cope with their diagnosis and to age successfully. For some, their spirituality was in connection to their Indigenous roots, whether that was learning about their culture and traditions for the first time or strengthening their connection, and for other participants their spirituality came from other sources. Regardless of the source of their spirituality or the motivation behind their spiritual recognition, it was apparent that their individual sense of spirituality had a positive effect on their health and well-being and was essential to their ability to age successfully.

"I find, I need, as I age, I need balance, holding this eagle's feather and smudging during ceremonies and just being with my brothers and sisters" (Dave).

"Understanding that I am a spiritual being and how I can connect with others is really important to me, and part of that is through being mindful, using mindful practices, meditation. And those things really ground me and make me realize that living in this world is not just about me" (Tom).

"One other thing, on the spirituality part, just because we are going through this whole transition and reclaiming our culture and getting our culture back. I think that is a very important part within my life, because I was raised as a Christian, but now I am learning more about my traditional background, and it's really helped me, I guess, in the aging process, to open my mind and to help me gain wisdom and be more mindful, be more aware, ugh, and take pride in who I was, to be proud to be Anishinabek" (Steve).

## Social Engagement

The importance of social engagement in participants' lives was extremely evident. Social engagement seemed to be the common thread that bound all dimensions together. Opportunities for social engagement could be clearly linked to physical, emotional, mental, and spiritual health and well-being. Participants spoke of how being connected with others had a positive impact on their well-being. Most often this connection to others occurred in teaching, in passing down their knowledge to youth. Many participants spoke about the obligation they felt to share their stories, to teach others about HIV, in hopes that its further spread in their communities could be stopped. Opportunities to share and teach contributed to participants' sense of generativity, which appeared to be an essential component to aging successfully with HIV/AIDS.

"Aging successfully for me is about meeting my needs and then my world gets better, right? Because I isolate if I am not feeling good, and I don't want to be around other people. And it is easy to chew through a year or 18 months of not feeling well, or at least it has been for me. And my world would get really small, right? And then out of desperation I would reach out for socialization, right? And friendship and company. And that would help my world get bigger, or feel bigger, right?" (Tony).

"I guess another thing that for me, around successful aging I guess, is really being connected to my community and with my brothers and sisters and sharing those stories and recognizing the similarities we have and acknowledging the differences. But seeing the similarities that we have in our journeys by communicating and talking is really important, because you find out things that ugh, and recognize that you are not going through it alone" (Steve).

While many participants demonstrated the interconnectedness of the dimensions of successful aging, some spoke about the significance of these dimensions in isolation from one another. Even then, it was clear how, if that apparently isolated dimension was not directly linked to another, at least it related to or led to another. For example, social activities may provide an opportunity to improve individuals' physical health, whether through a group physical activity such as going on a walk, or enjoying cultural foods at a community potluck. Attending ceremonies or church can also contribute to one's spirituality. Here individuals can learn from others and/or teach and share their knowledge with others, contributing to their mental health and well-being. Conversely, participants recognized emotional well-being as a prerequisite to be able to engage intimately with others in a social context. Ultimately, the decision to engage with some or all of these dimensions and to what degree lies within the individual. While these dimensions are all clearly interrelated and each can be seen as a component necessary to successful aging, it is up to the individual to find a balance between each domain in order to age successfully. In the end, there is no standardized approach or formula to achieve successful aging, at least not from within the lens of Indigenous world views.

*Barriers to Successful Aging*

While our sharing circles and interviews were focused primarily on participant strategies to "age successfully," these strategies were commonly formulated in response to commonly experienced barriers. Within our sharing circle with service providers for older Indigenous peoples living with HIV/AIDS, participants described poverty as a major barrier to successful aging for their clients. Similarly, the men and women in our sharing circles spoke about a lack of access to social determinants of health as a major barrier to successful aging. Interestingly, participants didn't seem to view HIV/AIDS itself as a barrier to successful aging. Instead, they found a lack of access to the basic social determinants of health as a barrier.

"Also another barrier is the high cost of living. You know, especially in, where I am now, there is so much mining going on so the rents have gone right through the roof. If our APHAs [Aboriginal peoples living with HIV/AIDS] are on a pension, you know, you decide whether or not you are going to have a roof over your head, or if you are going to have something to eat, you know? And, we have, further up north, we have the big diamond mine, big diamond mines coming up, a case of water, 24 [bottles] of water is $40. You know those little bottles of Fruitease are 99 cents, up there they are $9.99! Toilet paper, four-roll pack, is one time I saw it for $12 or something. You know, it's just outrageous, so I don't know how they're, how they do, choices between, you know, what you are going to get this month or whatever. Inadequate housing, if there even is housing" (Sara).

Participants' wish list for services and programs were quite basic. Opportunities for social participation were very important, as well as access to transportation, food, adequate income, and culturally sensitive (discrimination-free) care. Transportation seemed to be particularly important, as it could increase opportunities for social participation and access to food, health-care services, and other services for individuals living with HIV. These barriers need to be recognized as priorities in the federal response to HIV/AIDS in Canada.

## Policy and Research Recommendations

On the basis of our findings of what successful aging with HIV looks like through an Indigenous lens, we can begin to formulate recommendations for culturally resonant programs and policies that will enable older Indigenous peoples with HIV to age successfully.

The experience of aging with HIV for Indigenous peoples is not yet well understood. Although our review of the aging/HIV literature provided a substantial overview of major concepts and theories, it did not address differential experiences from the perspectives of Indigenous peoples. As such, we advocate for further aging/HIV research where the substantive focus is on Indigenous peoples. Such research would best be conducted using Indigenous methodologies. We believe that positive health outcomes for Indigenous peoples aging with HIV will be viable only insofar as they resonate with the localized and culturally defined, gendered, and age-appropriate experiences of Indigenous peoples. Although there appear to be similarities between the experience with HIV of Indigenous peoples and other cultural groups, health programs that are designed to be culturally malleable will more positively attend to and ground responses in specific and differing meaning attached to localized contexts through attention to traditions, customs, and local conditions specific to each person, family, and community.

Two-eyed seeing may offer researchers and policymakers a grounding in Indigenous knowledge that can support creation of health programs that are congruent with Indigenous world views. Developed as an Indigenous approach to providing culturally grounded educational opportunities for Indigenous students in Western academic settings, two-eyed seeing refers to seeing "from one eye with the strengths of Indigenous ways of knowing, and from the other eye with the strengths of Western ways of knowing, and to use both of these eyes together" (Hatcher and Bartlett 2010, 16). However, we recommend that two-eyed seeing be approached with care. We take seriously the notion that equal value can be given to Indigenous knowledge and the Western knowledge system. We are troubled with the use of two-eyed seeing in research or policy contexts, as it may inadvertently compromise or subvert Indigenous ways of knowing. To use two-eyed seeing successfully, it may be necessary to marry the approach to a basic precept of Indigenous knowledge that favours experiential knowing. As Battiste reminds us, "To acquire Indigenous knowledge [and then use it effectively in the context of health] ... one must come to know through extended conversation and experiences with elders, peoples, and places of Canada" (2008, 502). Perhaps our concerns about using two-eyed seeing will not be realized if researchers and policymakers commit to working with Indigenous peoples to develop an intimate and lived experience with Indigenous peoples.

## Conclusion

In order to meet the needs of this population and to prevent rising HIV/AIDS incidence in the older adult population, ageism needs to be confronted. Ageism, combined with HIV stigma, continues to contribute to the lack of education, prevention, and treatment targeted at the older population (Bhavan, Kampalath, and Overton 2008; Levy-Dweck 2005). This stigma and resulting lack of education can have devastating consequences, as it leads to under-testing and thus under-diagnosing of older adults with HIV. This lack of testing often results in older adults being diagnosed at advanced stages of the disease, making older adults more likely to progress to AIDS than their younger counterparts (Balderson et al. 2013). When older adults are diagnosed, they continue to face discrimination by their peers and service providers. This is extremely problematic, given that older adults tend to have smaller informal social networks, thus they often require additional support in managing and controlling the disease (Brennan-Ing et al. 2014; Levy-Dweck 2005). In addition to ageism, Indigenous peoples experience barriers to health care leading to inequitable access as a result of shortages of health-care professionals, geographic location of communities, lack of culturally competent care, lower levels of education and/or income, and experiences of racism and discrimination frequently encountered while navigating the health-care system (PHAC 2014). All of these issues highlight the importance of research that examines not only the social aspects of HIV and aging in education, prevention, and treatment but also research that recognizes the heterogeneity of the aging, HIV-positive, Indigenous population.

There is a need to examine the cultural histories and perspectives of older First Nations, Métis, and Inuit living with HIV and highlight the significant differences between these groups and the differences within them. This is particularly relevant for First Nations both on and off reserve, as well as rural and urban populations. It is also necessary to acknowledge how the experiences of older Indigenous women and men with HIV are similar and/or different and how this will affect future policies and programs. Future research that is grounded in Indigenous world views and ways of knowing may provide a more nuanced understanding of the ways aging is experienced by Indigenous peoples living with HIV. In this respect, methodological innovation is needed to draw on decolonizing and Indigenous methodologies. In this way we might begin to explore and understand aging and HIV from within the world views of peoples who experience it. When understanding is methodologically grounded in these ways, resulting programs and policy might be more respectful of self-determination and provide more culturally relevant care.

The majority of health-care practitioners who serve Indigenous peoples are non-Indigenous and have been educated within a Western biomedical model. Bernice Downey calls for "a reclamative and restorative process of acknowledging and integrating Indigenous knowledge" that can address this gap (2014, 35). We recommend that Indigenous peoples aging with HIV/AIDS enhance their self-care when culturally relevant approaches are available to them. This approach is in keeping with an Indigenous world view and one that will assist in the creation of an "Indigenous therapeutic relational space" between non-Indigenous health-care practitioners and their Indigenous patients (ibid.). For this recommendation to be more fully realized, however, further research is needed that explores aging with HIV from the perspectives of Indigenous peoples. It is imperative, from our perspective, that when this research is conducted it is grounded in and framed by using Indigenous knowledge. In other words, it is necessary (and morally and ethically sound) to create understanding from within the world views, perspectives, and value systems of a people who originally experienced the phenomena in the first place (McLeod 2007). The shift towards use of Indigenous knowledge – rather than relying solely on other interpretative, critical phenomenological, or constructivist frameworks – may also shift our understanding in ways that fully appreciate the culturally mediated experience of aging with HIV among older Indigenous peoples.

The call for more Indigenous grounded research – coupled with appreciation for other ways of knowing – is in line with principles of two-eyed seeing. In other words, two-eyed seeing may offer a new approach in research to mediate, and not resolve, the uncertainty and the irreconcilable ways Indigenous knowledge may ascribe to Western research methods. It also potentially offers a way to understand the ways in which participants – because of varied social location and cultural identity – may differentially describe experiences of aging with HIV/AIDS. Using two-eyed seeing, the research approach advocated here will strive for common ground, respect differences, avoid knowledge domination and assimilation, and rest on the principle that co-learning and appreciation of different ways of knowing is connected to culture and community processes (ibid.). However, use of two-eyed seeing in either policy or research context must be approached carefully and cautiously: does two-eyed seeing devalue Indigenous knowledge? The drive to use these principles may be failing to appreciate that Indigenous knowledge systems on their own can explore and know the world, and in doing so, arrive at rigorous and sound knowledge that is applicable in a contemporary health context dealing with Indigenous peoples.

REFERENCES

Adelson, Naomi. 2005. "The Embodiment of Inequity." *Canadian Journal of Public Health* 96 (1): 45–61.
Balderson, Benjamin H., et al. 2013. "Chronic Illness Burden and Quality of Life in an Aging HIV Population." *AIDS Care* 25 (4): 451–8. https://doi.org/10.1080/09540121.2012.712669.
Battiste, Marie. 2008. "Research Ethics for Protecting Indigenous Knowledge and Heritage: Institutional and Researcher Responsibilities." In *Handbook of Critical and Indigenous Methodologies*, ed. N.K. Denzin, Y.S. Lincoln, and L.T. Smith, 497–510. Thousand Oaks, CA: Sage. https://doi.org/10.4135/9781483385686.n25.

Beuthin, Rosanne E., Anne Bruce, and Laurene Sheilds. 2015. "Storylines of Aging with HIV: Shifts toward Sense Making." *Qualitative Health Research* 25 (5): 612–21. https://doi.org/10.1177/1049732314553597.

Bhavan, K.P., V.N. Kampalath, and E.T. Overton. 2008. "The Aging of the HIV Epidemic." *Current CIDS/HIV Reports* 5 (3): 150–8. https://doi.org/10.1007/s11904-008-0023-3.

Brennan, Mark. 2008. "Older Men Living with HIV: The Importance of Spirituality." *Generations (San Francisco)* 32 (1): 54–61.

Brennan-Ing, Mark, et al. 2014. "Substance Use and Sexual Risk Differences among Older Bisexual and Gay Men with HIV." *Behavioral Medicine (Washington, DC)* 40 (3): 108–15. https://doi.org/10.1080/08964289.2014.889069.

Canadian Aboriginal AIDS Network (CAAN). 2009. *Aboriginal Strategy on HIV/AIDS in Canada II: For First Nations, Inuit and Metis Peoples from 2009 to 2014.* Ottawa: CAAN.

Coates, K.S., and W.R. Morrison. 1986. *Treaty Research Report: Treaty Five (1875).* Ottawa: Indian and Northern Affairs Canada.

Cooke, M., et al. 2007. "Indigenous Well-being in Four Countries: An Application of the UNDP'S Human Development Index to Indigenous Peoples in Australia, Canada, New Zealand, and the United States." *BMC International Health and Human Rights* 7 (1). https://doi.org/10.1186/1472-698X-7-9.

Downey, Bernice. 2014. "Diaspora Health Literacy: Reclaiming and Restoring Nibwaakaawin (Wisdom) and Mending Broken Hearts." PhD diss., McMaster University, Hamilton, Ontario.

Duncan, Katrina, et al. 2011. "HIV Incidence and Prevalence Among Aboriginal Peoples in Canada." *AIDS and Behavior* 15 (1): 214–27.

Emlet, Charles A., et al. 2013. "Protective and Risk Factors Associated with Stigma in a Population of Older Adults Living with HIV in Ontario, Canada." *AIDS Care* 25 (10): 1330–9. https://doi.org/10.1080/09540121.2013.774317.

Emlet, Charles A., Shakima Tozay, and Victoria H. Raveis. 2010. "'I'm not going to die from the AIDS': Resilience in Aging with HIV Disease." *Gerontologist* 51 (1): 101–11.

Evans, Mike, et al. 2009. "Common Insights, Differing Methodologies: Toward a Fusion of Indigenous Methodologies, Participatory Action Research, and White Studies in an Urban Aboriginal Research Agenda." *Qualitative Inquiry* 15 (5): 893–910. https://doi.org/10.1177/1077800409333392.

Foster, Pamela Payne, and Susan W. Gaskins. 2009. "Older African Americans' Management of HIV/AIDS Stigma." *AIDS Care* 21 (10): 1306–12. https://doi.org/10.1080/09540120902803141.

Hampton, Melvin C., et al. 2013. "Religiousness, Spirituality, and Existential Well-being among HIV-Positive Gay, Bisexual, and Other MSM Age 50 and Over." *Journal of Religion, Spirituality and Aging* 25 (2): 160–76. https://doi.org/10.1080/15528030.2012.739992.

Hatcher, A., and Cheryl Bartlett. 2010. "Two-Eyed Seeing: Building Cultural Bridges for Aboriginal Students." *Canadian Teacher Magazine* 6 (5): 14–17.

International Indigenous Working Group on HIV/AIDS. 2006. *Toronto Charter: Indigenous Peoples Action Plan on HIV/AIDS*.

Jackson, R., et al. 2015. "The Seven Paths of Resilience: Findings from the Two-Spirit HIV/AIDS Wellness and Longevity Study (2SHAWLS)." Research findings presented at 24th Annual Canadian Conference on HIV/AIDS Research, Toronto.

Kahana, E., and B. Kahana. 2001. "Successful Aging among People with HIV/AIDS." *Journal of Clinical Epidemiology* 54 (12): S53–6. https://doi.org/10.1016/S0895-4356(01)00447-4.

Liang, Jiayin, and Baozhen Luo. 2012. "Toward a Discourse Shift in Social Gerontology: From Successful Aging to Harmonious Aging." *Journal of Aging Studies* 26 (3): 327–34. https://doi.org/10.1016/j.jaging.2012.03.001.

Levy-Dweck, Sandra. 2005. "HIV/AIDS Fifty and Older: A Hidden and Growing Population." *Journal of Gerontological Social Work* 46 (2): 37–50. https://doi.org/10.1300/J083v46n02_04.

Macintosh, Constance. 2006. "Jurisdictional Roulette: Constitutional and Structural Barriers to Aboriginal Access to Health." In *Just Medicare: What's In, What's Out, How We Decide*, ed. Colleen Flood, 193–215. Toronto: University of Toronto Press. https://doi.org/10.3138/9781442676459-010.

McLeod, Neal. 2007. *Cree Narrative Memory: From Treaties to Contemporary Times*. Saskatoon, SK: Purich Publishing.

Minore, Bruce, and Mae Katt. 2007. "Aboriginal Health Care in Northern Ontario: Impact of Self-Determination and Culture." *IRPP Choices* 13 (6): 1–22.

Onwuegbuzie, Anthony J., et al. 2009. "A Qualitative Framework for Collecting and Analyzing Data in Focus Group Research." *International Journal of Qualitative Methods* 8 (3): 1–21. https://doi.org/10.1177/160940690900800301.

Owen, Gareth, and Jose Catalan. 2012. "'We never expected this to happen': Narratives of Ageing with HIV among Gay Men Living in London, UK." *Culture, Health & Sexuality* 14 (1): 59–72. https://doi.org/10.1080/13691058.2011.621449.

Poff, Deborah C. 2006. "The Importance of Story-Telling: Research Protocols in Aboriginal Communities." *Journal of Empirical Research on Human Research Ethics: JERHRE* 1 (3): 27–8. https://doi.org/10.1525/jer.2006.1.3.27.

Poindexter, Cynthia Cannon. 2004. "Six Champions Speak about Being over 50 and Living with HIV." *Journal of HIV/AIDS & Social Services* 3 (1): 99–117. https://doi.org/10.1300/J187v03n01_08.

Psaros, Christina, et al. 2015. "Reflections on Living with HIV over Time: Exploring the Perspective of HIV-Infected Women over 50." *Aging & Mental Health* 19 (2): 121–8. https://doi.org/10.1080/13607863.2014.917608.

Public Health Agency of Canada (PHAC). 2004. *Federal Initiative to Address HIV/AIDS in Canada: Strengthening Federal Action in the Canadian Response to HIV/AIDS*. Ottawa: PHAC.

– 2010. *Population-Specific HIV/AIDS Status Report: Aboriginal Peoples*. Ottawa: PHAC.

– 2014. *HIV/AIDS Epi Updates: HIV/AIDS among Aboriginal People in Canada*. Ottawa: PHAC.

Roger, Kerstin Stieber, Javier Mignone, and Susan Kirkland. 2013. "Social Aspects of HIV/AIDS and Aging: A Thematic Review." *Canadian Journal on Aging / La Revue canadienne du vieillissement* 32 (3): 298–306. https://doi.org/10.1017/S0714980813000330.

Rothe, J.P., D. Ozegovic, and L.J. Carroll. 2009. "Innovation in Qualitative Interviews: 'Sharing Circles' in a First Nations Community." *Injury Prevention* 15 (5): 334–40. https://doi.org/10.1136/ip.2008.021261.

Sankar, Andrea, et al. 2011. "What Do We Know about Older Adults and HIV? A Review of Social and Behavioral Literature." *AIDS Care* 23 (10): 1187–207. https://doi.org/10.1080/09540121.2011.564115.

Siegel, Karolynn, Victoria Raveis, and Daniel Karus. 1998. "Perceived Advantages and Disadvantages of Age among Older HIV-Infected adults." *Research on Aging* 20 (6): 686–711. https://doi.org/10.1177/0164027598206004.

Siegel, Karolynn, and Eric W. Schrimshaw. 2002. "The Perceived Benefits of Religious and Spiritual Coping among Older Adults Living with HIV/AIDS." *Journal for the Scientific Study of Religion* 41 (1): 91–102. https://doi.org/10.1111/1468-5906.00103.

Strauss, Anselm, and Juliet Corbin. 1990. *Basics of Qualitative Research: Grounded Theory Procedures and Techniques*. Newbury Park, CA: Sage Publications.

Vance, David E., and F. Patrick Robinson. 2004. "Reconciling Successful Aging with HIV: A Biopsychosocial Overview." *Journal of HIV/AIDS & Social Services* 3 (1): 59–78. https://doi.org/10.1300/J187v03n01_06.

Vance, David E., Thomas C. Struzick, and James Masten. 2008. "Hardiness, Successful Aging, and HIV: Implications for Social Work." *Journal of Gerontological Social Work* 51 (3–4): 260–83. https://doi.org/10.1080/01634370802039544.

# 13 On the Experience of Pregnancy: Stories of HIV-Positive Refugee Women in Canada

TERESA CHULACH, MARILOU GAGNON,
AND DAVE HOLMES

Women from endemic countries, mainly African and Caribbean countries, account for more than half of the women living with HIV in Canada (Public Health Agency of Canada 2011). While research suggests they are more likely to want to have children and more likely to conceive, we know little about their experience of pregnancy (Loutfy et al. 2009). Canadian studies have focused primarily on prenatal screening for HIV, vertical transmission, fertility, intent to have children, mothering issues such as breastfeeding, and the type of antiretroviral therapy used to suppress the virus at birth (ibid.; Forbes et al. 2012; Kaida et al. 2009; Money et al. 2009; Wang et al. 2005). As a result, the experience of pregnancy remains largely overlooked in the Canadian literature, especially that of refugee women from endemic countries. HIV-positive refugee women find themselves in a unique situation when they are pregnant. They undergo a complex identity transformation that shapes and redefines how they view themselves as women, mothers, refugees, and persons living with HIV. They also face numerous challenges including social isolation, displacement, stigma, shame, and the loss of connections with customs, values, and belief systems. Most importantly, they have to navigate a foreign health-care system and a confusing web of policies that affect their ability to access housing, employment, social support, child care, health care, medications, and so forth (Chulach, Gagnon, and Holmes 2016). Access to health care for pregnancy may be further complicated by direct access issues (locations, hours, language barriers, consistency of providers), lack of resources (economic, informational, and practical), and failure to provide gender-specific, needs-specific, and culturally safe care (Almeida et al. 2014; Bokore 2013; Carter et al. 2013).

This chapter draws on qualitative data derived from a study of the experience of pregnancy among HIV-positive refugee women. As part of the Ottawa-based study, we interviewed Tulun, Mageti, and Chidimma (all pseudonyms). Their stories are unique, but they share common themes that can help us understand what pregnancy means for HIV-positive refugee women and the challenges this experience poses at the micro, meso, and macro levels. We begin by introducing their stories. We then propose an intersectional analysis of these stories based on the framework outlined by Guruge and Khanlou (2004). This type of analysis draws attention to the intersections of dimensions of identity and how they influence the ways in which HIV-positive refugee women define themselves and are defined by others. An intersectional analysis is particularly pertinent to understanding their experiences of pregnancy, as it provides a more inclusive view of women's experiences, encompassing not only the influences of gender, but also the dynamic, temporal, and geographic constructions of race, class, citizenship status, HIV status, and socio-economic status. Rather than viewing categories as static, unitary, or institutional, such analysis integrates the individual with the institutional, recognizing the social processes and organizational structures of society that influence formations of identity (Chulach and Gagnon 2013). At its most complex level, it moves the focus of the analysis beyond the person to shed light on social relationships and to see the broader context in which HIV-positive refugee women are located. Drawing on the work of Guruge and Khanlou, our analysis raises important questions about the ways in which dimensions of identity intersect during pregnancy, the strategies used by women to break the isolation and "manage" social relations during pregnancy, and the issues that women face as they navigate the healthcare and policy landscape in Canada. We conclude the chapter with key policy recommendations with particular emphasis on mandatory HIV-testing policy and the Interim Federal Health Program.

## Tulun's Story[1]

Tulun came to Canada from West Africa with her young adult son. Prior to landing in Canada, she spent several years in a refugee camp in a country that bordered her country of origin. Her first husband left her after he learned that he was HIV-positive. The only contact she had in Canada was a sister. Eight days after her arrival in Canada, she learned about her HIV-positive status. Subsequent to this news of her serological status, she experienced inappropriate disclosure of her status by a person within her ethnocultural community. This exposure led to her rapid relocation. Her son did not travel to her new location with her, nor did her sister. She maintained social contact (by phone) with her son and sister in the original point of entry, as well as with a brother in another country, and with family in her country of origin. She did not want to make friends in this new location, since she had experienced being "outed" in the previous setting in Canada. After learning about her serological status, she was unable to sleep, which had a negative impact on her mental health. This has affected her ability to work. As a result, she became dependent on social assistance as her source of income. This contrasted significantly with her economic and employment situation within her country of origin, where she had gainful employment. During her pregnancy, she experienced stigma and discrimination within the hospital setting, and had many concerns regarding her ability to attend medical appointments without transportation assistance.

## Mageti's Story

Mageti is a Muslim woman from East Africa who migrated to Canada with her infant son. Her first husband died in her country of origin after becoming sick. There were rumours about the reasons for his death, and she left because of this situation. En route to Canada, she passed through another country, where her residency was prohibited as a result of entry bans on persons with a positive HIV serological status. She had one relative in that country. When she arrived in Canada, she was afraid to meet new people because of her serological status. Finally, she became connected to a support group for HIV-positive women from African and Caribbean countries. Through this support group, she met her partner, who is HIV-positive. She also learned that it is possible to have a baby who is HIV-negative. She has one family member in Canada, but that person does not know her diagnosis, nor do her parents in her country of origin. This means that her husband is the sole family member who is aware of her HIV serological status. During her pregnancy, she was criticized for the choice of the hospital where she delivered the baby, as well as for her choice to bottle-feed rather than breastfeed her infant. She did not want people to visit her in the hospital. She made up stories to keep things private. She took the bus, bringing her school-age son with her, to attend medical appointments at the hospital. At the time of the interview, she was awaiting a decision on her refugee status.

## Chidimma's Story

Chidimma migrated from Central Africa to Canada with her husband and children. She spent time in a refugee camp in a neighbouring country. This is a second marriage for both her and her partner. She came from a big family in Africa, where she was surrounded by brothers and sisters. The loss and lack of family support she experienced in Canada was an extreme source of stress for her. Since moving to Canada, they have moved from an apartment into a town home. She talked about the shame she felt surrounding her HIV status, and about her fear of disclosure. As a newcomer, she found it difficult to navigate the transportation system within the city. She also was disturbed by quarantine measures (associated with a possible tuberculosis diagnosis) that were imposed on her husband when they first arrived in Canada. During her pregnancy, she identified her husband as the sole source of her support. She talked about the difficulty of having children and of being alone, with no friends around. She also revealed the postpartum isolation she endured, sometimes to the point that she did not eat during the day. When she bottle-fed her baby while at church, she experienced stigma from other members of her congregation. She also feared "exposure" and judgment while attending the HIV clinic at the hospital. She talked about the difference in culture between Canada and her country of origin. At the time of the interview, Chidimma had obtained landed immigrant status. She was attending school.

## What Can We Learn from the Stories of Tulun, Mageti, and Chidimma?

Three major themes surfaced from the stories of Tulun, Mageti, and Chidimma. The first focused on identity transformation and restoration. Pregnancy was described as a point of intersection where multiple dimensions of identity come together. It was also described as an opportunity to restore a sense of identity. The second theme was untangling isolation and "managing" relationships in order to maintain a certain level of social support. The third theme was traversing systemic barriers that affect the experience of pregnancy and how women move through Canadian society – including its health-care system. Each of these themes will be discussed further in the following sections using quotes from Tulun, Mageti, and Chidimma.

### Restoring Identity: A Micro-level Analysis

Tulun, Mageti, and Chidimma were born in the western, central, and eastern regions of Africa (specific countries of origin are not named in order to protect confidentiality). They ranged in age from thirty to forty-four years and all had an education level equivalent to a high school diploma. At the time of this interview, their immigration status was variable, although all of them left their countries of origin as refugees. The variability in their age, countries of origin, and immigration status resulted in similarities as well as differences among this group of women. Similarities were identified when participants talked about the rupture in identity they experienced as a result of both their refugee status and their HIV status. Once arrived in Canada, they set about restoring their identity. Pregnancy was integral to this restoration. The intersection of their identities as mothers, refugee women, and HIV-positive women was particularly salient in each of their stories. For analytical clarity, we discuss each identity separately. However, it is important to recognize that these identities interact in complex ways.

All three women connected strongly with motherhood, and saw it as a fundamental part of their identity. Being a mother was considered to be the "normal thing" to do. This was evidenced by the following quote:

> Back home, you get married. It is normal to have children ... it [having children] made it special. (Mageti)

Similarly, Tulun illustrated the value she placed on mothering and having children:

> [Back in Africa] I want to have another child ... I just have one ... I *love* children ... I want to have four ... Here [in Canada] I have two pregnancies ... two babies ... It's positive. (Tulun)

The identity as mother and the experience of being a mother brought meaning to their lives, and also became a bridge to integration within Canadian society. Pregnancy allowed them to re-establish their identity as good mothers and as women. Becoming a mother in the host country enhanced their self-esteem and identity as women, but it also provided them with a reason to be and a means of social survival.

Tulun, Mageti, and Chidimma also experienced a shift in their identity as mothers. This was evident in how they described the experience of pregnancy in their home countries, where their communities conferred an elevated status on them, as opposed to their experience in Canada, where no such status was bestowed.

> In my country ... You have a baby ... You are a princess ... The people are going to give you, the family, everybody ... food ... to eat ... Money ... At night everybody came with the food to help you to take the baby. (Tulun)

They experienced a loss of such status and recognition due to the absence of extended family members and different postpartum practices. This observation was made by Chidimma who described her postpartum time at home:

> To find myself in my bed where there is no one ... It's like, "Oh my God ... I am going to die ... What kind of life is this?"

Thus, the evolving micro and meso intersection of culture, social support, and sociocultural norms influenced their identities as mothers, and was particularly important because of the context in which they experienced pregnancy.

The importance of breastfeeding to their identities as mothers was a particularly salient finding in this study. For participants, not being able to breastfeed made them question their identity as mothers, and in turn this led to psychological distress:

> It's like something is broken between you and the kids ... I'm crying many, many times for this. (Tulun)

Similarly, Chidimma talked about how the experience of not breastfeeding altered her perception of herself as a mother, since it was so contrary to what was expected within her culture. She found the experience overwhelming in that it produced a feeling of separation between her and her child.

> Back in Africa ... there is no way you could have a child without breastfeeding ... Once you are not breastfeeding, you don't know that child ... you are like strangers.

As refugees, all three women were displaced several times while en route to Canada. There were considerable differences in their pathways to Canada, which influenced their subsequent sense of belonging and integration. On average, they spent between three to five years within the confines of a refugee camp. Once they arrived in Canada, their immigration statuses became more amplified, since other aspects of their identity such as race, religion, and language dialect potentially situated them as racially, culturally, and ethnically "different."

An intersectional analysis draws attention not only to the transitional circumstances of pregnancy and its impact on identity but also recognizes the effect of pre- and post-migration experiences. Pre- and post-migration experiences are important as they often occur as a result of systems of oppression, providing insight to relational processes, contexts of power, and the "new" identity that forms as a result of those intersections (Chulach and Gagnon 2013). Pre-migration experiences may include trauma or torture, while post-migration influences involve changes in employment and socio-economic status. For example, during Tulun's pre-migration phase, her identity changed from that of a married woman to that of a single mother, after her husband abandoned her while living in the refugee camp. Similarly, Mageti's husband became sick and died prior to her journey to Canada. At a relatively young age, her identity changed from married woman to widow. Both women subsequently migrated to North America on their own as single mothers with children.

Many refugee women experience both belonging and othering as they attempt to reconstruct their identities in Canada. The dynamic interplay between belonging and othering is illustrated in Mageti's case. As a refugee claimant, Mageti was still waiting to receive confirmation of her immigration status. The fact that she had not received valid status placed her in limbo and socially located her as "the Other" within her host country. However, she was able to reconstruct her identity as a woman in Canada when she remarried, became pregnant, and delivered her baby in the new context. In this way, she affirmed her sense of identity for herself and for her newborn, who, she stated, "will be a citizen of the country" and who belongs to the people of Canada.

Tulun experienced a significant shift in her identity as a result of her migration. As a refugee woman in Canada, she faced a significant change in social status, from that of a woman who had gainful employment and access to resources in her country of origin, to a person requiring social assistance and additional supportive services. She had attempted and wanted to work in Canada, but her health prevented her from sustaining meaningful employment. Such changes in employment and social status influenced how she viewed herself and what resources were available for her to look after herself and her family. Tulun maintained connections with her family in Africa, along with other relatives in North America, ensuring a sense of identity and continuity with her previous self.

Finally, Chidimma's alterations in identity formation took a different pathway. By the time of the interview, Chidimma had obtained her landed immigrant status. This enabled her to attend school, and she was formulating a new identity that might not have been available to her in her former home. Attending school introduced her to a new social status, role, and social network. School became a place of meaningful associations with the Canadian culture and an opportunity for Chidimma to construct a new social identity within this culture (Smith 2013). Married, with four children, she was continuing to affirm her identity as mother, while at the same time developing an additional aspect of her identity that would enable her to establish herself in the workplace in Canada.

For each woman, becoming HIV-positive could not be separated from the social world in which they lived. This social world included both the pre-migration contexts of their homeland, their cultural communities in the host context, and the larger socio-political context of Canada. This identity was profoundly shaped by experiences of HIV-related stigma before migration and after migration. For example, Mageti talked about the gossip that circulated in her country-of-origin community when her husband displayed signs of HIV infection. Such speculation about the illness discredited and devalued her as a woman and as a mother. The powerful stigma in her home country resulted in her becoming the object of gossip and community judgment (Rohleder and Gibson 2006).

> Back home, I was pregnant with my son. We both found out we were positive [my husband and me]. We were sick, he was sicker. He passed away. There are rumours back home [about the HIV diagnosis of her husband and how he contracted his illness].

Tulun talked about the perception of being "dirty" and about the experience of abandonment by her former husband when he learned of his own HIV diagnosis and blamed his diagnosis on her. She also carried expectations from her country of origin about the terminal nature of her illness. This influenced her expectations of her own health. In her own words, "In Africa ... it will kill you."[2]

Chidimma internalized some of the stigmatizing messages surrounding HIV from her home country; when she was first diagnosed, she blamed herself and saw HIV as a kind of punishment. She previously had distanced herself from ever being identified as an HIV-positive woman, and she described the difficulty she had incorporating this identity into her own self-image:

> It did not cross my mind that one day I'll be in that situation ... I thought maybe somebody else. I lived my normal life ... as a teenager. That's because in Africa ... once you have it ... people think you are sleeping around and having that kind of life. It was not my case ... so I thought ... Why? ... I didn't deserve this ... It made it very tough on me. I lived a really pure, I can say respectable life, and to be in that position was really tough. It was like unfair ... In Africa, you have it ... you deserve it. (Chidimma)

Participants incorporated their identity as HIV-positive women in various ways, depending both on other aspects of their identity and on their particular social contexts. The decision of how to manage information about HIV status, including when and to whom to disclose, was central to how they managed their identity after their HIV diagnosis. Often the process began with non-disclosure and secrecy related to fear of stigma and discrimination. This was the case for Mageti and Chidimma, who, upon learning about their diagnosis, kept the knowledge hidden from others and discussed it only with medical personnel. Non-disclosure allowed them to carry on with re-establishing and reformulating new identities in their post-migration contexts.

For all participants, HIV was a determining factor in how they viewed themselves along a continuum that ranged from being sick to being healthy. Being pregnant and HIV-positive made them feel "more sick." For example, Tulun experienced persistent nausea and vomiting from the combination of pregnancy and HIV medications. Tulun talked about how sick she felt, and how her feeling unwell made it difficult for her to walk:

> With pregnancy, I can't walk ... I just walk like this [gets down on the floor, and walks on her hands and knees]. It's so difficult. I'm very sick. When I am pregnant with HIV, I see a big difference ... weak ... more sick.

As such, it is important to consider the influences that intersect, for they may produce an entirely new identity for HIV-positive refugee women during pregnancy.

## Untangling Isolation: A Meso-level Analysis

Research has shown that, upon arriving in a host country, refugee women are often relocated to places where they have no support network and where they eventually feel isolated and outcast (Kitzinger 2004). Many refugee women are set adrift from their families, and they report a loss of social networks that protect women who experience life transitions (e.g., migration, pregnancy, illness) (Donnelly et al. 2011). This was true for Tulun, Mageti, and Chidimma. They all talked about the pervasive isolation they experienced as a result of their newness to Canada, which left them particularly vulnerable to mental health issues and put them at a disadvantage, especially during their pregnancy.

Chidimma described the stress she experienced upon first arriving in Canada:

> I remember ... when we came ... I was really in deep, deep stress. I remember I used to walk and cry by myself. I felt like ... We are lost ... What kind of life is this ... I could feel my heart pounding ... Like it would explode ... The stress started as soon as I put my feet on this land.

Chidimma migrated to Canada with her husband and family. For women who migrate alone or with their children, the isolation may be intensified further. Relocation stressors (including social isolation) and pre-migration experiences of possible trauma, torture, deprivation, and abuse (psychological and physical) often make the situation untenable, and affect refugee women to a point where many of them will develop symptoms of depression, post-traumatic stress disorder (PTSD), psychosis, and suicidal ideation (Carolan 2010; Reynolds and White 2010). Tulun talked about how isolation and relocation affected her mental health:

> You don't know nobody ... We didn't see one person who spoke my language ... Nobody ... We didn't know anybody ... School, I can't ... I can't do nothing ... I can't go out ... and depression ... I can't eat ... I can't sleep ... I can't wash ... I can't do nothing ... Just [stay] in the house ... Alone ... Depression is high.

For pregnant refugee women who have been diagnosed with HIV – most often upon their arrival in the host country – the situation of social isolation or exclusion may be amplified further. Women living with HIV are often isolated during pregnancy (Ingram and Hutchinson

2000; Sanders 2008). Their relationships with relatives and friends may be affected, and they may find themselves excluded from social networks that usually develop throughout the course of pregnancy (e.g., prenatal groups, support groups, social groups) (Ross et al. 2007). We found examples in all three stories when women talked about being "cut off" from cultural groups because they could not breastfeed.

HIV-related stigma in the context of pregnancy can lead to rejection by family members, eviction from the home, and special precautions (e.g., washing of kitchen utensils) within the family environment, or to other measures that attest to their families' irrational fear of transmission, which may limit and decrease contact with children and distancing of the spouse (Anderson and Doyal 2004). All three women talked about how they kept the knowledge of their serological status to themselves, shielding it from family members in their country of origin, as well as from family members in Canada. They did not disclose their status to their children. Their spouse was often one of the very few people who knew about their serological status. This imposed (yet strategic) silence resulted in emotional isolation and secrecy. Some relief from this secrecy was offered when they were able to join support groups, usually offered by AIDS service organizations (ASOs).

The immediate and extended family may have a positive or negative influence on pregnant HIV-positive women, serving as both a source of strength and of stress (Anderson and Doyal 2004). In this study, Tulun received negative messages from family members when she disclosed the news of her pregnancy. Mageti and Chidimma chose to keep the news within a tightly knit circle of contacts to maintain their privacy and to protect themselves from the judgments that could result from being pregnant and HIV-positive. HIV-positive refugee women are most often separated from family, and they report intensified social isolation during pregnancy (ibid.), hence, the importance of engaging in a meso-level analysis of social networks. This was the experience of all participants in this study.

As we examined the stories of Tulun, Mageti, and Chidimma through migration, pregnancy, and motherhood pathways, we found intersecting influences that contributed to their social isolation. Their stories illustrate how these forces affected their formal and informal networks, which in turn had implications for their health and well-being during pregnancy.

When we examine Tulun's story, we see a clearer picture of all the factors that contribute to her isolation as a refugee woman in Canada.

Before migration she lived in a refugee camp. Although Tulun never referred specifically to that experience, many refugee women experience pre-migration trauma that can subsequently affect their mental health, which in turn affects their ability to maintain and sustain social connections. The news of her serological status, and then her subsequent exposure, led to her rapid relocation away from the social support that she had in Canada. In her second location, Tulun had limited formal and informal social networks. She experienced depression and insomnia. Both made it difficult for her to maintain employment, further isolating her. Her small income, maintained by social assistance, limited her choices and opportunities for social engagement. Perhaps stigma and discrimination encountered within the health care system made her mistrustful of people, and led to additional isolation within the new context. Limited access to medical appointments made it difficult for her to maintain her health, and in turn that affected her ability to engage with others.

Throughout Mageti's story, we can see that pre-migration and post-migration experiences affected her social networks. Prior to coming to Canada, she lost her first husband. His death, associated with possible HIV and its stigma, caused her to leave family and friends and to start at new life where she perceived that she could have more opportunities. While en route to Canada, she experienced exclusion related to her HIV status. This led to further displacement. In Canada, her social network is composed of her brother (who does not know her HIV status) and a support group through an ASO. The fact that only a few people are aware of her diagnosis contributes to her emotional isolation. In turn, her isolation means there are limited resources to assist her to maintain her health. As a result, she travels by bus, along with her school-age son, to attend medical appointments. As her immigration status is still being decided, there is potential for more displacement, which in turn may also affect her social networks. At the time of the interview, Mageti was also considering leaving her current place of residence.

Chidimma's story reveals some of the circumstances that contributed to her social isolation. She had no extended family in Canada who were able to assist in her transition to a new geographical location. Stigma and shame associated with her HIV status kept her from sharing this information with anyone, limiting the number of people with whom she could discuss her concerns about her status. This lack of social support intensified during pregnancy and the postpartum period. When she returned home from the hospital, her lack of social support made it difficult for her to attend to her nutrition and to manage the pain she experienced. Thus, pre-migration experiences that associated pregnancy with a supportive family were at odds with her post-migration experience. Decreased community networks in her new context, HIV stigma, displacement, and lack of formal networks in the postpartum period shaped her experience of pregnancy, leaving her little relational and social support.

### Traversing a Web of Systemic Barriers: A Macro-level Analysis

Despite the fact that refugee women have complex health needs, they typically experience barriers in accessing health care (Gabriel et al. 2011). They also report considerable difficulties in accessing affordable housing, sustaining sufficient income to meet their most basic needs, and finding employment or training services (Danso 2001). For Tulun, Mageti, and Chidimma, access to health care and services during pregnancy was complicated by barriers such as locations, hours, language, insufficient economic resources to get to appointments, lack of adapted information and services, lack of cultural competencies, stigma in health-care settings, and breaches of confidentiality, to name just a few.

Tulun, Mageti, and Chidimma discussed how they were provided with recommendations for their health, but at times were unable to carry out those recommendations with their limited income. An example was nurses' suggestions to enhance nutritional status with certain foods when these foods were unaffordable. All three women talked about the difficulty of attending their appointments without transportation assistance. In addition, one woman talked about how having another health condition related to pregnancy made it necessary to attend additional appointments at the hospital. For two of the women, the lack of proximity to health appointments and of transportation assistance made them consider relocating in order to more easily attend health appointments. The importance of this assistance was emphasized by one participant when she declared that, if any assistance were to be offered to women living with HIV, transportation assistance to attend appointments would be the most helpful.

Tulun, Mageti, and Chidimma mentioned the effects of Canada's mandatory HIV-testing policy, which was implemented in 2002. This policy has caused many refugee women to discover their HIV status immediately before, or shortly after, their arrival in Canada (Bisaillon 2011). They talked about their experience during the immigration medical exam, when they were forced to undergo an HIV test. For some, test results were delivered within the first ten days of their arrival into Canada. Besides the experience of overwhelming shock, it immediately led them to question the timing of the transmission, and whether HIV had been transmitted to any of their children. Chidimma provides an example when talking about receiving knowledge of her status at the immigration medical exam:

> Oh wow, it was a shock ... by then I had my second child, who was only one year old ... my first thoughts went to him ... like, Oh my God ... What is this? ... For me, I thought it was like a kind of punishment ... Right away, I just pray and say ... "God, if this is like a kind of punishment, please let it be just on me and not my innocent son." ... It was very, very tough.

For other women who might have known earlier about their status, the HIV test administered in the immigration medical exam created fear and worry about their potential ability to remain within Canada. For example, Mageti did not disclose her HIV serological status freely during this exam out of fear of deportation, because she had passed through the United States en route to Canada at a time when the United States still banned persons living with HIV from entering the country (Ofori-Asneso 2013).[3] She already knew her serological status but was worried that she might face the same situation in Canada. Though Canada allowed refugees to remain in the country, she feared that her HIV serological status would subject her to specific forms of investigation and might influence the decision that determined whether she could remain in the country.

For Tulun, the revelation of her diagnosis at the immigration medical exam led to inappropriate disclosure of her status, and to her subsequent rapid relocation. Tulun talked about her experience of learning she was HIV-positive, her lack of knowledge surrounding the diagnosis, and her subsequent exposure:

> This is really, really difficult, because the doctor told me that I have HIV eight days after I came to Canada ... Just one week. And when I got [the news] ... I don't know anything about it ... A person came [a volunteer translator] to do the bloodwork ... He took me to the hospital ... To explain to the doctor ... That is so bad for me and my son ... This volunteer is African ... This volunteer had a sister in the same English school as me ... Just two weeks [after I came to Canada] *everybody* in the school who was an immigrant knew that I had HIV.

Although all three women were subsequently connected to some form of HIV care, they experienced adverse effects as a result of the mandatory HIV testing conducted during the immigration medical exam. This policy resulted in uninformed and suboptimal testing, increased their anxiety surrounding deportation, and contributed to further stigma and isolation caused by rapid relocation to another city in Canada.

Another federal policy that affected the health of all three women was the Interim Federal Health Program. This complex policy is difficult to navigate, and it often acts as a barrier to health care and services (Miedema, Hamilton, and Easle 2008). Although the policy was not specifically mentioned within the current study, both Mageti and Tulun referred to a time when the health coverage changed:

> Health coverage … Changed some things now as of June. People are not accepting the coverage … When things are going good, [you], don't need help. [You] only find out what is needed when things are not going good. (Mageti)

Tulun also echoed concerns about a time when everything suddenly stopped. This meant that she needed to seek out alternate resources and means of support in order to access health services.

It is relevant that the period referred to in these statements coincided with changes to the Interim Federal Health Program that were implemented on 30 June 2012. These changes resulted in the elimination of valuable health-care coverage for many refugees and refugee claimants, and decreased access to health-care services for most (Barnes and Wellesley Institute 2013). The funding cuts amplified confusion and administrative complexity, preventing refugee claimants from accessing health care, even if they had a disease that was a concern for public health (Barnes and Wellesley Institute 2013). For certain refugee populations, it meant that there was little funding for conditions such as pregnancy, diabetes, and mental health.

Attention to systemic barriers across the health-care system is another aspect of macro-level analysis. These barriers range from ethnocentric and biomedical practices to bureaucratic and administrative processes (Hancock 2007), as is evident in Tulun's story. She experienced barriers to care when she attempted to access the health-care system through the emergency department. She was first told that there was no place for her, and her experience resulted in a crisis. She also experienced barriers to care when it became necessary for her to take medication to relieve the nausea and vomiting during her pregnancy. In this case, she finally accessed the medication she needed. However, in the interim, she suffered and experienced a worsening of her HIV illness.

## Policy Recommendations

What is evident from the stories of these women is the psychological distress they experienced upon revelation of their HIV status during the immigration medical exam. Mandatory HIV screening of asylum seekers for HIV infection is against WHO's guiding principles of expanded HIV testing and counselling (World Health Organization 2003). Testing that is done only when clinically indicated would enable HIV-positive refugee women to learn of their diagnosis in a more appropriate setting, at a time that is suitable to them, when they may not be experiencing the additional challenges of immigration and entry. The following recommendations are therefore proposed:

- Re-evaluate the immigration HIV testing policy
- Ensure that HIV testing is conducted on a voluntary basis after obtaining fully informed consent
- Ensure that HIV testing includes pre- and post-test counselling done by trained and qualified staff with experience in the field of HIV
- Provide information, counselling, immediate linkage to care for all refugees who test positive
- Protect confidentiality and provide the necessary information to ensure that refugees understand their rights
- Provide translation for all services

The stories of Tulun, Mageti, and Chidimma are a testament to the challenges that they faced in securing their health during pregnancy. While reinstating the cuts that were made to the Interim Federal Health program is the first step to facilitate access to comprehensive benefits to women in such situations, additional measures are recommended.

To improve access to primary care for refugee clients:

- Provide transportation assistance that enables attendance at health and social services appointments
- Implement multidisciplinary clinics that provide a range of health services to clients including physiotherapy, nurse practitioners,

nurses, pharmacists, dietitians, and physicians and operate with a "care-based" philosophy rather than one that is totally bio-medically based
- Provide occupational assessment that assists people to integrate towards a level of occupational functioning comparable to that experienced in their country of origin

During pregnancy:

- Extend postnatal services in the home to promote continuity in care, particularly for those who may be recovering from the effects of Caesarean section and who often lack social support
- Provide ASOs and/or health centres funding for support groups specifically for HIV-positive pregnant women

**Final Remarks**

The experiences of HIV-positive refugee women during pregnancy are complex and intricately attached to their social identities, social relations, and context. They undergo significant alterations in their identities that may be attributed to the stigmas imposed as a result of refugee status, HIV status, and pregnancy, as well as to the processes undergone during migration and resettlement, such as racialization, gender-role adjustments, and lack of acknowledgment of educational credentials. Social support, an integral determinant of health, is altered, as refugees are so often separated from family and community, leaving them vulnerable to experiences that can adversely affect their spiritual, emotional, and mental health. Access to health services is often complicated and confusing. Pregnant, HIV-positive refugee women commonly experience not only language, discriminatory, financial, and transportation barriers when they attend health-care appointments, they may also be subject to perceptual barriers regarding their HIV care and to lack of caregiver knowledge about particular cultural practices, which directly affects their obstetrical experiences.

For Tulun, Mageti, and Chidimma, the revelation of their serological status during the mandatory immigration medical exam intersected with the micro and meso levels of their experience. It confirmed an identity that determined pathways through immigration and affected social interactions within their ethnic communities and Canadian society at large. An identity as an HIV-positive woman had connotations that they carried with them from their countries of origin, which in turn affected their self-concept and movement within the new geography of Canada. At times, their HIV status made them mistrustful of health-care providers or afraid to meet new people, while at other times, the illness left them feeling sick and weak. These overlapping influences produced persistent isolation, which often was interrupted only when women were able to connect with other HIV-positive women in similar situations. These connections often became a source of information sharing and mutual support. The HIV serological status connected them to a health-care system that identified them as "HIV-positive," assigning them to lifelong surveillance. The other macro-level force was the Interim Federal Health Program, which determines the type of health coverage to which refugee women with HIV have access during their pregnancy.

The stories presented in this chapter provide insight into the experience of HIV-positive refugee women during pregnancy. Such knowledge provides a more nuanced picture that enables us to improve the care and services delivered to this population. It compels us to be cognizant of the transitional and contextual nature of identity and the challenges faced by HIV-positive refugee women. It also brings to light the isolation that is part of this experience and how isolation affects the health and well-being of women and their children. Assistance in the form of programs and services to mitigate this isolation is paramount if the well-being of HIV-positive refugee women is to be fostered and supported – especially during pregnancy. Lastly, the findings revealed the effects of government policies, such as mandatory HIV testing policy and the Interim Federal Health Program. These policies have far-reaching effects for HIV-positive refugee women and should be reformed to ensure the full protection of women's rights to informed and consensual HIV testing and optimal access to proper health-care and services – especially during pregnancy.

NOTES

1 Here and throughout the chapter, some details in these stories have been altered to protect participants' privacy.
2 Women's lower socio-economic status, unequal access to education and employment, gender-based violence, stigma, and greater physiological

susceptibility contributes to women's vulnerability to HIV; this can be especially acute in a developing country. Access to treatment is also often more limited.

3 That ban was subsequently lifted in January 2010, after it was recognized that HIV infection does not pose a risk to public health, because it is preventable and is not spread through casual contact (CDC 2009).

## REFERENCES

Almeida, Ligia Moreira, et al. 2014. "Migrant Women's Perceptions of Healthcare during Pregnancy and Early Motherhood: Addressing the Social Determinants of Health." *Journal of Immigrant and Minority Health* 16 (4): 719–23. https://doi.org/10.1007/s10903-013-9834-4.

Anderson, Jane, and Lesley Doyal. 2004. "Women from Africa Living with HIV in London: A Descriptive Study." *AIDS Care* 16 (1): 95–105. https://doi.org/10.1080/09540120310001634001.

Barnes, Steve, and the Wellesley Institute. 2013. "The Real Cost of Cutting the Interim Federal Health Program." Wellesley Institute: A Health Equality Impact Assessment. http://www.wellesleyinstitute.com/wp-content/uploads/2013/10/Actual-Health-Impacts-of-IFHP.pdf.

Bisaillon, Laura. 2011. "Mandatory HIV Screening Policy and Everyday Life: A Look inside the Canadian Immigration Medical Examination." *Aporia: The Nursing Journal* 3 (4): 5–14.

Bokore, Nimo. 2013. "Suffering in Silence: A Canadian-Somali Case Study." *Journal of Social Work Practice* 27 (1): 95–113. https://doi.org/10.1080/02650533.2012.682979.

Carolan, Mary. 2010. "Pregnancy Health Status of Sub-Saharan Refugee Women Who Have Resettled in Developed Countries: A Review of the Literature." *Midwifery* 26 (4): 407–14. https://doi.org/10.1016/j.midw.2008.11.002.

Carter, Allison J., et al., and the CHIWOS Research Team. 2013. "Women-Specific HIV/AIDS services: Identifying and Defining Components of Holistic Service Delivery for Women Living with HIV/AIDS." *Journal of the International AIDS Society* 16 (1). https://doi.org/10.7448/IAS.16.1.17433.

Centers for Disease Control and Prevention (CDC). 2009. *Removal of HIV Entry Ban from Immigration Medical Screening*. Atlanta: CDC.

Chulach, Teresa, and Marilou Gagnon. 2013. "Rethinking the Experience of HIV-Positive Refugee Women in the Context of Pregnancy: Using an Intersectional Approach in Nursing." *Research and Theory for Nursing Practice* 27 (4): 240–56. https://doi.org/10.1891/1541-6577.27.4.240.

Chulach, Teresa, Marilou Gagnon, and Dave Holmes. 2016. "The Lived Experience of Pregnancy among HIV-Positive Refugee Women: A Qualitative Study." *Advances in Nursing Science* 39 (2): 130–49.

Danso, Ransford. 2001. "From 'There' to 'Here': An Investigation of the Initial Settlement Experiences of Ethiopian and Somali Refugees in Toronto." *GeoJournal* 55 (1): 3–14.

Donnelly, Tam Truong, et al. 2011. "If I was going to kill myself, I wouldn't be calling you. I am asking for help: Challenges Influencing Immigrant and Refugee Women's Mental Health." *Issues in Mental Health Nursing* 32 (5): 279–90. https://doi.org/10.3109/01612840.2010.550383.

Forbes, John C., et al., and the Canadian Pediatric AIDS Research Group. 2012. "A National Review of Vertical HIV Transmission." *AIDS (London, England)* 26 (6): 757–63. https://doi.org/10.1097/QAD.0b013e328350995c.

Gabriel, Patricia S., et al. 2011. "Refugees and Health Care – The Need for Data: Understanding the Health of Government-Assisted Refugees in Canada through a Prospective Longitudinal Cohort." *Canadian Journal of Public Health* 102 (4): 269–72.

Guruge, Sepali, and Nazilla Khanlou. 2004. "Intersectionalities of Influence: Researching the Health of Immigrant and Refugee Women." *Canadian Journal of Nursing Research* 36 (3): 32–47.

Hancock, Ange-Marie. 2007. "When Multiplication Doesn't Equal Quick Addition: Examining Intersectionality as a Research Paradigm." *Perspectives on Politics* 5 (1): 63–79. https://doi.org/10.1017/S1537592707070065.

Ingram, Deborah, and Sally A. Hutchinson. 2000. "Double Binds and the Reproductive and Mothering Experiences of HIV-Positive Women." *Qualitative Health Research* 10 (1): 117–32. https://doi.org/10.1177/104973200129118282.

Kaida, Angela, et al. 2009. "Antiretroviral Adherence during Pregnancy and Postpartum among HIV-Positive Women Enrolled in the Drug Treatment Program in British Columbia, Canada." *Canadian Journal of Infectious Diseases & Medical Microbiology* 20 (SB): S236–8.

Kitzinger, Sheila. 2004. "Sheila Kitzinger's Letter from Europe: Pregnant Asylum Seekers: The Dispossessed." *Birth (Berkeley, Calif.)* 31 (3): 236–8. https://doi.org/10.1111/j.0730-7659.2004.00310.x.

Loutfy, Mona R., et al., and the Ontario HIV Fertility Research Team. 2009. "Fertility Desires and Intentions of HIV-Positive Women of Reproductive Age in Ontario, Canada: A Cross-Sectional study." *PLoS One* 4 (12): e7925. https://doi.org/10.1371/journal.pone.0007925.

Miedema, Baukje, Ryan Hamilton, and Julie Easle. 2008. "Climbing the Walls: Structural Barriers to Accessing Primary Care for Refugee Newcomers to Canada." *Canadian Family Physician / Médecin de famille canadien* 54 (3): 335–6.

Money, Deborah, et al. 2009. "Impact of Type of Antiretroviral Therapy on Virologic Suppression at Birth in HAART Treated Pregnant Women." *Canadian Journal of Infectious Diseases & Medical Microbiology* 20 (SB): 24B.

Ofori-Asneso, Richard. 2013. "HIV-Related Travel Restrictions: A Focus on US and Canada." *Internet Journal of World Health and Societal Politics* 8 (1): 1–10.

Public Health Agency of Canada. 2011. "Summary: Estimates of HIV Prevalence and Incidence in Canada." http://www.acch.ca/resources/Summary%20HIV%20Prevalence%20and%20Incidence%20in%20Canada,%202011.pdf.

Reynolds, Becky, and Judy White. 2010. "Seeking Asylum and Motherhood: Health and Wellbeing Needs." *Community Practitioner* 83 (3): 20–3.

Rohleder, Poul, and Kerry L. Gibson. 2006. "'We are not fresh': HIV-Positive Women Talk of Their Experience of Their 'Spoiled Identity.'" *South African Journal of Psychology / Suid-Afrikaanse Tydskrif vir Sielkunde* 36 (1): 25–44. https://doi.org/10.1177/008124630603600103.

Ross, Ratchneewan, et al. 2007. "The Lived Experiences of HIV-Positive Pregnant Women in Thailand." *Health Care for Women International* 28 (8): 731–44. https://doi.org/10.1080/07399330701465218.

Sanders, Lorraine B. 2008. "Women's Voices: The Lived Experience of Pregnancy and Motherhood after Diagnosis with HIV." *Journal of the Association of Nurses in AIDS Care* 19 (1): 47–57. https://doi.org/10.1016/j.jana.2007.10.002.

Smith, Ripley L. 2013. "Female Refugee Networks: Rebuilding Post-Conflict Identity." *International Journal of Intercultural Relations* 37 (1): 11–27. https://doi.org/10.1016/j.ijintrel.2012.04.011.

Wang, Fu-Lin, et al. 2005. "Potential Factors That May Affect Acceptance of Routine Prenatal HIV Testing." *Canadian Journal of Public Health* 96 (1): 60–3.

World Health Organization. 2003. "The Right to Know: New Approaches to HIV Testing and Counselling." https://extranet.who.int/iris/restricted/handle/10665/68131.

# 14 HIV and Hepatitis C Co-Infection: Pathways to Care, Pathways to Advocacy – A Conversation with Colleen Price

COLLEEN PRICE

My name is Colleen Price. I am a 53, a survivor of trauma, addictions, HIV, and hepatitis C (HCV). I have an academic background in psychology and sociology, and as a social service worker. The following narrative is based upon my unique experiences, my personal perspectives, and the various lessons I have learned over the past 10 years – a decade in which I was an advocate for access to HCV treatment, care, and support for people living with HIV/HCV co-infection. Over time, I have experienced the distinct stigma attached to three communities: (1) when I was HCV mono-infected in 1997, I became familiar with the world view of mono-infected persons, and treatment access and judgments based upon HCV diagnosis; (2) when I became co-infected with HIV in 2000, I shared in the unique set of experiences associated with that group of people, experiencing dual HIV/HCV stigma and marginalization; and (3) after successful HCV treatment (2004 and 2005), I assumed the identity of a woman living with HIV.

On the one hand, I have experienced first-hand the lack of available services and programs for HCV and HIV/HCV co-infected people, the lack of integration of services, and the silos of people, communities, and diseases. On the other hand, I have also experienced incredible support from my diverse communities. Long-term survivors taught me about resiliency, hope, and perseverance – to never give up on advocating for effective programs, better policy, ethical research, and meaningful support to improve the quality of life and health outcomes of people living with HIV and/or hepatitis C.

## Diagnosis and Pathways to Care

*What was it like living with HCV, then HCV and HIV co-infection, and now, with HIV?*

When I was first diagnosed with HCV in 1997, treatment was not evolved: treatments were harsh and had limited success in those days. I had a low fibrosis score, so treatment was not encouraged; a "watch and wait" for better treatment was recommended. I was told it would be 20 to 30 years before it became a problem, if it did. I put it to the back of my mind and didn't tell anyone due to the stigma, especially with HCV's links to injecting drug use, which I had tried a few times in my early 20s, knowing nothing about harm reduction or dangers of sharing needles. I blamed myself, internalized the stigma, and continued risk taking.

Three years later, in 2000, I was diagnosed with HIV, making me HIV/HCV co-infected. When my long-time GP told me, I saw a skull and crossbones, I thought I was double dead. The HIV stigma overwhelmed me. I remember him asking me if I was OK, and mumbling, "Yes, sure." I walked out and relapsed worse than ever. My drinking and cocaine use was extreme. My partner Sandie knew something was wrong. I was so stigmatized having both HCV and HIV and so afraid. I could not tell her, and as I was infected by a man, I was afraid of losing her. I ended up bringing her to my GP (whom we both see) as I hadn't told her for six months and said she had to see him with me. As we were about to go in she asked, "What do you have, HIV?" I broke down and we saw him. Her knowing was better, but my behaviour spun out of control, culminating in a DUI in 2000. This was my wake-up call. Grateful that no one was hurt, I knew I could not continue the way I was. Shortly after, I went into the Jean Tweed recovery house in Toronto and started to think and learn about addressing trauma and addictions and HIV. While I relapsed, the things I learned did stick, and I was able to functionally manage my addictions, in that I entered recovery from hard drugs in 2001 but was still drinking.

My pathway to clinical HCV care in 2004 was via an Ottawa GP (with HIV speciality) who told me I was worrying too much about my HIV, that I needed to think about my drinking and my HCV, and that HCV treatments had improved. With his referral, in 2004 I entered into HCV clinical care and a 48-week HCV treatment as an outpatient at the Ottawa Hospital. I was grateful that the specialist took a chance on me, even though I was drinking. I quit drinking entirely for treatment. I wanted the treatment to work and I wanted to make some positive changes to my behaviour, regardless of treatment outcome. These changes improved my life and have been sustained.

The treatment was the hardest thing I have ever done due to the side effects, but I was so very fortunate to have cleared the HCV, as at that time, HIV/HCV co-infected clearance rates were about 25 per cent. Post–HCV treatment my mental health improved, as I was now a woman living with HIV, a chronic manageable disease. I am living well with HIV, with an undetectable viral load, and am in clinical care at the Ottawa Hospital for my HIV.

A heartfelt thanks to Drs Don Kilby, Curtis Cooper, Bill Cameron, and Phillip Townsend for long-term HCV and HIV care. Entering into clinical care and treatments was a catalyst for me. In engaging in my health, I learned to care about myself and to embrace life. As an HIV-positive woman, I am strong and resilient and I refuse to be stigmatized. I am more than my HIV, and HIV does not define me.

Critical to my emotional recovery and engagement in my HIV and HCV communities was the support of long-term survivor friends that I took training with, conferenced with, that supported me, and that have helped me to support others. They mentored me; thank you Jack Haight, Donald Turner, Nicola Diliso, Louise Binder, and Ron Rosenes. I no longer feel the shame, and that's the biggest part of healing. It's my peers, long-term survivors, who taught me that: to feel no shame, to be resilient, and that we have to help each other. My partner Sandie, my parents, friends, and colleagues were also critical to my getting through HCV treatment, the side effects, living well with HIV, and moving towards a life with meaning, passion, and joy.

*What challenges did you experience when you were first diagnosed and seeking services?*

One of my greatest challenges wasn't at the time of my HCV diagnosis, but rather when I decided to treat my HCV as an HIV/HCV co-infected woman. I had been working as a travel agent (my dream job) specializing in the Caribbean and Europe, and travelling frequently, but I became increasingly fatigued and sick, and I had liver pain. As HCV treatment had improved, I decided to start HCV treatment in 2004. The first hurdle was when I went to my employer and told him I had HCV. He was shocked, asked how I'd acquired it, and rather than find ways for me to stay at work, we decided long-term disability was best. This was without telling him I also had HIV. While he didn't intend to stigmatize – he was a good boss – I did feel stigmatized by his reaction. I realized during treatment, though, that this really was the best choice, as I endured debilitating side effects of mood, cognition, and sleep.

Looking back, I definitely experienced gaps in services. There was a hospital HCV peer group for people on treatment, which I benefited from. At first it was scary, as I saw the side effects they were experiencing, but we helped each other with support and ideas on managing side effects. It helped that there were others in the group; we were not alone and it helped de-stigmatize my internal stigma about HCV. On the whole, back in 2004 there were no dedicated support services or programs for people living with HCV, pre-, during, and post-treatment. I ended up getting much of my support from a U.S.-based website where people shared their experiences and strategies for dealing with side effects, and gave each other hope. There were people on the site 24 hours a day, and I will forever be grateful for the peer support that I received. I was also supported by Ron L., a liver transplant recipient and survivor of HCV; he would meet with me, give me support that I could and would get through treatment, that there was hope and that advocacy was important for access to treatment, as many were denied. This one-on-one peer support from Ron would impact my life and future. I vowed to give back and to help others on or in need of HCV treatment.

Back in 2004, the AIDS Service Organizations (ASOs) had mandates focusing only on HIV, and that combined with a lack of knowledge and much misinformation meant that they were not equipped or trained to assist people living with HIV/HCV co-infection. I was able to access some support and services for my HIV, but not my HCV. There were no dedicated HCV organizations that I knew of back then, and limited information was available. There was no place for people living with HIV/HCV co-infection that recognized the unique challenges of dual infection, the weight of living with dual infection, dual stigma, dual treatments, and the need for peer support and sharing of lived experiences and knowledge. And there was always a big divide between mental health and addictions services. I endured that, despite having concurrent disorders of mood and addictions.

Mental health support, based on my own experiences during my HCV treatment, was never there when I needed it. It wasn't immediate. By the time I had an appointment, I'd forgotten whatever the problem was. They really did nothing. I had an assessment at one hospital, and my distress was chalked up to treatment side effects and deemed temporary. Regardless, I had to fend for myself. I was lucky that I had long-term survivor friends who helped me through this. When I was on HCV treatment, it had these "mind-melting" side effects, and there was an immediacy. The crisis was then and there, not nine-to-five. That was the biggest single problem: services were nine-to-five. If I had to tell policymakers anything, what I really wanted them to do, I'd want them to make services more accessible: overnight and over the weekends. You take care of people Monday to Friday, and then what? You let them fall apart over the weekends or at night? If I had a crisis, I'd have to wait, probably a couple of weeks, and even then it seemed impossible to see the hospital psychologist and even longer to see a psychiatrist. If I wanted to see a psychologist immediately outside of the hospital, I knew I couldn't afford the fees. I didn't want to have to see a psychiatrist just because they were free; they would only prescribe pills, and I was already on enough pills. Mental health and addiction services need to be integrated and available. There need to be more recovery programs of longer duration. Lastly, health-care professionals, frontline professionals, peers – everybody needs to be trained and cross-trained in HCV and HIV to be able to effectively impact the epidemic and to positively impact quality of life, and access to treatment, care, and support.

*What was it like to access HCV treatment services?*
*What made a positive difference for you?*

Back when I did my HCV treatment in 2004, as a co-infected person, I had 25 per cent odds of a cure. There was so little hope, so little hope among the co-infected. But I wanted to stop the liver fibrosis progression and the symptoms of HCV, and my HIV was well managed, so I decided to treat, despite the odds, undergoing 48 weeks of HCV treatment with the assistance of a multidisciplinary care team at the Ottawa Hospital.

I felt very lucky to have had access to these medications when so many did not. So many of us were denied because success rates were low for people who had past or current issues of addiction or mental health. Back then, they didn't treat anybody who used drugs, and I was an alcoholic right up to the day I started treatment – and then I quit. My HCV specialist took a chance on me. It was Dr Curtis Cooper who gave me the faith that things were going to be OK, that I was in the driver's seat, it was no one but me. Dr Cooper has long supported people with mental health and addictions issues, saying that they deserve the right to treatment. He was so supportive, he believed in the chance of the cure and believed in me. This is what motivated me to engage in HCV treatment. I trusted his expertise, and he and his team of nurses sustained me throughout a difficult treatment.

Working with a multidisciplinary team, engaging in clinical care was the first time I cared about my health. It was a catalyst for me. I never cared about my health in the past, but I wanted the HCV treatment to work, and I did everything I could to get healthy, including exercise and nutrition. It was the first time I prioritized my health over my addictions and I learned new ways of coping. In those 48 weeks, I made behavioural changes that are sustained, and I reinvested in myself, and in life, in training, in conferencing, in building my knowledge about HCV, HIV, and HIV/HCV co-infection.

In 2005, I was told I was cured of my HCV, and my mental health skyrocketed. I went from feeling "double dead" to "only" living with HIV, a chronic manageable disease that remains well maintained all these years later. My HCV treatment, the people who helped me, helped me to develop resiliency. Post-treatment, I vowed to advocate for the rights of people living with HIV/HCV co-infection to access treatment, care, and support, and for integrated care and service provision that focused on the whole person, holistic health.

**Pathways to Advocacy**

*How did you become a spokesperson and advocate for people living with HIV and HIV/HCV co-infection? What sort of work have you done?*

I became an advocate because of the barriers I faced, and because I lost people to HCV and HIV/HCV co-infection. My pathway to advocacy started with training in the pilot group of the Ontario AIDS Network Positive Leadership Development Institute, where I learned skills in leadership and governance and made lifelong friendships with peers in the program. In 2006, I joined the Canadian Treatment Action Council (CTAC), and with the guidance and support of my mentors Louise Binder and Ron Rosenes I started and chaired the HIV/HCV co-infection portfolio for six years. As a board member, I appealed to the board to include HCV, and it was approved, changing the HIV mandate to include HCV.

Since joining CTAC, I've supported greater involvement of people living with HIV/HCV co-infection in projects ranging from a working group, to an Ontario think tank, an HIV/HCV co-infection documentary film, and the first Canadian HIV/HBV/HCV Co-infection Research Summit in 2010, which I co-chaired with Dr Marina Klein and Randy Jackson. The outcome of this summit was the Roadmap of HIV/HCV Co-infection Research Recommendations. After the summit, I wanted to develop a knowledge transfer and exchange (KTE) project to share this information nationally, and to develop the capacities of people living with HIV/HCV co-infection in peer facilitation, evaluation, and dissemination.

With the assistance of Louise Binder and Leah Stephenson, we created the CTAC Co-infection KTE and Capacity-Building Project. People living with co-infection were the drivers of this project, integral to the development, implementation, and dissemination of HIV/HCV co-infection research through webinars to community, frontline, and other stakeholders. We saw new champions who are living with HIV/HCV co-infection emerge in this group: it really fostered leadership, KTE, and capacity building, and we presented results at several HIV research conferences.

In 2013, I joined the board of the Interagency Coalition on AIDS and Development and enjoyed my volunteer work with this international board. A highlight was initiating and working with a remarkable group of women to hold the Canadian Association of HIV Researchers ancillary event, the National Women, Trans People, and Girls HIV, Hepatitis C, and Co-infection Health Research Summit in 2015. This event brought together community members, frontline service providers, epidemiologists, clinical and social scientists, and community-based researchers to share current research and lived experiences and to address gaps in clinical care, services, support, research, and policy as they relate to cis and trans women and girls. It was a multi-sectoral dialogue and led to the development of a Sex and Gender-Specific Research Roadmap that outlined key issues and action items as they relate to the diverse issues and needs of cis and trans women and girls affected by HIV and/or HCV in Canada.

Today, I am a member of numerous working groups, research teams, and committees on HIV and HCV. I have been a member of the Ontario Advisory Committee on HIV/AIDS since 2009 and am a long-term member of the Ontario HIV Treatment Network Ontario Cohort Governance Committee. I also volunteered with the Ottawa Hospital hepatitis C social worker and peers to run a six-week women's HCV peer group and a mixed-gender group for ten weeks to provide information and linkages to treatment, care, and support.

*On the basis of your experiences and advocacy, what do you want policymakers and the public to understand about the challenges of co-infection? Why is it important for policymakers to pay attention specifically to HIV and HCV co-infection?*

Challenges with co-infection are throughout the lifespan, and they differ in your 20s, 30s, 40s, and 50s, as you age. It's complex, and it's degenerative. If left untreated, HCV is the number one killer in people with HIV, so if it isn't treated, there will be increased hospitalizations, kidney disease, cardiovascular disease, and complex comorbidities related to both HIV and HCV. The government needs to take concrete action to treat anyone with HCV, universally, not only when they are at a liver fibrosis of F2 score. This is currently a barrier to access, and cost can also be a barrier to access for some. Testing and treating HCV among people who use drugs, as well as one-time testing of all baby boomers, is critical to impacting the epidemic.

   People living with HCV and/or HIV are somebody's mother, father, brother, son, daughter. It's important to treat everyone as individuals, not as part of a marginalized group. Challenges to effective treatment, care, and support are that so many are undiagnosed. About 40 per cent do not know their HCV status, and others remain outside health-care or organizational supports. I was tested three times for HCV before I was diagnosed – in 1997 they finally had a test that accurately measured me. So it's quite possible that people have tested for HCV before, in the 1990s, and think they're fine. It is important to know our current HCV status and to have confirmatory testing. We also need specific programs for prevention, harm reduction, and peer support.

*What would those programs look like?*

We need InSites, supervised injection facilities, across the country, in every major city. It *will* save lives. If people overdose inside InSite or other facilities, there are nurses there who can revive them. And they're in a safe, clean, sterile environment. They aren't in high-risk situations with others or alone. These programs save lives and can help moderate use. Users of these services may time their drug use around their visits, so it might be a bit of behaviour modification. And at InSite, they give counselling and help people into treatment programs, at that moment in time, if they wish. We also need harm reduction in prisons – and access to medications while in prison. We'll never stop this epidemic unless we have adequate harm reduction across the country, including in prisons. We also need longer duration, comprehensive recovery programs, and more of them, to be effective. Waitlists for recovery programs hamper harm reduction efforts.

Programs would also have to involve counselling and mental health. Mental health is nowhere to be seen in the HCV response. Of all the social determinants of health, the one that I think we can have the greatest impact on, the one where we've invested the least, is in mental health, and in peer support. Mental health is the link. It threads through HCV, HIV, and HIV/HCV co-infection. Investing in mental health is the single biggest thing we can do to help. If I look at the social determinants of health, if your mental health is strong enough, you can live in a drug-filled city housing project and be OK, and be able to maintain your recovery, if your mental health is solid, if that is your goal. If your mental health isn't solid, you're just going to drown. Mental health is the foundation. And trauma is the first link in the vulnerability chain: it's what made me an addict, it's what made me take a lot of risks. There are few programs for trauma-based therapy and compound mental and physical challenges that are faced by people living with HCV, HIV, or HIV/HCV co-infection. Mental health is key, because with it you can overcome so much. It's what helps people care about themselves, their health, healing, and prevention. And it's what gives self-esteem; in fact, really, mental health wipes out stigma. When you regain yourself and you reach a point of mastery and coping, you're solid, resilient.

Peer support remains, in my eyes, one of the most valuable but underfunded resources that we have to improve testing, treatment uptake, retention, adherence, and treatment outcomes. The value of peer support is the lived and shared experiences that we have in common. Other people's experiences helped me through my HCV treatment and dealing with side effects. They provided support in making it to the end of treatment. And in lieu of psychologists or psychiatrists or any kind of mental health care, they provided support to help keep me stable. They weren't therapeutic sessions, but still, the support in and of itself, and being with other people who had been through it made a world of difference. Peer support from people that I have trained with, and co-infected people that I have worked with in peer projects and research, both sustain and motivate me. And this relationship is based in mutuality, trust, and confidentiality. Peer support is an area where many people living with HCV or co-infection would like to be meaningfully involved, but it requires substantial investment in people, training, and organizations. With dedicated funding and training, peer support builds not only capacities, but also resiliency. It improves our health and our quality of life.

Gender-specific services are important too. Gender, poverty, and marginalization intersect, and multi-layered stigma adds to complexities. Women-only spaces are important. If women are isolated or kept quiet because of their families, it's hard for them to find a voice. Often their voices are stifled. In women-only groups, they have the opportunity to say how they feel, without being judged. The energies of women when they're alone is different from when they're in a mixed-gender population. Also of importance to programming is the need for LGBTQ services and support for people living with HCV, HIV, and HIV/HCV co-infection. There needs to be recognition that prevention needs are different in different populations.

*What messages do you have specifically for policymakers in government?*

My message to my government is that all people living with HCV, HIV, or HIV/HCV co-infection have the right to be treated, to access clinical care and treatments, and they deserve to be treated the same as anyone else, to not be judged and to be treated as individuals and with respect.

What do I want my government to do? I want them to invest in mental health and peer supports for people living with HIV and/or HCV. I want them to pump money into HCV-specific prevention programs, and programming for HCV mono-infected and HIV/HCV co-infected people. The government needs to make substantive investments in HCV programming, services, prevention, research, and support. This funding needs to be equitable and sustainable. It remains to be seen, with HIV, HCV, and STBBIs now being under one funding umbrella, whether this will benefit people living with HCV and/or HIV. We are lagging behind other countries and have no national HCV strategy. The government must accept responsibility and put into place a strategy to address the epidemic and the lives impacted. There is a promising HCV strategy from Glasgow that should be evaluated for transferability and applicability to the Canadian context.

And about the government argument about the high cost of HCV medication, this so-called economic barrier that means we can't afford to treat all the people living with HCV, that if we encouraged universal HCV testing, we aren't prepared and it's going to break the health-care system. Well, my HCV treatment was about $30,000, but then I think about how much my HIV treatment will cost over my lifetime, and I think about all the other diseases out there with expensive medications, and I do not buy this argument. HCV is one of the number one problems in Ontario, and in Canada. Friends have died because treatment didn't work, or they didn't get it in time because they were diagnosed late, or because their liver disease was too far gone. Now, the new medications are very promising, even for people in quite dire shape. Treatment side effects are minimal, treatment durations are far shorter, and success rates for clearing the virus are very high. The challenge, with the new medications, is 100 per cent access. They should do the one-time birth cohort testing, I firmly believe in that. I don't believe that if suddenly everybody knew their HCV status, they would go running to their doctors and break down the health-care system. What I do believe is that if people were aware of their HCV infection and they were properly counselled, and did things like quitting drinking which could mitigate fibrosis, and accessed support services, they'd be better informed and could prepare for treatment. I mean, it's true, yes, we don't have enough doctors. There will be challenges, and there will be complications. But of those people tested, then first treat those who need it most and it will save a lot of lives. Treatment should not be denied to anyone with HCV who wants to treat it, regardless of fibrosis score. Current guidelines state that you should have an F2 fibrosis score before treatment is paid for. That means likely you will be experiencing symptoms rather than being proactive and treating early if you want to.

Our government also needs to provide services, and I don't mean the traditional services we have, because they aren't working. Organizations are over-stretched, they're under-funded, under-staffed, and sometimes under-trained when it comes to HCV and co-infection. And ASOs, for the most part, don't provide HCV services. They used to. A few years ago there was a little bit of money, and we actually had HCV workers in ASOs in Ontario. But how many HCV mono-infected people do you think ever walked into an ASO? So I commend the ASOs, because they help a lot of people, but why isn't there the same service for HCV? Why isn't there an HCV centre in every town, in every city? Why aren't there agencies? There's no national HCV agency, no national HCV strategy or co-infection strategy. We have silos of strategies when in fact they should be integrated. I personally believe that it's beneficial that governments are starting to move them all together, that they're integrating HIV and HCV services, because the shared transmission routes, the vulnerabilities, the facilitators and barriers are all so very similar. So I hope this new federal HIV/HCV/STBBI integration will address the problem more cohesively, because what we've been doing hasn't worked.

Our services need to be integrated, to provide whole-systems care, from counselling to harm reduction to housing. The first step is to bring people into care. Integrated, holistic care. They may not be ready for treatment: they may need mental health care, they may need harm reduction, whatever care they need. We have come so very far in the clinical management of HIV and HCV, but there are still challenges in accessing integrated mental health and addictions services, in linking and engaging people in care.

What's critical, in any strategy, is the involvement of community members living with HIV and HCV. We are the experts in the barriers, gaps in care and support, gaps in social and health-care systems, missed opportunities. It is essential that we be included in the design, implementation, and evaluation of programs, service provision, and policy decision-making processes.

*What would you say to other people who are co-infected?*
*What misconceptions would you like to see addressed?*

I want people living with HIV and HCV to know that they're more than their diseases. That they don't deserve to be marginalized and stigmatized and judged. That they have the same rights as any other person, the right to mental health and any other services, and especially to treatment.

Misconceptions about access to HCV treatment that I have encountered include that people who use drugs or other substances including alcohol or methadone, or who have mental health issues, will not be eligible for treatment. The old guidelines did have a lot of restrictions. HCV treatment was long denied to people living with HIV/HCV co-infection due to the serious side effects of HCV treatment, or existing or previous addiction or mental health issues. These issues can be managed today, given the tolerability of new HCV medications. With these new highly effective, short-duration treatments with fewer side effects,

HCV treatment is tolerable for all populations, including people living with HIV, including people who use drugs, including people with mental health issues. The new treatments are as effective in these populations as any other, and the rate of success in clearing HCV is close to 100 per cent. Treating a co-infected person has the same rate of efficacy as treating an HCV mono-infected person. But this misconception still persists about who is eligible, who will be covered.

Also, some people think, "I have HIV, what does it matter that I have HCV?" It matters a lot because of accelerated fibrosis in the liver caused by dual infections. HCV is a leading cause of death in people living with HIV. Your HCV should be as prioritized as your HIV. People also think, "I can wait until my HCV becomes a problem and then I will do treatment," that they feel fine and will do it when they feel like they have to. But the symptoms of HCV are silent, often manifesting only after liver damage has occurred, and in many cases when liver damage is severe. Treating HCV early is beneficial, just like treating HIV.

We need a community. The co-infected community is very splintered, there is no group, there is no true community. It's held together by threads, over the Internet and the odd support group, but government has really failed to develop an infrastructure that can support the number of people in the population that have HCV.

The great challenge to HIV/HCV integration is silos of communities, of disease, of stigmas. All of us – community, frontline staff, researchers, clinicians, and government – have critical roles in the development, implementation, evaluation, and funding of programs and services with real life impact for individuals and populations. For integration to work, we need to focus on our similarities, not our differences. The siloing of people, populations, and diseases has to stop.

# 15 AIDS Activism: Remembering Resistance versus Socially Organized Forgetting

GARY KINSMAN

## Effective AIDS Activism: Epp = Death

*An effigy of the Canadian health minister in flames. It was May 1988 and AIDS ACTION NOW! engaged in a series of actions at the third Canadian Conference on AIDS[1] directed at the inaction and neglect of the federal government, and the federal minister of health, Jake Epp, on AIDS. We organized a die-in to dramatize what government policies were leading to. I helped unfurl a banner reading "Epp = Death" when the representative of the minister spoke, and at the demonstration at the end of the conference hundreds of people took to the streets in a march concluding with the burning of an effigy of Epp.*

*This activist intervention was successful in developing a broader composition of struggle, drawing into action members of the Canadian AIDS Society (CAS), and others, given the widespread frustration with the lack of AIDS action by federal state agencies. We heard that Prime Minister Brian Mulroney called Jack Epp into his office demanding to know why people were so angry with him that his effigy was being burned in the streets of Toronto. This action disrupted consensual relations between AIDS groups and the federal government, creating pressure for change, helping to set the stage for a new health minister (Perrin Beatty) taking office, and creating the situation where the government had to develop a National AIDS Strategy both to respond to community-based AIDS groups and AIDS activists and to attempt to manage them.*

I start with this narrative of highly effective AIDS activist intervention into Canadian state relations and public policy formation, to which state agencies were forced to respond. This demonstrates how activism can bring about transformations that open up more possibilities for addressing the needs of people living with AIDS/HIV (PLWA/HIV) and AIDS groups. At the same time, these activist gains have been largely forgotten, so we can no longer remember the important part AIDS activism played in challenging and transforming state and social responses to AIDS – and the part that activism could play in addressing the situations we currently face. These histories of activism are covered over in official AIDS documents, as activism is "disappeared" in official textual time (Smith 1990, 74; Smith and Turner 2014; Kinsman 1997) and is largely forgotten within AIDS service organizations (ASOs) as well. In particular the critical approaches to state relations in early AIDS activism have been forgotten. This social amnesia produces major problems for reigniting AIDS activism in the present.

As the diverse chapters in this book make clear, the AIDS/HIV crisis is very much a bringing together of social relations. This is far more than the story of a virus and very much about social organization, including the social construction of knowledge about what came to be called AIDS and HIV – including both the homosexualization of AIDS and "African AIDS" (Patton 1990); the resulting organization of stigmatization and discrimination along sexual, racializing, drug use, and other lines; problems with the social organization of health care; problems created by the for-profit capitalist organization of drug companies; and more. AIDS/HIV cannot be fully addressed without contending with sexuality, gender, racialization, class, poverty, global underdevelopment, and the capitalist and professional organization of health care and the pharmaceutical industry. While AIDS/HIV has its own specific features that must be addressed, it is also organized through these broader social relations. To use Himani Bannerji's expression (1995), drawing on dialectical theorizations of mediation, AIDS is both autonomous and specific but also simultaneously mutually constructed through these broader relations.

Public policy and state agencies that have the task to protect "public health" have only begun to address some aspects of these relations and all too often focus on regulating PLWA/HIVs and AIDS organizing as social problems. One feature of this approach is constructing PLWA/HIVs as the problem to be addressed, especially those "irresponsible" PLWA/HIVs who cannot or do not wish to follow medical and state regulation regarding treatment, or disclosure of HIV status – whether for lack of resources or knowledge, or for other reasons (Kinsman 1996, 1997). Overwhelmingly, as chapters in this book point out (see chapters by Alex McClelland, Adrian Guta, and Nicole Greenspan, and by Marilou Gagnon and Christine Vezina, among others), these "irresponsible" PLWA/HIVs are people of colour, Indigenous people, sex workers, injection drug users, and people living in poverty. There is a division between the "responsible" PLWA/HIV who is "self-regulating," following medical and state regulation (including the advice of ASOs, which can also become sites of regulation) and those "irresponsible" PLWA/HIVs who do not, and this often falls along class and race lines.

In this chapter I reflect on the AIDS activism that changed the world in the 1980s and early 1990s that has often been forgotten, for remembering this activism can offer insights and resources for addressing current AIDS-related struggles in the context of a more consolidated neoliberal capitalism, especially regarding cuts to social assistance, and health care, and criminalization. We can also see the initial formation of the distinction between the responsible/irresponsible PLWA/HIVs in these years that continues to inform our historical present.

This exploration is informed by my own experiences as an AIDS activist in the 1980s and early 1990s largely in Toronto, but also in St John's, Newfoundland, and in Nova Scotia, and by my memory work (Frankenburg 1993; Haug 1992) based on this. This chapter focuses more on my experiences with AIDS ACTION NOW! (also see McCaskell 2016) and this produces a rather Toronto- and Ontario-centric focus. This is intended only as a starting point and needs to be added to in recovering AIDS activist histories in other regions. I also draw on the work of historical recovery that the AIDS Activist History Project (AAHP) is engaged in for the late 1980s up to 1996 in "Canada" (AAHP 2017). Throughout this chapter I draw upon some of the interviews that are available on the AAHP website.[2]

As Patrizia Gentile and I argue, one of the ways that ruling takes place is through the systematic social organization of forgetting the struggles and forms of resistance of the past. We are denied access to the social and historical literacies that would allow us to feel and hear the struggles of people that won us gains that are currently being cut and curtailed. If we do not remember this organizing, we forget the origin of these gains and how we can harness these capacities for resistance and transformation in the present. We forget how AIDS organizing from below created support for PLWA/HIVs, combatted discrimination, opened up greater treatment access, and developed safer practices and harm reduction approaches. The struggles of people in the past are not being actively remembered within many current ASOs, and certainly not in mainstream state and public policy discussions. In the official texts and documents addressing AIDS policy, the impact of AIDS organizing and activism is systematically disappeared. The necessary antidote

to the social organization of resistance is the resistance of remembering the struggles and resistance of the past (Kinsman and Gentile 2010,
21–2, 37–8).

The bulk of this chapter focuses on what AIDS activism can teach
us about our historical present and future. This history from below
(Thompson 1968; Kinsman and Gentile 2010, 27–8), which rewrites history from the vantage point of the oppressed, produces a history not
of elites but of grassroots organizing. After a brief survey of earlier
AIDS activism, this chapter suggests ways in which this history remains crucial for current organizing.

## Clarifying the Contested Terrain

Before diving into remembering aspects of these histories, we need
clarification of the terrains we encounter in this exploration.

Inspired by the feminist health movement that extended feminism
from reclaiming control over bodies, sexualities, and reproductive capacities, to reclaiming control over health, early AIDS organizing attempted to develop a notion of "health from below," in contrast to the
"health from above" that dominates in ruling state, medical, and pharmaceutical relations. Health from above is the hegemonic social form[3]
of health in a capitalist society. Health from below challenges the professional power/knowledge relations in the medical profession, which
establishes doctors and other officials as the "experts" so that the rest
of us are only "patients" who can display and narrate "symptoms" but
have no knowledge or control ourselves. In suggesting that people can
have knowledge about their bodies and health and can collectively
seize control over their own health, this points towards a different social form of health. This approach also informed the PLWA/HIV self-
empowerment movement and the treatment-based AIDS activism in
North America that often led in the late 1980s and early 1990s to individual PLWA/HIVs knowing more about AIDS/HIV and treatments
than their primary-care physicians. AIDS activists also developed
their own treatment agendas and participated in community-based research initiatives, and argued for changes in drug trials and research,
which also challenged the research and drug company establishments
(Epstein 1998). This challenged professional and state power/knowl-
edge relations, which are central to health from above.

From its inception, AIDS organizing confronted state relations and
has often been managed by state agencies. People often refer to "the

state" as if it were an external "thing" or "structure." I prefer to describe this as state relations or state formation (Corrigan and Sayer 1985) to clarify that these relations are not a reified object but a social power relation produced by people. But at the same time this is a particular social form of "power over" relation (Holloway 2005) that attends to ruling and managing people's lives. It is characterized by top-down relations, the separation of the "political" realm from people's everyday lives, the hegemony of bureaucrats, professionals, and "experts" over people's lives, including in relation to health, and a "democracy" that is at best a limited indirect, representative form. It is not a social relation that facilitates liberation and freedom from oppression, but instead organizes the relations of oppression and marginalization that many people face, including PLWA/HIVs. This is a particular capitalist and oppressive form of social organization (ibid.).

At the same time, as a social relation produced by people, it needs to be engaged with, even though it is a difficult terrain of struggle that is not on the side of oppressed and exploited people. Activism and organizing can win important gains from state agencies (Corrigan and Sayer 1981), including regarding AIDS/HIV, but at the same time state formation is invested in health from above and capitalist and oppressive health relations. At the very same time that AIDS groups often need the resources that only state funding under current circumstances can provide, it is this very funding and the regulations that come with it that often manage AIDS groups away from needed activism and advocacy work (Kinsman 1997). This sets up a series of dilemmas for AIDS groups. While state funding is often needed, it also can lead to regulation and the transformation of community-based groups into state-managed groups. At times this means getting funding and resources while actively resisting state regulation. Other groups like AIDS ACTION NOW! reject state funding because of the restrictions this presents for AIDS activism. Activism will often be needed against state relations themselves. We need to organize both within and against state relations, but health from below comes only from a direction of struggle that ruptures with and moves beyond state formation to build towards a different social form of health. As Holloway (2005, 2016) suggests, we need to organize simultaneously within, against, and beyond state relations.

In this light there is a problem with "common-sense" liberal pluralist theories of state relations that assume that state relations are simply a plural, consensual balance between different social forces. This approach traps us into simply engaging within state relations and does not lead to understanding the major non-consensual aspects of state formation. It also blurs how social power relations operate in and through state relations, even if sometimes in a contradictory fashion. This liberal pluralist approach often implicitly informs ASOs and their operation with and within state relations and much public policy discourse. Instead AIDS activism requires a far more critical approach to state relations.

Related to state formation is public policy formation regarding AIDS, which involves state agencies, social agencies, and at times community groups. This can be a contested terrain involving AIDS activist groups challenging public policy, such as quarantine measures against people living with AIDS/HIV in the late 1980s in BC (Craik 2017; Banner 2017; Guinan 2017) and the early 1990s in Ontario. It can be the activist campaign organized by AAN! that led to the creation of a Trillium drug-funding plan in Ontario for people in catastrophic situations (Southin 2017; Brown 2017) or the campaign for treatment funding in Quebec (Hendricks and LeBoeuf 2017) initiated by ACT UP Montreal. And it can also be much more internal to state relations and professional relations, perhaps with some "consultation" with ASOs. Often state regulation and public policy formation occur through forms of textual regulation (Smith 1990) such as in the National AIDS Strategy, which in response to activism laid out new conceptual practices for ruling, including neoliberal notions of "consultation" and "participation," which allow community-based groups to be managed by state and professional relations. In the current period, "integration" (see chapter by Richard Elliot) is one of these conceptual strategies attempting to consolidate more programs in specific agencies in the context of social program cuts with hopes of cost-saving and "downloading" more work onto non-state bodies.

Neoliberalism, despite its different currents and contradictions, is the capitalist strategy that informs current state formation (Drucker 2015; Kinsman 2017b, 139–41) and began to take shape in the Canadian state context in the 1980s. This strategy is directed against the power that social struggles, workers, and the oppressed were able to exert in the 1960s and early 1970s. While certainly an attack on social programs, the social wage, and Keynesian perspectives, this was centrally an attempt to weaken the composition of struggle that workers (in a broad sense) and the oppressed had been able to develop in the 1960s and early 1970s. Neoliberalism leads to cuts in spending on social programs, which intensifies reproductive and domestic labour largely assigned to women, but also to an expansion of spending on disciplining the poor and working class, on "law and order," and the tightening of borders against people of colour from the "Global South" (Kinsman and Gentile 2010, 436–8; Kinsman 2016, 2017b). It also opens the door to the further globalization of capitalist relations through various "free-trade" agreements, which are really charters for the rights of corporations (McNally 2006).

In relation to state and public policies regarding AIDS/HIV, it has led to spending cuts and viewing ASOs as more "cost-effective" ways of delivering services than through direct state provision, regulatory strategies of "consultation" and "partnership," the individualization of the response to AIDS/HIV, and the criminalization of some people living with AIDS/HIV. Neoliberalism is now the major capitalist strategy; AIDS groups need to understand what it is and how to combat its influence in state and public policy formation.

Early on neoliberalism had a moral conservative form and was overtly anti-gay and anti-PLWA/HIV, but feminist, queer and other struggles opened up the space for non-moral conservative forms of neoliberalism to emerge which support limited rights for PLWA/HIVs and queers, and at least some funding for AIDS programs (Kinsman 2016, 2017b). Both neoliberal approaches, however, are united in supporting the criminalization of PLWA/HIVs, assigning "responsibility" for transmission issues only to HIV-infected persons.

## A Brief Historical Sketch of AIDS Activism and the Management of AIDS Organizing

AIDS organizing of the early 1980s developed in response to state inaction and indifference, major problems with the response of the medical profession, and social discrimination against gays, Haitians, Indigenous and other racialized people, injection-drug users, and sex workers. Years were wasted in the development of research and social policy, since AIDS/HIV was often addressed by those in positions of power as only affecting "expendable" populations. Community-based support and educational groups were set up in the early and mid-1980s based largely in gay communities (but also including lesbians and women involved in the feminist health movement) when no one else was addressing these needs. It is important to remember that community groups stepped in to meet the needs that were not being addressed by state agencies, health officials, and the medical profession. At first only job-creation funding was provided for these groups, but this was extended by the mid-1980s to include streams of health funding (Kinsman 1997).

State and public policy was dominated in the mid- to late 1980s by "public health" and to a certain extent by palliative care. Regarding public health it is always important to ask which public and whose health is being protected through public health practices. During these years the central focus of public health was protecting the "general population" from infection. This was "protecting" people from the affected communities and what were often still referred to as "high-risk" groups. This term was taken from epidemiological discourse but was shifted in public health and mass media discourse to make these groups a "threat" (Patton 1990). This meant that PLWA/HIVs, gays, Haitians, injection drug users, sex workers, and others were excluded from the "general population." The communities most affected by AIDS and people living with AIDS were written out of the "general population" and instead became "threats" and "risks" to others. This general population was defined as being heterosexual, largely white, and often middle class. This built on earlier public health responses to STIs, which involved a social course of action going from contact-tracing to possible quarantine (Brandt 1987), especially in BC (Craik 2017; Banner 2017; Guinan 2017) and Ontario (Brown 2017). The focus on "public health" and transmission questions also meant there was little official focus on treatment and the survival of PLWA/HIVs (Smith 1995, 2006). While there have been important modifications to public health practices, this historical legacy continues to create problems. The focus on palliative care, while important, viewed AIDS/HIV as a death sentence and therefore mandated comfort while dying, with no attention to the survival of PLWA/HIVs. There is currently more of a focus on aging with HIV, as discussed elsewhere in this book.

Out of this early community-based AIDS organizing came a focus on safe practices. Regarding safe/safer sex, this was based on eroticizing practices that would not lead to the transmission of HIV, or at least were at a lower risk of transmission (Patton 1985, 1996). This was extended to safe injection-needle use, including the distribution of clean needles, the setting up of injection sites, and early harm-reduction work (Barnett 2017), which led to a lowering of transmission in many areas. Engaging in safe practices was a collective responsibility; there was no space in this view for focusing only on the responsibility of those who knew they were HIV-positive.

For a time, this organizing shifted erotic practices and showed that sex practices are socially made. Among gay men, for instance, who were not generally using condoms, since they did not usually engage in reproductive sex, many gay men took up and eroticized using condoms as part of their regular sexual repertoire. This was shifted and sanitized in public health measures that often pushed abstinence, monogamy (mostly understood as serial monogamy, which is not necessarily safe) or, if all else fails, use a condom. This safe-practice organizing was a challenge to neoliberal individualizing of the PLWA/HIV, but was also reshaped by public health discourse and within some AIDS groups to emphasize that individuals are rational actors calculating the risk associated with certain practices, like good, neoliberal subjects (Patton 1985, 1996). This shift was also used to undermine the collective and social character of early safe-practice organizing.

Community-based AIDS groups formed in the early and mid-1980s through uneven state funding and regulation became managed by state and professional relations and transformed into AIDS service organizations (ASOs). These forms of reorganization and management include the need for more professionalized staff, boards of directors, executive directors, incorporation, and charitable tax status (Kinsman 1997). As one illustration, after the AIDS Committee of Toronto incorporated and received charitable tax status in 1983, with its prohibition on activism and advocacy work, it no longer supported the pro-choice reproductive rights movement, even though before this the connections between the AIDS struggle and the pro-choice movement were well accepted. ASOs moved from organizations being driven by membership to being driven by boards and sometimes by staff. This shifted groups away from activism and towards top-down forms of organization that replicate the form of organizing in the corporate and state worlds (Ng 1996). Through this transformation, ASOs are influenced by and become part of social power relations. As a result, despite the forms of solidarity they develop, they often come to perpetuate forms of social exclusion of people of colour and women, helping to create the basis for the later emergence of new AIDS groups addressing these concerns.

In the period from 1986 to 1987 a number of Persons with AIDS Coalition groups were set up in Vancouver (Kozachenko 2017), Halifax (Smith 2017), Toronto, and elsewhere as PLWA/HIVs increasingly felt that their needs were not being addressed by the mainstream ASOs (Smith 2017), whose funding often focused on prevention education rather than the survival and treatment needs of PLWA/HIVs. Many felt they were being left to die and not enough was being done around their survival in the ASOs. Some formed their own groups based on the self-organization of PLWA/HIVs. They challenged the language of "AIDS victim" and focused on the possibility of survival. They contested the official focus only on public health and palliative care. The Vancouver Persons with AIDS Coalition initiated the first treatment-based activism in 1986 (Kozachenko 2017).

This shift was expressed early on in the 1983 Denver Principles statement from people with AIDS and was continued and made more global in the Montreal Manifesto, which was also known as the Declaration of the Universal Rights and Needs of People Living with HIV Disease, that AAN! and the AIDS Coalition to Unleash Power (ACT UP) NYC produced for the 1989 International AIDS conference in Montreal. Later this was taken up in more limited organizational forms relating to employment within ASOs as Greater Involvement of People Living with AIDS/HIV, and Meaningful Involvement of People with HIV/AIDS.

The self-organization of PLWA/HIVs, and this focus on survival, set the stage for the explosive emergence of treatment-based AIDS activism in the later 1980s. Following the emergence of ACT UP in New York and other centres across the United States, AIDS ACTION NOW! was formed in Toronto and ACT UP groups emerged in Vancouver (Kozachenko 2017; Kaleta 2017; Craik 2017), Montreal (Hendricks and LeBoeuf 2017), and Halifax (Smith 2017; Allan 2017; Petty 2017). These groups emerged out of the contradiction between knowing that there were treatments that could extend people's lives – especially against opportunistic infections, which is what people were actually dying of – and state and drug company policies that denied it. These groups were based on direct action politics, which did not focus on lobbying or meeting with government officials or playing by the official rules, but instead on more disruptive and often confrontational tactics where people put their bodies on the line: moving needed drugs across borders, and engaging in die-ins, occupations, and effigy burnings (as we saw earlier). This direct-action focus won significant victories in expanding treatment access that extended people's lives and improved people's quality of life. *This is crucial to remember.*

Activists confronted the drug trial for aerosolized pentamidene (AP) to prevent the development of *Pneumocystis carinii* pneumonia, which was a major killer of people with AIDS during these years. The trial employed a double-blind placebo, which meant some people got no treatment at all and there were "clinical end points" (deaths) as a result. In response, activists focused on the difference between the organization of research, and the social relations of treatment and the need for everyone who wanted to access treatment to be able to have it (Smith 1990, 2006). AAN! aided in getting AP across the border from Buffalo for people in the Toronto area who needed it. There was early success in getting the Emergency Drug Release Program (EDRP) to release AIDS/HIV treatments on compassionate grounds. At the same time there were problems here as well. Even when the EDRP approved the release of the antiviral drug ddI, Brystol-Myers Squibb, who "owned" the drug, refused to release it to people who could not tolerate AZT. A blockade of their office, which led to the arrests of seven AAN! activists (myself included), and other organizing around this was required before ddI was released (Kinsman 2017a).

This activism produced expanded treatment access, including treatment arms in clinical trials, and began to point towards the possibilities of AIDS/HIV becoming a chronic, manageable condition. AIDS activists attempted to put in place the social basis for this to become a reality through these campaigns. At the same time, in the 1990s some medical and state officials were able to use the rhetoric of AIDS now being "a chronic, manageable condition," even though the material basis for it had not been produced, in order to de-prioritize the concerns of people living with AIDS/HIV and to deny needed supports (Kinsman 1996). It is also important to remember that while this activism and organizing created greater treatment access, often very unevenly for many (but not all) in the "Global North," it did not in the "Global South."

This wave of AIDS activism led to PLWA/HIVs being included on more state and medical committees addressing AIDS concerns. AIDS activists took over the opening session of the International AIDS Conference in Montreal in 1989, produced the Montreal Manifesto, and engaged in other activism at the conference. This altered the character of these medical- and state-dominated conferences, creating more space for PLWA/HIVs within them. The Montreal Manifesto raised the need to transfer resources from the "Global North" to the "Global South" if AIDS was going to be adequately addressed in most of the world.

The protest I started this chapter with focused on "Epp = DEATH." The resulting disruption of consensual relations between AIDS community groups and state agencies set the stage for AIDS groups making limited but significant gains and for the articulation of the National AIDS Strategy. These struggles led to gains but were combined with a new regulatory strategy to contain AIDS organizing. While valuable time was wasted on these discussions, this strategy embodied important gains in access to treatment information and representation for PLWA/HIVs, as well as developing a new neoliberal strategy of "consultation" and "participation" for managing AIDS groups. Amid these unequal social power relations, state agencies defined this process of "consultation" and "partnership" (Kinsman 1997).

Aside from a commitment to include PLWA/HIVS on all committees addressing AIDS, there was also support for setting up a treatment information registry, which would provide PLWA/HIVs and their doctors with vital information on possible treatments. This was pushed for in particular by AAN! Despite the bureaucratic and professional nightmare created around the establishment of the registry, it was housed eventually at CATIE which grew out of the Treatment Information Exchange (TIE) Project of AAN! and provided a major treatment information resource for PLWA/HIVs (McCaskell 2017; Brown 2017; Hosein 2017).

Simultaneously and interwoven with this wave of AIDS activism there was an explosion of organizing by groups of people affected by AIDS/HIV beyond gay men, including organizing by women (Taylor 2017; Allen 2017) people of colour (Bernard 2017; Falconer 2017; Mohamed 2017; Stewart 2017) and Indigenous people, sex workers, drug users, prisoners (Barnett 2017) and in relation to the blood supply, including by hemophiliacs. This expanded the social and political response to AIDS to address gender relations and women, racism and colonialism, the prisons and the blood supply (Dryden 2015). Again we are reminded that to fully address the social impact of AIDS/HIV we need to view it as a condensation of social relations, including relations of class, racialization, and state. This led to the emergence of specific groups (including ASOs) that addressed these specific needs, funded by the Ontario AIDS Bureau and other state agencies. This includes groups like the African and Caribbean Council on HIV/AIDS in Ontario. At the same time all too often addressing these concerns as central to AIDS politics was forgotten in more mainstream ASOs.

Some AIDS groups also began to address poverty and class relations, as so many PLWA/HIVs were living in poverty, or were thrown into poverty after their diagnosis. George Smith and Eric Mykhalovskiy explored the unpaid "hooking up work" people have to do to access social assistance and how this work is affected by people's different class, gender, and racialized social locations (Mykhalovskiy and Smith 1994; Mykhalovskiy 2017). This focus on the need to address poverty and class has unfortunately not been consistently carried forward in AIDS organizing, with many ASOs coming to be dominated by white, middle-class perspectives. The notion of "hooking-up work" has been extended into explorations of the health work that PLWA/HIVs and others have to engage in to manage and produce their own health (Mykhalovskiy and McCoy 2002; Mykhalovskiy 2008). This view preserves the activity and agency of PLWA/HIVs and also makes visible people's skills and knowledge that can be useful in developing capacities for health from below.

One area where relations of class affect PLWA/HIVs is in accessing expensive treatments when most people do not have access to drug plans. This exposes a major limitation of the supposed universal health-care "system" in Canada, since getting needed drugs and treatments into the bodies of people who need them is seldom covered. AAN! waged a major campaign against the NDP government in Ontario in the early to mid-1990s that included meetings, an occupation of the health minister's office, and the threat to burn Premier Bob Rae in effigy in the streets of Toronto. This persistent activism created the Trillium Drug Plan, which provided access not only to AIDS/HIV drugs but to other drugs needed by people in catastrophic situations (Southin 2017; Brown 2017). In Quebec campaigning by ACT UP Montreal and other groups led to funding for treatments and for coverage under pharmacare in 1995 (Hendricks and LeBoeuf 2017). In other jurisdictions, struggle led to different funding arrangements. The federal/provincial division of labour in state formation on health funding and support does not guarantee people who need it funding for necessary treatments.

By the mid-1990s, however, state management of AIDS groups through funding and regulations was largely successful, and the wave of AIDS activism subsided as the new "drug cocktails" became available and some of the urgency of the AIDS crisis seemed to lessen. This shifted ASOs further away from "health from below" and back to reliance on medical and other middle-class "experts" and professionals, especially as the terrain of treatment became more complex. Some who had educated themselves in medical discourse were able to become part of a new "expert" strata, while many of those who were on the boards of directors of ASOs were part of the professional and managerial middle class. For those groups tied into gay community formation, this was also related to the emergence of a new white middle-class elite who came to speak for the "community," to project their interests as the "community" interests, and in some respects to stand over the working class, people of colour, and poorer people in queer communities (Kinsman 2016, 2017b; Higgins 2011).

Hopefully this brief and selective sketch of early AIDS organizing and activism allows for a better grasp of where we have come from and provides some grounding for how activism has been and can be useful in our historical present. I now move to explore how remembering these activist histories can assist AIDS activists in our current struggles.

## Current AIDS Organizing, Neoliberalism, and Capitalist Globalization

The current context of public policy formation on AIDS/HIV is shaped by the hegemony of neoliberalism and capitalist globalization and the broader attacks on working-class, poor, and oppressed people they are producing. These policies have a major impact on health funding, social assistance policies, drug policies, and more. There is a need to defend social funding, and to forge alliances with anti-poverty groups and with health-care and social assistance workers who are also opposed to these cuts. This is also why AIDS organizing needs to include a central challenge to neoliberal capitalism in Canada and on a global scale. At the same time that there is an urgent need for activism on these questions, ASOs have largely been successfully managed and moved in very non-activist directions, while some groups are experiencing important threats to their funding. While current activism on AIDS is at a low level, it needs to be developed extensively. Beginning to undertake activist initiatives in these areas, even on a small scale, will play a part in rebuilding an AIDS activist movement. This new activism also needs to face the changing nature of the epidemic that has been described in this book. Here I address some aspects of neoliberalism and current responses to AIDS, suggesting ways that the history of activism described earlier is still relevant and necessary, and can still be very effective.

Central to neoliberalism has been the tearing apart of the social wage and the "welfare state" and the forms of social solidarity built around them. These are also residues of the struggles of people in the past, even though these services have been delivered to people in bureaucratic and disempowering ways. Cuts to social programs, social assistance, and health care directly affect PLWA/HIVs and the communities of people affected by AIDS/HIV. One example is the major cuts and shifts in social assistance policies to PLWA/HIVs and many others. For instance, in Ontario there are medical reviews directed at those who receive Ontario Disability Support Program (ODSP) benefits who are deemed to be only "temporarily disabled," including people living with AIDS/HIV (OCAP 2015). These reviews can result in people being pushed off ODSP, which should be of concern to AIDS groups. In Ontario there were official suggestions to merge ODSP into Ontario Works (basic social assistance, which provides significantly less support), which could have a devastating impact on people living with disabilities (OCAP 2014). There is a need for AIDS groups to join with anti-poverty groups in opposing these reviews and cuts. AIDS groups need to develop a consistent anti-poverty activist approach and alliances with such groups as the Ontario Coalition Against Poverty (OCAP). It is important to avoid being trapped within a defensive strategy of defending what we used to have, but to both expand these services and to challenge the social form of these programs so that people have more control over their health and lives.

In this context there have been significant shifts in the funding and regulation of AIDS groups. The first was to merge funding for AIDS/HIV and hepatitis C, which is being expanded to include all "blood-borne infections." As discussed in this book, while this can be useful, it can also mean that the specificities of addressing AIDS/HIV needs and concerns may be undermined. This is part of the new state focus on "integration" of services and programs. Part of its purpose is to promote cost cutting and to provide more services that are not provided directly by the state. There have also been important tensions between how "integration" is used within more community-based AIDS groups and by state funding and regulatory agencies (Mykhalovskiy et al. 2009). This can have a major differential impact on AIDS groups. Larger AIDS groups may be able to deal with this more easily than smaller and more focused groups that already receive insufficient funding to carry out their activities. This can seriously harm smaller AIDS groups that address the needs of people of colour, a point that was raised by participants at a conference on AIDS organizing in Toronto in October 2014.[4] Regarding "integration" we need to ask whose integration, and integration on whose terms.

Neoliberalism focuses on cutting back on social funding but also increases funding and support for "law and order" and for disciplining workers and the poor. This has included opposition to the distribution of clean needles and safe injection sites. Neoliberal approaches worked over and undermined community and social responsibility for engaging in safe practices developed by earlier AIDS activism to focus instead on individual responsibility, and especially on the individual responsibility of the HIV-positive person. This opened the door for the growing criminalization of people living with HIV (at least 181 cases since 1989) and for Supreme Court decisions moving in this direction, as has been detailed in chapters in this book (also see Mykhalovskiy, Betteridge, and McLay 2010; Mykhalovskiy and Betteridge 2012; Mykhalovskiy 2011). This criminalization, as mentioned previously, often has a class and racialized dimension (Mykhalovskiy et al. 2016). The stigmatization, isolation, and lack of adequate treatments facing HIV-positive people in prisons points to many of the problems with the prison complex and is one reason why many AIDS activists working on prison issues are also prison abolitionists (Fink 2015).

Opposition to this criminalization of PLWA/HIVs is central to current AIDS activism. The criminalization of PLWA/HIVs builds on the construction of some PLWA/HIVs as "bad" or "irresponsible" PLWA/HIVs who do not follow medical regulation, are "non-compliant" with treatments, and do not always tell their partners they are HIV+ (Kinsman 1996; Mykhalovskiy, McCoy, and Bresalier 2004). On the other hand, "responsible" PLWA/HIVs follow medical regulation, are compliant with their treatments, always disclose their HIV status, and don't cause other problems for state and medical officials. As was demonstrated in earlier AIDS activism, it is vital to break down this distinction between "good" and "bad" PLWA/HIVs and in opposing this focus on the individual PLWA/HIV as the "criminal," to push for a return to a more collective and social responsibility for safer practices.

On a global scale, capitalist globalization and various "free trade" agreements have imposed structural adjustment programs on people in the "Global South" while making it easier for capital to move around the world (McNally 2006). Pharmaceutical corporations that will release and sell their drugs only if they can make a profit have led to many people in the "Global South" being denied access to treatments that can prolong their lives. The irrationality of the capitalist organization of treatment research and delivery is clear when people who cannot afford these drugs are left to die in the "Global South." The Trans-Pacific Partnership would have made it even more difficult for people to access generic drugs and would have denied many people in the "Global South," and poorer people, access to badly needed treatments. While some health and AIDS groups have spoken out against this denial of access (Global Treatment Access Group 2013), AIDS groups more generally need protest such agreements and act to create the conditions for expanded treatment access for people in the "Global South," defying the profit motivation of the pharmaceutical corporations. This activism continues the spirit of the 1989 Montreal Manifesto.

In order to effectively challenge neoliberalism and "health from above," we require not simply lobbying and polite meetings with state, corporate, and professional officials but a return to grassroots activism and building alliances with other communities and movements in the new contexts we face. This involves resisting bureaucratization and "professionalization," strategies of "consultation" and "partnership," and state and professional forms of regulation. As much as possible, this requires a commitment to grass roots activism and organizing. Given the low level of current AIDS activism and mobilization, we need to start with smaller initiatives that begin to move us in the direction of remaking an AIDS activist movement. Some of the direct action tactics that I described earlier will be useful in the current contexts we face, but organizing needs to be always related to the concrete social relations of struggle we are engaged in – the social forces lined up against us as well as the social composition of struggle we can mobilize (Kinsman 2006). The effigy burnings and die-ins mentioned earlier will therefore not always be effective in pushing the struggle forward. At the same time, AIDS ACTION NOW! did a highly successful banner drop during the 2016 Pride parade in Toronto directed at the Ontario premier against the criminalization of people living with HIV infection (Greyson 2016). Like with the demonstration and effigy burning in 1988 with which I started this chapter, there remain ways to actively withdraw our consent from, and to challenge, state and professional regulation in the present to bring about gains for the communities of people most affected by AIDS/HIV.

We need to strategize ways to resist cuts and get badly needed funding and resources, while avoiding strategies of regulation and containment. Clearly some service-oriented groups require social resources for the important work they do, and require state funding. The trick is to get this funding with as few strings attached as possible. Other smaller and more activist groups can survive, as AIDS ACTION NOW! does, without state funding. We need to open up discussion on these questions. For instance, groups need to start weighing the benefits and limitations of state funding. If the imposed limits are too high, perhaps state funding should be refused and other sources of funding located. If state funding must be accepted, strategies to more collectively resist state regulation need to be developed. This requires critically addressing state and class relations as central to the social response to AIDS.

Remembering our earlier histories of AIDS organizing which I focused on earlier in this chapter is therefore crucial for AIDS activism in the present. It is only by resisting the social organization of forgetting and remembering our own resistance that we can rebuild badly needed AIDS activism in the current situations we face. As mentioned, this activist project requires holding together in our organizing working within, against, and beyond state and capitalist relations (Holloway 2005, 2016). It means not getting trapped into playing by their rules within ruling relations but also entails resisting these rules and policies and building alternatives to them. This requires an activist direction for shifting from the practices of "health from above" towards a "health from below" that meets the needs of people affected by AIDS/HIV and all oppressed and exploited people.

## NOTES

1   This conference was co-sponsored by the Canadian Public Health Association, the Federal Centre for AIDS, and the Canadian AIDS Society.
2   These are designated with the name of the person interviewed, and all can be located at the AAHP website, https://www.aidsactivisthistory.ca/interviews.html.
3   On social forms see Corrigan and Sayer (1985) and Holloway (2005). Social forms are not "natural" and they all have a social and historical character and can therefore be socially transformed.
4   This was at a conference titled Where Do We Go from Here? AIDS Organizing, Services, Bureaucracy, and the State, held in Toronto on 17 October 2014. Information on the conference and some of the presentations can be found at Where Do We Go from Here?, http://aidsorganizing.ca/.

## REFERENCES

AIDS Activist History Project (AAHP). 2017. https://aidsactivisthistory.ca/.
Allan, R. 2017. Interview transcript. Nova Scotia. https://aidsactivisthistory.files.wordpress.com/2016/06/aahp_-_robert_allan.pdf.

Allen, J. 2017. Interview transcript. Nova Scotia. https://aidsactivisthistory
    .files.wordpress.com/2016/06/aahp_-_jane_allen.pdf.
Banner, R. 2017. Interview transcript. Vancouver. https://aidsactivisthistory
    .files.wordpress.com/2016/06/aahp_-_richard_banner.pdf.
Bannerji, H. 1995. *Thinking Through: Essays on Feminism, Marxism and Anti-
    Racism.* Toronto: Women's Press.
Barnett, J. 2017. Interview transcript. Toronto. https://aidsactivisthistory.files
    .wordpress.com/2016/06/aahp_-_julia_barnett.pdf.
Bernard, K. 2017. Interview transcript. Halifax. https://aidsactivisthistory
    .files.wordpress.com/2016/06/aahp-kim-bernard1.pdf.
Brandt, A. 1987. *No Magic Bullet: A Social History of Venereal Disease in the
    United States since 1880.* Oxford: Oxford University Press.
Brown, G. 2017. Interview transcript. Toronto. https://aidsactivisthistory.files
    .wordpress.com/2016/06/aahp_-_glen_brown.pdf.
Corrigan, P., and D. Sayer. 1981. "How the Law Rules? Variations on Some
    Themes in Karl Marx." In *Law, State and Society,* edited by B. Fryer, 21–53.
    London: Croom Helm.
– 1985. *The Great Arch: English State Formation as Cultural Revolution.* Oxford:
    Basil Blackwell.
Craik, P. 2017. Interview transcript. Vancouver. https://aidsactivisthistory
    .files.wordpress.com/2016/06/aahp_-_paul_craik.pdf.
Drucker, P. 2015. *Warped: Gay Normality and Queer Anticapitalism.* Chicago:
    Haymarket Books.
Dryden, O. 2015. "'A Queer Too Far': Blackness, 'Gay Blood,' and Transgressive
    Possibilities." In *Disrupting Queer Inclusion: Canadian Homonationalisms
    and the Politics of Belonging,* edited by O. Dryden and S. Lenon, 116–32.
    Vancouver: UBC Press.
Epstein, S. 1998. *Impure Science: AIDS Activism and the Politics of Knowledge.*
    Berkeley: University of California Press.
Falconer, D. 2017. Interview transcript. Toronto. https://aidsactivisthistory
    .files.wordpress.com/2016/11/aahp-dionne-falconer.pdf.
Fink, M. 2015. "Don't Be a Stranger Now: Queer Exclusions, Decarceration,
    and HIV/AIDS." In *Disrupting Queer Inclusion: Canadian Homonationalisms
    and the Politics of Belonging,* edited by O. Dryden and S. Lenon, 150–68.
    Vancouver: UBC Press.
Frankenburg, R. 1993. *White Women, Race Matters: The Social Construction
    of Whiteness.* Minneapolis: University of Minnesota Press.
Global Treatment Access Group. 2013. "Don't Trade Away Health: Brief
    to Canada's Minister of International Trade regarding the Trans-Pacific
    Partnership Negotiations and Access to Medicines." http://www.aidslaw

.ca/site/wp-content/uploads/2014/05/GTAG-TPP_MedAccessBrief-
July2013-ENG.pdf.

Greyson, J. 2016. "Wynnetario." https://vimeo.com/174574621.

Guinan, D. 2017. Interview transcript. Vancouver. https://aidsactivisthistory.
files.wordpress.com/2016/06/aahp_-_dan_guinan.pdf.

Haug, F. 1992. *Beyond Female Masochism: Memory Work and Politics*. London:
Verso.

Hendricks, M., and R. LeBoeuf. 2017. Interview transcript. Montreal. https://
aidsactivisthistory.files.wordpress.com/2016/10/aahp-michael-hendricks-
and-renc3a9-leboeuf-eng.pdf.

Higgins, R. 2011. "La Régulation Sociale de l'Homosexualité: De la Répression
Policière a la Normalisation." In *La Régulation Sociale des Minorités Sexuelles:
L'inquiétude de la Différence*, edited by P. Corriveau, and V. Daust, 67–102.
Quebec: Presses de l'Université du Québec.

Holloway, J. 2005. *Change the World without Taking Power: The Meaning of
Revolution Today*. London: Pluto.

– 2016. *In, Against and Beyond Capitalism: The San Francisco Lectures*. Oakland,
CA: PM.

Hosein, S. 2017. Interview transcript. Toronto. https://aidsactivisthistory.files
.wordpress.com/2016/06/aahp_-_sean_hosein.pdf.

Kaleta, J. 2017. Interview transcript. Vancouver. https://aidsactivisthistory
.files.wordpress.com/2016/06/aahp_-_janis_kaleta.pdf.

Kinsman, G. 1996. "'Responsibility' as a Strategy of Governance: Regulating
People Living with AIDS and Lesbians and Gay Men in Ontario." *Economy
and Society* 25 (3): 393–409. https://doi.org/10.1080/03085149600000021.

– 1997. "Managing AIDS Organizing: 'Consultation,' 'Partnership,' and
'Responsibility' as Strategies of Regulation." In *Organizing Dissent: Contemporary Social Movements in Theory and Practice*, edited by William Carroll,
2nd ed., 213–39. Toronto: Garamond.

– 2006. "Mapping Social Relations of Struggle: Activism, Ethnography, Social
Organization." In *Sociology for Changing the World: Social Movements/Social
Research*, edited by Caelie Frampton et al., 133–56. Halifax: Fernwood
Publishing.

– 2016. "From Resisting Police Raids to Charter Rights: Queer and AIDS
Organizing in the 1980s." In *A World to Win: Contemporary Social Movements
and Counter-Hegemony*, edited by W. Carroll and K. Sarker, 209–32. Winnipeg:
ARP Books.

– 2017a. Interview transcript. Toronto. https://aidsactivisthistory.files
.wordpress.com/2016/06/aahp_-_gary_kinsman.pdf.

– 2017b. "Queer Resistance and Regulation in the 1970s: From Liberation to
Rights." In *We Still Demand! Redefining Resistance in Sex and Gender Struggles*,

edited by Patrizia Gentile, Gary Kinsman, and Pauline Rankin, 137–62. Vancouver: UBC Press.

Kinsman, G., and P. Gentile. 2010. *The Canadian War on Queers: National Security as Sexual Regulation.* Vancouver: UBC Press.

Kozachenko, J. 2017. Interview transcript. Vancouver. https://aidsactivist history.files.wordpress.com/2016/06/aahp_-_john_kozachenko.pdf.

McCaskell, T. 2016. *Queer Progress: From Homophobia to Homonationalism,* Toronto: Between the Lines.

– 2017. Interview transcript. Toronto. https://aidsactivisthistory.files .wordpress.com/2016/06/aahp_-_timmccaskell.pdf.

McNally, D. 2006. *Another World Is Possible: Globalization and Anti-Capitalism.* 2nd ed. Winnipeg: Arbeiter Ring.

Mohamed, A. 2017. Interview transcript. Toronto. https://aidsactivisthistory .files.wordpress.com/2016/10/readytobepostedaahp-anthony-mohamed.pdf.

Mykhalovskiy, E. 2008. "Beyond Decision Making: Class, Community Organizations and the Healthwork of People Living with HIV/AIDS. Contributions from Institutional Ethnographic Research." *Medical Anthropology: Cross-Cultural Studies in Health and Illness* 27 (2): 136–63. https://doi.org/10.1080/01459740802017363.

– 2011. "The Problem of 'Significant Risk': Exploring the Public Health Impact of Criminalizing HIV Non-disclosure." *Social Science & Medicine* 73 (5): 668–7. https://doi.org/10.1016/j.socscimed.2011.06.051.

Mykhalovskiy, E. 2017. Interview transcript. Toronto. https://aidsactivist history.files.wordpress.com/2016/06/aahp_-_eric_mykhalovskiy.pdf.

Mykhalovskiy, E., and G. Betteridge. 2012. "Who? What? Where? When? And with What Consequences? An Analysis of Criminal Cases of HIV Non-disclosure in Canada." *Canadian Journal of Law and Society* 27 (1): 31–53. https://doi.org/10.3138/cjls.27.1.031.

Mykhalovskiy, E., G. Betteridge, and D. McLay. 2010. *HIV Non-disclosure and the Criminal Law: Establishing Policy Options for Ontario.* Toronto: Ontario HIV Treatment Network.

Mykhalovskiy, E., and L. McCoy. 2002. "Troubling Ruling Discourses of Health: Using Institutional Ethnography in Community-Based Research." *Critical Public Health* 12 (1): 17–37. https://doi.org/10.1080/09581590110113286.

Mykhalovskiy, E., L. McCoy, and M. Bresalier. 2004. "Compliance/Adherence, HIV/AIDS and the Critique of Medical Power." *Social Theory & Health* 2 (4): 315–40. https://doi.org/10.1057/palgrave.sth.8700037.

Mykhalovskiy, E., et al. 2009. "Conceptualizing the Integration of HIV Treatment and Prevention: Findings from a Process Evaluation of a Community-Based, National Capacity-Building Intervention." *International*

*Journal of Public Health* 54 (3): 133–41. https://doi.org/10.1007/s00038-009-8078-5.

Mykhalovskiy, E., et al. 2016. "'Callous, Cold and Deliberately Duplicitous': Racialization, Immigration and the Representation of HIV Criminalization in Canadian Mainstream Newspapers." Available at SSRN: https://ssrn.com/abstract=2874409.

Mykhalovskiy, E., and G.W. Smith. 1994. *Getting Hooked Up: A Report on the Barriers People Living with HIV/AIDS Face Assessing Social Services*. Toronto: Ontario Institute for Studies in Education/CATIE.

Ng, R. 1996. *The Politics of Community Services: Immigrant Women, Class and the State*. Halifax: Fernwood.

Ontario Coalition Against Poverty (OCAP). 2014. "Wynne Government Backs Away from Plans to Merge ODSP and OW." http://update.ocap.ca/node/1147.

– 2015. "Official Raise the Rates Campaign Statement on ODSP Medical Reviews." http://www.ocap.ca/node/1225 (accessed June 2015).

Patton, C. 1985. *Sex and Germs: The Politics of AIDS*. Boston: South End.

– 1990. *Inventing AIDS*. New York: Routledge.

– 1996. *Fatal Advice: How Safe-Sex Education Went Wrong*. Durham, NC: Duke University Press.

Petty, M. 2017. Interview transcript. Nova Scotia. https://aidsactivisthistory.files.wordpress.com/2016/10/aahp-mary-petty1.pdf.

Smith, D. 1990. *Texts, Facts, and Femininity*. London: Routledge. https://doi.org/10.4324/9780203425022.

Smith, D., and S. Turner, eds. 2014. *Incorporating Texts into Institutional Ethnographies*. Toronto: University of Toronto Press.

Smith, E. 2017. Interview transcript. Nova Scotia. https://aidsactivisthistory.files.wordpress.com/2016/06/aahp_-_eric_smith.pdf.

Smith, G. 1995. "Accessing Treatments: Managing the AIDS Epidemic in Ontario." In *Knowledge, Experience and Ruling Relations: Studies in the Social Organization of Knowledge*, edited by Marie Campbell and Ann Manicom, 18–34. Toronto: University of Toronto Press. https://doi.org/10.3138/9781442657502-004.

– 2006. "Political Activist as Ethnographer." In *Sociology for Changing the World: Social Movements/Social Research*, edited by Caelie Frampton et al., 44–70. Halifax: Fernwood Publishing.

Southin, B. 2017. Interview transcript. Toronto. https://aidsactivisthistory.files.wordpress.com/2016/06/aahp_-_brent_southin.pdf.

Stewart, D. 2017. Interview transcript. Toronto. https://aidsactivisthistory.files.wordpress.com/2016/10/aahp-douglas-stewart.pdf.

Taylor, D. 2017. Interview transcript. Toronto. https://aidsactivisthistory.files
.wordpress.com/2016/06/aahp_-_darien_taylor.pdf.
Thompson, E.P. 1968. *The Making of the English Working Class*. Harmondsworth,
UK: Penguin Books.
Where Do We Go from Here? http://aidsorganizing.ca/.

# Conclusion

SUZANNE HINDMARCH, MICHAEL ORSINI,
AND MARILOU GAGNON

We began this collection by exploring the many meanings of "seeing red" in the context of HIV/AIDS politics and activism: from early activist mobilization in the face of state indifference (and sometimes outright hostility) to the people and populations most affected by HIV/AIDS, to Indigenous mobilization, to the cautious optimism of the early post-Harper years. We have suggested that these mobilizations, and the resulting complex interactions among PHAs, activists, ASOs, and multiple levels of government, work in combination with formal, top-down policy mechanisms to produce HIV/AIDS policy. Our understanding of "policy," then, is capacious and encompasses diverse actors: policy is not simply something that is done to PHAs, ASOs, and communities, but rather is intersubjectively created through our collective actions, interactions, and inaction. We all are, or have the potential to be, policy actors and agents of policy and political change.

This does not mean, of course, that all policy actors have equal power to shape HIV/AIDS policy. As contributors to this collection have shown, there are persistent inequities in whose voices and perspectives dominate the policy process, and in whose needs are most likely to be meaningfully addressed by federal, provincial, and ASO policies. This creates gaps, silences, exclusions, and a patchwork of policy interventions that have produced significant variation, across jurisdictions, populations, and sectors, in the extent and nature of service provision to PHAs. The result is an HIV/AIDS policy landscape characterized by persistent marginalization and inequity, in which we are still struggling, some thirty years into the epidemic, to meaningfully address the ultimate drivers of HIV that leave some people and communities, through complex processes of social exclusion, more vulnerable to HIV. At the same time, the policy landscape has evolved with medical advances in treatment and the resulting cohort of people aging with HIV; the emergence of PrEP and "treatment as prevention" strategies; resurgent social movement activism, including Indigenous and trans* activism; and with changing norms and laws relating to sex work, supervised injection sites, and other forms of harm reduction that are so critical to addressing the epidemic.

In this concluding chapter, we explore some of the challenges and opportunities that contributors have identified in this evolving policy landscape; draw out common themes of the collection; and discuss the implications of this analysis for policy actors. To be clear, our aim is not to propose definitive solutions to the myriad HIV-related policy challenges that have been explored in this collection. As is evident from the range of perspectives in this volume, even within "the" HIV/AIDS community there are deep disagreements about which policy interventions should be pursued, and about the extent to which activists ought to engage with, against, and beyond the state in seeking policy change. Nevertheless, all contributors share a commitment to HIV/AIDS policy that centres the needs, voices, and perspectives of those living with and most directly affected by HIV/AIDS, and it is this shared commitment that unites the diverse voices and analyses presented here. Reflecting the structure of the book, this concluding chapter explores themes and implications by level of analysis. We begin with populations, that is, the impact of policies "on the ground" for some of the people living with, vulnerable to, and affected by HIV/AIDS. We then explore what contributors suggest about how HIV/AIDS services currently work, and how they might be improved. Finally, we turn to the systems level to unpack the potential benefits and limitations of the conceptual and theoretical frameworks that structure HIV/AIDS policy and activism, as well as our analyses of this policy and activism.

## Populations

The "Populations" section asked how people and communities interact with, mobilize in response to, shape, and are shaped by policy decisions at "the point where [power] becomes capillary ... in its most regional forms and institutions ... [and] is embodied in techniques and acquires the material power to intervene, sometimes in violent ways" (Foucault 2003, 27–8).

In reading these population-level analyses, as well as the reflective chapters by Ibáñez-Carrasco and Rosenes, we were struck, first, by the persistent fragmentation of identities by state and service providers.

Policy variation across sectors, jurisdictions, and levels of government has created a landscape in which state and community-based providers require people to prioritize different aspects of their identity, and perform different aspects of self (Goffman 1959) in order to cobble together, as individuals or communities, a comprehensive set of support services. PHAs need to become "mess managers" (Duchesne, chapter 10), navigating a complex network of policies that structure services in such a way that addictions services are often separated from mental health services, which are distinct from HIV services, which in turn are separated from HCV services (Price, chapter 14), pregnancy services, and settlement services (Chulach, Gagnon, and Holmes, chapter 13). Despite a rhetorical commitment to the importance of comprehensive services that cut across silos, the very organizing of social services and health-care services reinforces these divisions. The resulting need to fragment, bracket, or prioritize various aspects of one's identity in order to receive services can significantly affect how and from whom PHAs are able to access services and care. This is perhaps especially acute for Indigenous populations, whose state-imposed identities, via the Indian Act, as "status" or "non-status," are a primary determinant of where and from whom Indigenous PHAs are able to access care (Gabel, Jackson, and Ryan, chapter 12). All of this can be understood as a manifestation of structural violence (Galtung 1969; Farmer 2003), but also, following Foucault, as a form of policy violence, in which individuals' complex, multifaceted identities are truncated, delegitimized, silenced, or erased in the course of seeking medical and social services. This violence is especially problematic for groups or collectivities that have also experienced the direct, material violence of colonialism, and state attempts to "civilize" them and their ways of knowing.

These contributions also point to the need to rethink the links between identity and HIV. Identities evolve and shift by location and life stage, including pregnancy, migration (Chulach, Gagnon, and Holmes, chapter 13), and aging (Gabel, Jackson, and Ryan, chapter 12). Further, as Prentice et al. suggest, the social meaning of Indigeneity, and of living with HIV as an Indigenous person, may be better understood as a journey, rather than a static, fixed identity. Similarly, Chulach, Gagnon, and Holmes highlight that being a refugee and living with HIV intersect in various ways during pregnancy. Furthermore, the stories featured in this chapter clearly show that identity is not defined by one fixed attribute – i.e., being a refugee, being HIV-positive, being a woman, being a mother, and so on. Yet there appears to be little room in dominant ways of thinking about HIV for approaches that contextualize an HIV diagnosis in this way. Instead, an HIV diagnosis is assumed to be transformative: it is expected to become central to an individual's identity and mobilize them to take charge of their illness, structuring their life around "managing" their HIV (and increasingly around maintaining an undetectable viral load not only for their own health, but to proactively "protect" the broader public health).

But as Duchesne observes in the context of trans* populations, because many people living with HIV confront multiple, intersecting forms of exclusion, their sero-status is not always the most salient aspect of their identity, nor is access to HIV-specific services always as pressing as the need for other forms of support, including income supports (Rosenes, chapter 7), housing, access to gender-confirming surgery (Duchesne, chapter 10), or food and transportation (Chulach, Gagnon, and Holmes, chapter 13). A singular focus on the "HIV-ness" of people's identities can then render less visible the complex, overlapping, and intersecting forms of social exclusion that produce barriers to service provision. At the same time, if they are not attuned to the particular needs and life circumstances of people living with HIV (PHAs), non-HIV-specific services can end up excluding PHAs from much-needed forms of care and support.

Furthermore, as McClelland, Guta, and Greenspan (chapter 9) suggest, even efforts to meaningfully centre people living with HIV in policy and program development via GIPA initiatives may depoliticize PHA identities, transforming PHAs into "resources" whose capacity must be "developed" in ways that support efficient, smoothly functioning services within neoliberal regimes, while leaving intact structural inequities. In other words, the PHA identities produced by GIPA are ones that, for McClelland, Guta, and Greenspan, are compliant with and deferential to the state, rather than facilitating more radical, oppositional expressions of identity. The "PHA voice" produced through these strategies may not reflect the diverse voices and perspectives of many people living with HIV. A similar point is made by Ibáñez-Carrasco, who provocatively argues that the "biomoral imperative" of public health aims to produce compliant, depoliticized, and deradicalized PHAs, rather than enabling expressions of resistance and "radical disability." In sum, HIV/AIDS policy constructs a set of behavioural expectations for the "good PHA," most of which emphasize individual self-regulation rather than systems and structural transformation, and require the performance of "compliant," "adherent" selves.

Contributors to this section also demonstrate that many marginalized social groups are always/already deeply enmeshed in and entangled with the state. For the refugee women discussed by Chulach, Gagnon, and Holmes (chapter 13), immigration policies requiring mandatory HIV testing mean that even before they enter Canada, these women are monitored and surveilled by the Canadian state; but this does not always result in transition to appropriate support services upon arrival in Canada. As Prentice et al. show in chapter 11, in the case of Indigenous women, entanglement with the state includes pathologizing policies and practices that reproduce unequal power relations that can actually increase vulnerability to HIV, while simultaneously failing to recognize the strengths of Indigenous women and communities.

Implicit in these analyses, and as explicitly discussed by Kilty (chapter 3) in her consideration of carceral syndemics, syndemic conditions play a significant role in, first, enmeshing some people and communities in state relations of surveillance, domination, and control long prior to an HIV diagnosis, and second, heightening their vulnerability to HIV. Syndemics entail "the interaction between two or more diseases [or conditions], which by the nature of that interaction, serves to elevate negative health outcomes … The term syndemic also recognizes the influence of variables such as poverty, health disparity, and stress on the course of illness" (Eisenberg and Blank 2014). In sum, conditions, including mental health challenges, substance use, childhood adversity and abuse, interact with other forms of structural and policy violence to heighten HIV vulnerability and exacerbate the impact of HIV-related illness. While conceptually similar to social determinants, structural violence and structural stigma (Gagnon and Vézina, chapter 2), the notion of "syndemics" is useful when considering how policies are experienced by people and communities "on the ground" precisely because it draws attention to the *interactive*, multiple, and simultaneous forms of vulnerability and exclusion that drive the HIV epidemic, and that produce persistent, severe inequity, including inequitable access to care and support.

What emerges through these analyses is the need for policies that recognize the whole person, that are strengths- rather than deficit-based (Prentice et al., chapter 11), that enable peer as well as professional and paraprofessional support (Price, chapter 14), and that are premised on an understanding that identities are multiple, overlapping, and complex. For academics, practitioners, and policymakers alike, these analyses reaffirm the importance of intersectional analyses that recognize the interlocking nature of oppression, and that move us beyond a simplistic, reductive focus on "risk groups" that are defined by and reduced to a single identity marker (gayness, blackness, etc.), and then treated as categorically distinct, non-overlapping, and internally homogeneous.

Beyond intersectionality, these chapters illuminate that in the context of the Canadian settler colonial state, there is a need for decolonizing approaches that are grounded in Indigenous ways of knowing. These may pose more fundamental challenges to state-organized categories of and knowledge about Indigenous PHAs (Gabel, Jackson, and Ryan, chapter 12; Prentice et al., chapter 11). Similarly, the ways in which state policies produce, regulate and pathologize some populations also indicate, for some contributors, the importance of radical modes of community expression "against the state," in opposition to public health paternalism (Ibáñez-Carrasco, chapter 4; Kinsman, chapter 15).

Through these contributions, we additionally see that the challenges faced by HIV-affected and vulnerable populations are produced, in large part, by fragmented service provision, itself a result of a complicated patchwork of federal and provincial policies that vary by sector and by region.

### Services

This brings us to the book's second section, "Services," which examined trends and challenges in service provision, mainly from the "middle level" of community-based service providers who often find themselves caught between competing needs and demands of state funders and of the PHA communities that providers (and the state) ostensibly exist to support. The section reflects the growing attention to aging with HIV, as well as the move towards approaching HIV as an episodic disability.

As Rosenes (chapter 7) powerfully illustrates, successfully living and aging with HIV is still heavily dependent on individual good fortune, rather than comprehensive state supports: those whose employment provides access to private long-term disability and other insurance coverage are better able to mitigate the financial burdens associated with HIV, and access to jobs that provide this coverage is, in turn, significantly influenced by one's socio-economic status. As Porch and Yates (chapter 8) illustrate, people without access to private coverage, or whose HIV-related illnesses create gaps in their education and work histories, can find themselves caught in a spiral of poverty, illness, and limited social assistance. Income supports, including essential medicines coverage, vary significantly by province; they are often exacerbated by punitive policies that claw back earnings of people who are living on social assistance.

In part, this patchwork of policies is an inevitable result of Canada's federal system, in which considerable power and responsibility for social policy is devolved to the provinces. The resulting federal-provincial coordination challenges are complex and somewhat beyond the scope of this book, but they do point to the need to shift our attention somewhat from an exclusive, privileged focus on the federal government as a locus of power and towards provincial, municipal, and regional forms of authority (Boychuk 1998; Béland and Daigneault 2015; Rice and Prince 2013), as well as to the individualizing, responsibilizing nature of self-governance that is characteristic of neoliberalism. This does not mean ignoring what is happening at the federal level: as Murzin and Furlotte (chapter 5) argue, this policy patchwork also reflects a continued lack of federal leadership on essential medicines pricing and coverage, a federal seniors' strategy, integrated strategies to support healthy aging, and other policy interventions that would ensure equitable service coverage and access for all PHAs, regardless of their province of residence. It does mean, however, looking beyond the federal government to the places and spaces where, in practice, innovative policies, practices, and programs often originate.

For example, in spite of and perhaps in response to this lack of policy coherence, Greenspan shows that community-based service providers are increasingly being asked to help governments understand HIV through intensified monitoring and evaluation. These evaluation techniques reflect a growing pressure to demonstrate effectiveness, efficiency, and returns on investment in a climate of neoliberal austerity. But Greenspan's analysis, read in conjunction with Murzin and Furlotte and Porch and Yates' discussion of policy fragmentation and incoherence, also suggests the extent to which, when it comes to HIV policy, "seeing like a state" (Scott 1998) poses challenges for funders and government policymakers alike. That is, in spite of increased surveillance, monitoring, and data collection, there still appears to be a lack of state knowledge and understanding about how HIV policies are implemented and experienced at the community level – and more fundamentally, an underlying tension between the forms of knowledge that are *recognized* as knowledge by state versus community-based actors. Both the fragmentation of policies into discrete categories, sectors, and jurisdictions, and efforts to collect increasingly fine-grained, detailed monitoring and evaluation data, reflect and reproduce an approach to HIV in which complexity becomes a problem to be managed, and a barrier to comprehensive knowledge about, surveillance of, and control over HIV. Moreover, a focus on surveillance and the need for better data to reflect the changing demographics of the epidemic can divert attention from persistent structural problems, such as poverty and social exclusion, which are more challenging for governments to address.

The lack of pan-Canadian policy coherence, and tensions between the forms of knowledge and evidence valued by community-based service providers and their government funders, point to a larger set of questions about how, at a systems and conceptual level, we should understand HIV/AIDS and policy responses to the epidemic.

**Systems**

This brings us to the line of inquiry taken up in the "Systems" section, where contributors explored how legal, political, and economic systems structure the HIV response and construct different categories of PHAs. These contributors show that, first, notwithstanding a potential move towards integration of HIV into a larger sexually transmitted and blood-borne infections (STBBI) context, the HIV response continues to be marked by exceptionally stigmatizing practices, including criminalization (Gagnon and Vézina, chapter 2) and punitive carceral practices (Kilty, chapter 3). PHAs, especially those marked as "deviant" because of other stigmatized social identities, modes of drug consumption (Ibáñez-Carrasco, chapter 4; Kilty, chapter 3), or failure to adhere to hegemonic public health "safer sex codes" (Ibáñez-Carrasco, chapter 4) are still constructed as Other, in need of state surveillance, monitoring, and regulation, but not deserving of full inclusion in mainstream social and political communities. The concepts of structural stigma (Gagnon and Vézina, chapter 2) and the iatrogenic effects of health policy (Ibáñez-Carrasco, chapter 4) offer two powerful new analytical frameworks for understanding these enduring exceptionalisms and the fragmented policies and selves that they produce, even as they erase or render less visible their many problematic effects.

What emerges from these analyses, therefore, is an imperative to move beyond the silos and exclusions produced by some forms of exceptionalism (such as criminalization of HIV non-disclosure), while advancing the human rights of the people and communities most

vulnerable to HIV – who are vulnerable, in large part, precisely because of these punitive legal and policy regimes. Elliott's call (chapter
1) to treat HIV as an exceptional human rights and social justice challenge, one that highlights the pernicious effects of social exclusion and
socio-economic inequities, is a forceful reminder of the importance of
heeding the lessons of HIV/AIDS organizing. For Elliott, this means
preserving the "human rights core" of HIV/AIDS activism. In this
analysis, one largely shared by Kilty, and Gagnon and Vézina, the law
can and should be used to extend and deepen the rights of PHAs and
populations disproportionately affected by HIV, and engaging with the
state on legal terrain remains a vital task of HIV/AIDS activism.

Kinsman (chapter 15), while also urging us to remember the lessons
of early HIV/AIDS activism, is less persuaded that the enduring socio-
economic drivers of HIV can be meaningfully addressed by working
in and within the state; rather, he calls for resistance to and transformation of state-civil society relations. This is an approach that would
have important implications for how we think about the role of ASOs,
and especially for the tensions inherent in their potential to both maintain and disrupt state-civil society relations. Despite radical beginnings
with ACT UP in Montreal and Vancouver and AIDS Action Now! in
Toronto, the landscape of HIV/AIDS organizing is now dominated by
organizations that do not challenge state authority directly (and, not co-
incidentally, are increasingly reliant on increasingly scarce state funding). Yet this disruptive potential remains; for some it is a problem to be
managed, for others, a potential opportunity to be nurtured.

In these divergent perspectives of state–civil society relations in the
HIV/AIDS response, we see precisely the productive tensions, debates,
and multiple modes of community mobilization that have animated
HIV/AIDS activism from its earliest days, and that bring us to the
question: in light of the persistent challenges and limitations of HIV/
AIDS policies uncovered in this volume, how should we respond?

## Policy Research, Policy Action

Contributors to this book have suggested several potential paths for
policy research and action to address the emerging and the enduring
complexities of HIV.

With respect to research, as Mykhalovskiy and Rosengarten (2009,
188) argue, in the move towards evidence-based health policy, "evidence" has often been interpreted in narrow biomedical terms, or

reduced to simplistic quantitative metrics. This has "introduce[ed] a hierarchy of evidence that privileges ... in the realm of 'social' research, epidemiology and positivist social science." The contributors to this collection, though, suggest that both academics and policymakers need to pay greater attention to the importance of narratives as evidence. From the mess-managing trans* women in Duchesne's discussion (chapter 10), to the forms of tacit knowledge uncovered by Greenspan (chapter 6), to the artwork created by the women in Prentice et al (chapter 11), there is a need to recognize the voices, perspectives, and experiences of those who actually live with policies as valid, valuable, essential sources of evidence, not merely as add-ons to other, more legitimate forms of knowledge.

This in turn suggests a need to draw on research methods encompassing interviews, ethnography (Duchesne, chapter 10; Chulach, Gagnon, and Holmes, chapter 13), storytelling, photovoice, and sharing circles (Prentice et al., chapter 11; Gabel, Jackson, and Ryan, chapter 12), and of critical and decolonizing methodologies that destabilize some of the assumptions governing what we know about HIV. Some of the earliest work on HIV and intravenous drug use, for instance, recognized that in order to understand what was driving the epidemic in these communities, it was necessary to mobilize different kinds of knowledge. Ethnographic work with people who use drugs was helpful in describing the "risk environments" that supported unsafe drug-injecting practices (Rhodes 2002, 2009), and was instrumental in supporting the policy change that enabled supervised injection sites and other forms of harm reduction.

More broadly, and beyond mere research methods, it is clear that narratives, stories, emotions, and affect have been central to individuals' and communities' efforts to make sense of their lived experiences with HIV and HIV policy – and central to activist mobilization, which has been fuelled by grief, anger, empathy, love, and hope as much as, if not more than, by quantitative metrics demonstrating the impact of HIV. This raises very difficult questions about the meaning of evidence itself, and the role that emotions do and should play in policy development and advocacy. On the one hand, we are reminded that emotion-driven policy can be tremendously misguided and dangerous, as we have seen in punitive conservative approaches, rooted in fear and hatred of the Other, to drug use, sex work, and homosexuality. But an approach to evidence, activism, and policy that fails to wrestle with the emotional core of HIV/AIDS will overlook that, for people living with HIV, the meaning of HIV and the effectiveness of HIV-related policies cannot be extricated from what it *feels like* to live with HIV and HIV policies. And as Gould (2009) reminds us in her seminal study of ACT UP, it is virtually impossible to understand the history of radical AIDS activism unless one appreciates the role that emotions such as anger, shame and pride played in structuring a response to the unfolding epidemic. Moreover, appreciating the role of emotions and affect in the field of HIV means recognizing that there are no "good" and "bad" emotions at work: just as anger can be productive and empowering for PHAs, empathy and compassion can be mobilized in ways that reproduce problematic paternalistic assumptions about people's capacities and identities.

Finally, the collection as a whole also indicates the importance of interdisciplinary and intersectoral analysis that examines HIV from the perspective of disciplines including law, public health, political science, gender and feminist studies, social work, nursing and other health sciences, among others. Just as intersectional analysis supports investigation of multiple intersecting identities, so too do interdisciplinary efforts, which are necessarily collective, allow us to study HIV from multiple disciplinary viewpoints simultaneously.

## Policy Action

Following from these policy analyses, contributors have advanced several options for policy research and action. Some of these are specific policy prescriptions: reforms to income, pension, and other financial supports for PHAs (Rosenes, chapter 7; Murzin and Furlotte, chapter 5; Porch and Yates, chapter 8); reform of immigration HIV-testing policies and practices, and comprehensive, multidisciplinary services for pregnant women living with HIV (Chulach, Gagnon, and Holmes, chapter 13); development of strengths-based approaches grounded in Indigenous ways of knowing (Gabel, Jackson, and Ryan, chapter 12), that focus on HIV protective rather than HIV risk factors (Prentice et al., chapter 11); and harm reduction programming in prisons (Kilty, chapter 3). Others have focused less on specific policy reforms than the *nature* of those reforms: the need for a rights-based approach to policymaking that meaningfully advances social and economic rights and reduces structural inequities (Elliott, chapter 1); or for critical reappraisal of how GIPA principles are implemented in ways that may silence rather than amplify PHA voices (McClelland, Guta, and Greenspan, chapter 9).

We have seen some promising moves by the Liberal government elected in 2015, which may partially undo the punitive HIV-related policies that had activists "seeing red" under Harper. These include restoring the Harper government's cuts to refugee health benefits; rebuilding the federal government's nation-to-nation relationship with Indigenous communities (though this commitment has been more evident in rhetoric than in practice); and a more supportive stance on harm reduction. Yet significant change is still needed, and the mere election of a non-Conservative government cannot undo the enduring structural drivers and inequities that have characterized the epidemic from the outset. As the history of the HIV/AIDS response has taught us, such change is usually catalysed in large part by civil society mobilization. For some of our contributors, such as Kinsman (chapter 15), this means organizing against and beyond the state, mobilizing political communities capable of transforming state–civil society relations and building "health from below." For others, it means engaging with federal and provincial governments, pushing them to provide more and better support. Ultimately, we expect that a combination of both modes of organizing are needed; we cannot prescribe a single best mode of mobilization for policy change, which in any case is deeply dependent upon context.

Instead, we have sought to encourage a more expansive and inclusive dialogue about policy, one that encompasses diverse categories of policy actors from PHAs to academics to practitioners, and that explores policy design, implementation, and outcomes across multiple sectors, jurisdictions, and levels of government. We have sought to begin a conversation, recognizing that no single collection can represent all views and voices. We recognize, for example, that youth voices, the perspectives of ethno-racial communities and of Francophones are largely absent from this collection (though, to reiterate, we are cautious of simple, additive approaches to identity). Similarly, there are relatively few contributors from outside Ontario, and from smaller communities. The geographic overrepresentation of Ontario reflects, in part, that most of the largest HIV research institutes and ASOs are in Toronto and southern Ontario; this in turn reflects that in absolute numbers, the majority of people living with HIV in Canada live in this region. But we are also aware that knowledge, policies, and expertise are not simply produced in the centre and then exported to Canada's peripheries; readers must therefore be cautious in assuming that these analyses travel to, or represent the experiences of people living in cities and smaller communities, especially in the Atlantic provinces, the Prairies, and the North.

## Conclusion

We hope this collection will not be the last word about HIV policy in Canada, but will instead provide the grounds for further dialogue and deliberation, with PHAs' needs and perspectives at the centre of these discussions. We have sought to encourage discussion of policy outside the usual academic and government policy circles, and in so doing, to not only encourage a rethinking of HIV policy, but also to enlarge our conception of who can and should "count" as a policy actor.

Three decades into the epidemic, some have suggested that we are entering a period "after the exception" (Ingram 2013), when governments no longer regard HIV as an urgent priority requiring an exceptional response and funding; instead, the HIV response is being folded into neoliberal discourses of austerity and resource scarcity. As this collection has attempted to demonstrate, such complacency is sorely misplaced. We must continue to "see red": to recognize the social and structural inequities that underpin and facilitate the spread of HIV, and the persistently inadequate policy response to these inequities. Red, in addition to signifying the anger that characterized early AIDS activism, also symbolizes passion – a word that, in its original sense, refers to bodily suffering both caused by and borne by love. It is a word and a sentiment rarely associated with public policy. But the persistent limitations, exclusions, and gaps in HIV policy compel us all, as policy actors, to recover and rediscover this sense of passion and to channel it towards creating a more comprehensive, compassionate, effective, and ethical response to HIV.

REFERENCES

Béland, D., and P.M. Daigneault, eds. 2015. *Welfare Reform in Canada: Provincial Social Assistance in Comparative Perspective*. Toronto: University of Toronto Press.
Boychuk, G.W. 1998. *Patchworks of Purpose: The Development of Provincial Social Assistance Regimes in Canada*. Montreal: McGill-Queen's University Press.

Eisenberg, Marlene M., and Michael B. Blank. 2014. "The Syndemic of the Triply Diagnosed: HIV Positives with Mental Illness and Substance Abuse or Dependence." *Clinical Research in HIV/AIDS* 1 (1): 1006.

Farmer, Paul. 2003. *Pathologies of Power: Health, Human Rights and the New War on the Poor*. Berkeley: University of California Press.

Foucault, Michel. 2003. *"Society Must Be Defended": Lectures at the Collège de France 1975–1976*. Translated by D. Macey. New York: Picador. Original edition, 1997.

Galtung, Johan. 1969. "Violence, Peace and Peace Research." *Journal of Peace Research* 6 (3): 167–91. https://doi.org/10.1177/002234336900600301.

Goffman, Erving. 1959. *The Presentation of Self in Everyday Life*. New York: Anchor Books.

Gould, Deborah B. 2009. *Moving Politics: Emotion and ACT UP's Fight against AIDS*. Chicago: University of Chicago Press. https://doi.org/10.7208/chicago/9780226305318.001.0001.

Ingram, Alan. 2013. "After the Exception: HIV/AIDS Beyond Salvation and Scarcity." *Antipode* 45 (2): 436–54. https://doi.org/10.1111/j.1467-8330.2012.01008.x.

Mykhalovskiy, Eric, and Marsha Rosengarten. 2009. "HIV/AIDS in Its Third Decade: Renewed Critique in Social and Cultural Analysis – An Introduction." *Social Theory & Health* 7 (3): 187–95. https://doi.org/10.1057/sth.2009.13.

Rhodes, Tim. 2002. "The 'Risk Environment': A Framework for Understanding and Reducing Drug-Related Harm." *International Journal on Drug Policy* 13 (2): 85–94. https://doi.org/10.1016/S0955-3959(02)00007-5.

Rhodes, Tim. 2009. "Risk Environments and Drug Harms: A Social Science for Harm Reduction Approach." *International Journal on Drug Policy* 20 (3): 193–201. https://doi.org/10.1016/j.drugpo.2008.10.003.

Rice, James J., and Michael J. Prince. 2013. *Changing Politics of Canadian Social Policy*. 2nd ed. Toronto: University of Toronto Press.

Scott, James C. 1998. *Seeing like a State: How Certain Schemes to Improve the Human Condition Have Failed*. New Haven: Yale University Press.

# Contributors

**Elizabeth Benson** was diagnosed on 12 March 1995 and connected with organizations that provided her support services. In April 1995 she applied to be on the Board of Directors for the Positive Women's Network and was there for four years, where she learned to stand up and give voice to health needs for Aboriginal women living with HIV. In 2008, Elizabeth's active voice was recognized by the Canadian Association for Health Research with a Community Scholar Certificate. To further her involvement in the HIV community she participated in several HIV/AIDS research projects for better health care of Aboriginal women living with HIV. Elizabeth is from the Gitxsan territory in northern BC. Her name is Mountain Grass in the House of Ten Mountains. Her ancestral home is Gitanyow, north of Kispiox, BC.

**Teresa Chulach**, RN, NP, PhD, is a nurse practitioner working with individuals living with or at risk of HIV, hepatitis C, and/or substance use disorder in Ottawa, Canada. Her specific research and clinical interests include the health of marginalized populations with a specific emphasis on social justice and equity. She has devoted particular attention to the concepts of culture and place and how they influence health and health-care delivery. Her doctoral work focused on the lived experience of pregnancy among HIV-positive refugees arriving in Canada and used a critical postcolonial and intersectional lens. She has collaborated with First Nations and Inuit Health Branch (Canada) in guideline development, as well as municipal and territorial organizations in the management of health-care delivery. She has presented her work at local, national, and international conferences. Within her clinical practice she is actively involved in teaching and mentoring.

**Natalie Duchesne** holds a doctorate from the Centre for Interdisciplinary Studies in Society and Culture of Concordia University. Her PhD research examined how trans people interact with public policies, with a special focus on housing, social assistance, and migration. Today, Natalie works as consultant at Connect2Knowledge.

**Richard Elliott**, BA Honours (Queen's), LLB (Osgoode), LLM (Osgoode), is a lawyer and the executive director of the Canadian HIV/AIDS Legal Network, engaged in research, education, and advocacy for the human rights of people living with or particularly affected by HIV. He appears frequently in the media as an expert and advocate on HIV and human rights. He has written numerous reports, papers, and articles on a range of such issues, appeared before legislative committees, served as an expert resource to UN agencies, taught or lectured at several law schools, and presented extensively on HIV and human rights across the country and internationally. He served for six years on the Ministerial Council on HIV/AIDS (the advisory body to Canada's minister of health), and as a member of the Technical Advisory Group of the Global Commission on HIV and the Law and a member of the Expert Advisory Group to the UN Secretary General's High-Level Panel on Access to Medicines. He is a member of the International Advisory Committee of the International Centre for Human Rights and Drug Policy. He is the recipient of a Queen Elizabeth II Diamond Jubilee Medal for his contributions to the advancement of human rights related to HIV.

**Charles Furlotte** is a registered social worker at Stonechurch Family Health Centre, part of the McMaster Family Health Team, and assistant clinical professor (adjunct) in the Department of Family Medicine at McMaster University. Charles is also a PhD candidate in the School of Social Work at McMaster. Their doctoral research addresses perspectives of gay men who are growing older with HIV. Charles was the lead investigator on the community-driven project HIV and Aging: An Environmental Scan of Programs and Services in Canada, and is a past fellow of Universities without Walls, a strategic training program for the next generation of HIV researchers funded by the Canadian Institutes of Health Research.

**Chelsea Gabel** is Metis from Rivers, Manitoba. She holds a Canada Research Chair in Indigenous Well-Being, Community Engagement, and Innovation, and is currently the director of the McMaster Indigenous

Research Institute. She is an assistant professor in the Department of Health, Aging and Society and Indigenous Studies Program at McMaster University. Her research discusses and evaluates processes and institutional structures that influence relationships between Indigenous communities and government in the development, implementation, and evaluation of health policy.

**Marilou Gagnon** is an associate professor at the School of Nursing, Faculty of Health Sciences, University of Ottawa, and director of the Unit for Critical Research in Health. Her fields of study focus on the care of marginalized individuals, the management of risk, bodies, and behaviours, and structures that produce inequities and injustices. As a member of the University Chair in Forensic Nursing, she is working on a number of projects on HIV criminalization, HIV-related stigma and discrimination in health-care settings, and human rights. She served on the board of directors of the Canadian Association of Nurses in HIV/AIDS Care (CANAC), and was expert advisor, Research, Policy and Advocacy for CANAC from 2013 to 2016. She also served on the board of the Bureau Régional d'Action Sida and joined the Canadian HIV/AIDS Legal Network's board of directors in 2013. She is the founder and editor of the blog Radical Nurse. In addition to her scholarly publications, she has published in a number of newspapers, magazines, and blogs, including the *Globe and Mail*, the *Ottawa Citizen*, the *Georgia Straight*, *Le Devoir*, *Remaides*, *Impact Ethics*, and *Volteface Magazine*.

**Nicole R. Greenspan** is a researcher at St Michael's Hospital, in Toronto, Canada. She earned her PhD in Health Services Research from the University of Toronto in 2015 and completed a postdoctoral fellowship at the Memorial University of Newfoundland. Her research has focused on programs and services offered by community-based AIDS organizations, and ethical issues in providing medical care for people living with HIV. In her research, she draws on her experience from holding multiple professional roles at AIDS service organizations, government funders, and research institutions.

**Adrian Guta**, MSW, PhD, RSW, is an assistant professor in the School of Social Work at the University of Windsor. Adrian is an interdisciplinary health scholar with training in social work, medical sociology, public health, and bioethics, and conducts research with marginalized communities to advance knowledge and practice in primary care and population and public health. He is undertaking a series of related projects examining the social and ethical dimensions of HIV treatment and prevention technologies, and the health access needs of people living with HIV and who use drugs.

**Suzanne Hindmarch** is an assistant professor of political science at the University of New Brunswick. Her research sits at the intersection of international relations, critical global health, and critical security studies, with a focus on the processes through which health, disease, and other social policy problems come to be seen in security terms, and the policy and political consequences that this has for health, security, and structurally marginalized populations, communities and regions. She is the author of *Securing Health: HIV and the Limits of Securitization* (Routledge 2016).

**Dave Holmes** is professor and university research chair in Forensic Nursing at the School of Nursing, Faculty of Health Sciences, University of Ottawa. He is associate researcher at Institut Philippe de Montréal (Montreal) and research affiliate at the Center for Positive Sexuality (Los Angeles). Most of his work, comments, essays, analyses, and research are based on the poststructuralist works of Deleuze and Guattari, and Michel Foucault. He is co-editor of *Critical Interventions in the Ethics of Health Care* (Routledge, 2009), *Abjectly Boundless: Boundaries, Bodies and Health Care* (Routledge, 2010), *(Re)Thinking Violence in Health Care Settings: A Critical Approach* (Routledge, 2011), *Power and the Psychiatric Apparatus* (Routledge, 2014), and *Radical Sex between Men* (Routledge, 2017).

**Francisco Ibáñez-Carrasco**, PhD (Education, SFU 1999), is the director of education and training at the Ontario HIV Treatment Network and the eLearning for HIV Research program Universities without Walls (www.universitieswithoutwalls.ca). Francisco has lived in Canada and lived with HIV since 1986 and specializes in the role of education in research using new media and technologies. His research focuses on HIV in the contexts of rehabilitation, aging, stigma, and mental health. His fiction and non-fiction have been widely published, and his latest book is *Giving It Raw: Nearly 30 Years with AIDS* (Transgress, 2015).

**Randy Jackson** is Anishinaabe from Kettle and Stony Point First Nation in Ontario. He is a lecturer in the Department of Health, Aging, and Society and in the School of Social Work at McMaster University. Randy's research focuses on Indigenous peoples confronting HIV and AIDS. Drawing on Indigenous perspectives and values, he has explored a variety of HIV-related issues, including resiliency among two-spirit men, experiences of depression, stigma, and relational care.

**Kerrigan Johnson** is an HIV-positive 2-spirited mother of four. She has worked within her community for over 15 years in various roles. She is currently the executive director for 2 Spirited People of the 1st Nations. She has also worked with Prisoners HIV/AIDS Support Action Network as the Women's Community Program coordinator, the Aboriginal Program coordinator, and the Treatment Access coordinator. She has also worked in research for Women's College Research Initiative and McMaster University as a research assistant.

**Jennifer M. Kilty** is associate professor in the Department of Criminology at the University of Ottawa. Her research focuses primarily on gender and different aspects of criminalization, including the social construction of dangerous girls and women, the medicalization/psychiatrization of criminalized women, self-harming behaviours, drug use, and more recently the criminalization of HIV nondisclosure. In addition to numerous articles and book chapters, she has edited two books: *Within the Confines: Women and the Law in Canada* (Women's Press) and *Demarginalizing Voices: Commitment, Emotion and Action in Qualitative Research* (UBC Press), both published in 2014. Her latest book, *The Enigma of a Violent Woman: A Critical Examination of the Case of Karla Homolka* (Routledge), was co-authored with Sylvie Frigon in 2016.

**Gary Kinsman** is a professor emeritus in sociology at Laurentian University and queer liberation, AIDS, anti-poverty, and anti-capitalist activist on Indigenous land. He is currently involved in the AIDS Activist History Project and was involved in AIDS ACTION NOW!, the Newfoundland AIDS Association, and the Valley AIDS Concern Group. He is also the author of *The Regulation of Desire: Homo and Hetero Sexualities*, co-author (with Patrizia Gentile) of *The Canadian War on Queers: National Security as Sexual Regulation*, and editor of *Whose National Security? Sociology for Changing the World* and *We Still Demand! Redefining Resistance in Sex and Gender Struggles*. His website is radicalnoise.ca.

**Kecia Larkin** is a full-blooded Indigenous AIDS activist, who publicly disclosed her HIV status in July 1990. During two and a half decades she has been involved with some of Canada's most remote communities to educate youth and community about HIV. She has a nationally distributed award-winning video called *Kecia: Words to Live By*. Kecia has contributed to many projects, including AIDS service organizations, committees, conferences, education, and peer support, and she continues to commit to the HIV community. In 2016 Kecia won the AccolAIDS Kevin Brown's Award for her contributions.

**Renée Masching** is First Nation and works as the director of research and policy with the Canadian Aboriginal AIDS Network. Her research interests focus on community-based research frameworks, Indigenous knowledge, and community health, with emphasis on HIV and AIDS. She has dedicated her professional energies to Aboriginal health and earned her master's in social work in 2003. Renée has contributed to Aboriginal HIV and AIDS work with dedication and determination since 1995.

**Alex McClelland** is a writer who is working on a doctorate at the Interdisciplinary Centre on Culture and Society, Concordia University, under the supervision of Drs Viviane Namaste, Martin French, and Amy Swiffen. His work focuses on the intersections of life, law, and disease and encompasses sociological analysis, critical criminology, surveillance studies, and the social organization of knowledge. He has developed a range of collaborative and interdisciplinary writing, academic, artistic, and curatorial projects to address criminalization, sexual autonomy, surveillance, drug liberation, and the construction of knowledge on AIDS.

**Kate Murzin** specializes in HIV and its impact on older adults in Canada. Kate is health programs specialist at Realize and provides secretariat support to the National Coordinating Committee on HIV and Aging. In both roles, Kate is a catalyst and a capacity builder, bringing together stakeholders from the HIV, chronic illness, and aging sectors and fostering engagement in research, policy, education, and programming initiatives on HIV and aging. Kate has a master's in public health, with a specialty in health promotion, from the University of Toronto.

**Michael Orsini**, PhD, is full professor in the School of Political Studies and vice-dean, Graduate Studies, in the Faculty of Social Sciences at the University of Ottawa. A specialist in health policy and politics with a specific interest in social movement politics, he has published in journals such as the *Canadian Journal of Political Science, Critical Policy Studies, Policy and Society, Social and Legal Studies, Social Policy and Administration*, and *Sexuality Research and Social Policy*, among others. He is co-editor of one of the first edited collections to inaugurate the field of "critical policy studies" (UBC Press, 2007) and co-edited one of the first interdisciplinary collections on the social study of autism (*Worlds of Autism*, University of Minnesota Press, 2013). Twice a recipient of a Fulbright Visiting Research Chair (in 2009 at the University of Washington and in 2017 at Vanderbilt University), he has received prizes for journal publications, including in the *Canadian Journal of Political Science*, and a co-authored piece in the journal *Critical Policy Studies*. He has also written op-eds and commentaries in a number of newspapers and online venues, including the *Globe and Mail*, the *Toronto Star*, the *Ottawa Citizen*, the *Winnipeg Free Press*, and *Impact Ethics*.

**Doris Peltier** is a 60-year-old HIV-positive Anishinaabe AIDS activist from Wikwemikoong First Nations. As a community person with "lived experience," she has consistently championed the embracing of assets-based, strengths-based community-based research (CBR) in Indigenous research, and has advocated for strengthening meaningful engagement of women living with HIV and AIDS (MEWA) "in research." Her interests are in health research that supports the self-determination and autonomy of Indigenous women living with HIV and their families. Since her diagnosis in 2000, she has participated on numerous national committees related to HIV and is fluent in Anishinaabemowin. Her fluency in her language brings a wealth of Indigenous knowledge that is grounded in an Indigenous world view into all her work. In 2012, she received the Queen Elizabeth II Diamond Jubilee Medal for her dedicated service to community.

**Wendy Porch** is the manager, Episodic Disabilities Initiatives at Realize (formerly the Canadian Working Group on HIV and Rehabilitation). Wendy has been working in the field of accessibility, disability, human rights, and education for close to twenty years and is the chair of the national Episodic Disabilities Forum. Wendy has an MEd in counselling psychology from the Ontario Institute for Studies in Education at the University of Toronto.

**Tracey Prentice** is a community-based health researcher and a postdoctoral fellow at the School of Public Health and Social Policy, University of Victoria. Her interests include women's health, Indigenous health, and participatory research frameworks. She is particularly interested in arts-informed and strengths-based approaches to health and wellness, including collaborative visual methodologies. She has been engaged in the national and international response to HIV and AIDS since 2002, working primarily for and with Indigenous peoples. She received her PhD in population health from the University of Ottawa in 2015.

**Colleen Price** resides in Ottawa and is trained in psychology, sociology, and as a social service worker. A survivor of trauma, addictions, HIV, and hepatitis C, she is a committed advocate for testing, access to treatment, and program and policy development for people living with HIV and/or hepatitis C. She also advocates that harm reduction, mental health, and peer support services become part of integrated whole-health care to improve health outcomes, to help mitigate social determinants of health, and to improve our quality of life. Colleen currently serves on several advisory committees and research teams.

**Ron Rosenes**, BA (Hon.), MA, LLD (Hon.), CM, has been living with HIV for over 30 years and became an active volunteer member of the HIV community in Toronto in 1991. Ron has served in governance roles as the board chair of ACT, founding board member of the Sherbourne Health Centre, and a member of the Steering Committee of the Canada AIDS Russia Project and vice chair of AIDS2006 Toronto Local Host. In 2011 he stepped down as vice chair of Canadian Treatment Action Council after 14 years. Ron serves on numerous advisory committees, including a CIHR Working Group on Ethics in Patient Engagement in Research. Ron has received numerous awards for his community work, including an honorary doctorate from Carleton University and the Order of Canada.

**Chaneesa Ryan** is a health policy and programs coordinator at Pauktuutit Inuit Women of Canada. She is a recent graduate from the Department of Health, Aging, and Society at McMaster University. Chaneesa's thesis explored Indigenous people's experiences of aging with HIV/AIDS, highlighting the strength and resiliency within the aging HIV-positive Indigenous population.

**Krista Shore,** a 34-year-old Nêhiya (Cree), and mother of four, belongs to the Peepeekisis First Nation. She has been involved in the HIV movement and has accomplished much since her diagnosis in 2007. Her interests are in community engagement and nation-building that is grounded in Indigenous belief systems and ceremony; she is a remarkable visionary for the people for whom she dedicates much of her work; this is inclusive of youth, women, and their families who are living with or affected by HIV. She is also a strong voice in speaking to the issues around Missing and Murdered Indigenous Women (MMIW), an issue that has impacted her at a personal level. Krista is no stranger to the determinants of health and has risen above systematic barriers to be a leader for HIV-positive Indigenous Women in her community. In 2010, Krista was recognized by the Assembly of First Nations with the Young Eagles Challenge Award for her passion, dedication, and commitment to the HIV movement in Canada.

**Christine Vézina** is an assistant professor at Université Laval, where she teaches constitutional law and human rights. She is interested in implementing economic, social, and cultural rights in contexts of social exclusion and marginalization, and she considers these questions from a sociological standpoint using empirical research methodologies. Her publications focus on human rights challenges in the fight against HIV/AIDS; the links between legal culture and justiciability of economic, social, and cultural rights; mobilization of law and activism and research.

**Tammy C. Yates** is the executive director of Realize. Tammy's résumé includes over a decade of senior management, administration, and communications experience in the non-profit and international development sectors in gender, sexual and reproductive health, and HIV/AIDS.

# Index

Note: PHAs refers to people living with HIV/AIDS, and GIPA refers to greater involvement of people living with HIV/AIDS.

Lightning Source UK Ltd.
Milton Keynes UK
UKHW040411100119
335321UK00002B/307/P